PRIMARY HEALTH CARE OF THE OLDER ADULT

PRIMARY HEALTH CARE
OF THE OLDER ADULT

May Futrell, *Ph.D., R.N.,*
University of Lowell

Stephen Brovender, *M.D.,*
University of Lowell

Elizabeth McKinnon-Mullett, *Ph.D., R.N.,*
University of Connecticut

H. Terri Brower, *Ed.D., R.N., F.N.P.,*
University of Miami

DUXBURY PRESS   North Scituate, Massachusetts

Notice: Medical and nursing management information, including drug therapy, presented in this text represents the authors' approach to care. Because approaches vary, the reader is cautioned to check information in other readily available sources.

PRIMARY HEALTH CARE OF THE OLDER ADULT was produced by the following people:

Copy Editor: *Jacqueline M. Dormitzer,* Interior Designer: *The Book Department,* Cover Designer: *Joanna Prudden Snyder,* Cover photograph by: *Louis B. Dovner,* Interior photographs by: *Louis B. Dovner,* except 6.1, 6.4, 6.8, 6.11, 6.13 by *Oel Futrell,* and 6.22, 6.39, 6.58 by *Donald Anderson,* Chapter opening illustrations by: *Irene Roman,* Line drawings and graphs by: *B. J. & F. W. Taylor,* Production Coordinator: *Sylvia Dovner.*

Duxbury Press
A Division of Wadsworth, Inc.

Library of Congress Cataloging in Publication Data

Main entry under title:
PRIMARY HEALTH CARE OF THE OLDER ADULT.

Includes index.
1. Geriatric nursing.
2. Aged—Care and hygiene.
I. Futrell, May DiPietro.
RC954.P75   610.73'65   79-15816
ISBN 0-87872-236-X

Printed in the United States of America
1 2 3 4 5 6 7 8 9 – 84 83 82 81 80

AUTHORS

MAY FUTRELL, PH.D., R.N., Professor and
Graduate Coordinator, Department of Nursing,
University of Lowell, Lowell, Massachusetts

STEPHEN BROVENDER, M.D., Adjunct
Associate Professor, Department of Nursing,
University of Lowell, Lowell, Massachusetts

ELIZABETH McKINNON-MULLETT, PH.D.,
R.N., Professor, School of Nursing, University of
Connecticut, Storrs, Connecticut

H. TERRI BROWER, ED.D., R.N., F.N.P.,
Professor, School of Nursing and School of
Medicine, University of Miami, Miami, Florida

CONTRIBUTORS

DONALD ANDERSON, M.S., R.N., G.N.P.,
Department of Nursing, University of Lowell,
Lowell, Massachusetts

SUSAN CROCKER HOUDE, M.S., R.N., G.N.P.,
Department of Nursing, University of Lowell,
Lowell, Massachusetts

DOROTHY KARPOWICH, PH.D., R.N.,
formerly Assistant Professor, Department of
Nursing, University of Lowell, Lowell,
Massachusetts

WILLIAM O'ROURKE, PH.D., Coordinator,
Gerontology Program, Northern Essex
Community College, Haverhill, Massachusetts

To our older clients,
to our students, and
to the nursing profession
for its acceptance and
promotion of the expanded
role of the nurse—
all provided the necessary
stimulation for this text.

CONTENTS

PREFACE   xiii

I
INTRODUCTION   1

II

GERONTOLOGICAL NURSING PROCESS   59

III

GERONTOLOGICAL NURSING MANAGEMENT   265

IV
RESOURCES 445

INDEX 460

PREFACE

Although interest and concern for the health and well-being of all persons seem to be growing, social enlightenment with regard to health matters of persons over 65 years of age has not kept pace with that of other age groups. Even those in the health care professions of medicine, nursing, and social work tend to focus on the acute illnesses of the young and middle-aged rather than on the health problems of the older individual.

The authors have long been concerned about the inequality of health care as it relates to the elderly. With the expansion of the nurse's role in primary health care, nurses have an opportunity to improve the health of the elderly. Promotion of health and prevention of illness can now be given the attention needed for a high level of "wellness."

Most nursing textbooks concerned with the over-65 age group are oriented toward either physical or psychosocial aspects of care. This text includes both of these aspects and focuses particular attention on health promotion, prevention of illness, health assessment, and nursing management of the health problems that are more common to older adults.

The book is organized into four sections. Part I, the "Introduction," offers theories of aging and facts and figures in the cognitive areas of gerontology, health, nursing, and social welfare. Health care needs, health promotion, counseling, and patient education for self-management of health problems in the well elderly are also discussed. The expanded role of the gerontological nurse is described. Part II, "Health Appraisal of the Older Adult," discusses the nursing process, history taking, physical and mental health assessment, and recording of the data.

Part III, "Nursing Management of Health Problems in the Older Adult," explores systematically the pathophysiology, nursing assessment, diagnostics, and nursing management of health problems in the elderly. Particular attention is paid to health promotion, concepts of teaching, counseling, nutrition, and pharmacology. Part IV, "Resources," discusses community resources and includes criteria for selection of a nursing home.

The text will be particularly helpful for nurses who wish to update their knowledge and skills in gerontological nursing, for nurses who are participating in nurse practitioner programs and/or graduate programs, and for students in undergraduate nursing programs where gerontological nursing is integrated into or is a separate entity of the curriculum. Other professionals such as social workers, physical therapists, and occupational therapists should also find this text useful either in part or in total.

During the writing of this text, three of the principal authors were supported by federal projects of DHEW, Health Manpower Resources, Division of Nursing. Futrell and Brovender were supported by grant number 1 D24 NU 00075-01. Brower was supported by grant 1 D24 NU 00060-01.

We would like to express our gratitude to the following individuals who stimulated and encouraged us in this endeavor: Gertrude Barker, Jacqueline Brovender, Lee Brower, Oel Futrell, Eleanor Gill, Gloria Holmes, George S. Moran, John Maroney, and Eleanor Shalhoup.

Our thanks also go to Ed Murphy, Editor at Duxbury Press, for his contributions and support during the development of this text.

Our appreciation for their expertise and critique in the substantive portions of the management of health problems sections goes to Robert Boucek, M.D., Robert Boyette, M.D., Howard Duchon, D.D. Gunter Kahn, M.D., David Kudzma, M.D., Rona Levitt, R.N., Roy Maletz, M.D., Richard Pratt, M.D., Jack Skigan, M.D., and Sheldon Zane, M.D. In addition, we received helpful comments from Dolores M. Alford, R.N.; Irene M. Burnside, R.N., M.S., San Jose State University; Ruth P. Fleshman, R.N., Ph.D., President, Nursing Dynamics Corporation; Laurie M. Gunter, R.N., Ph.D., Pennsylvania State University; Ann Marie Yurick, R.N., M.A., University of Pittsburgh; Monica M. Bossenmaier, R.N., M.A., University of Minnesota; and Marilyn J. Wood, R.N., Dr.P.H., University of California at Los Angeles.

We would like to thank the staff and clients of the following facilities for their cooperation and assistance in allowing us to take the photographs for this book: D'Youville Manor Nursing Home and Day Care Center, St. Joseph's Hospital, and Smith Baker Senior Center—all in Lowell, Massachusetts—and South Shore Hospital in South Weymouth, Massachusetts.

Finally, our special thanks to Pauline Singer and Helen Pevey for their tireless and cheerful efforts in helping us put this book together.

MAY FUTRELL
STEPHEN BROVENDER
ELIZABETH McKINNON-MULLETT
H. TERRI BROWER

PRIMARY HEALTH CARE OF THE OLDER ADULT

To Age or to Grow Old

Am I caught up in a quilt
of reminiscence—a patchwork,
touch of red, scrap of green,
a used-up yesterday,
a sound grown thin . . . .
Have I let myself grow old?

Tomorrow beckons fresh, a gift.
Will I hear the vibrancy
beating in my universe,
feel myself a child,
see beyond my limitations, fears,
shed my disappointments?
Let the grown-up in me laugh . . .
grow old?

Let there be time—
time enough for aging,
but little time allowed
for growing old.

Betsy H. Woodman
Newburyport, Mass.
1979

I

INTRODUCTION

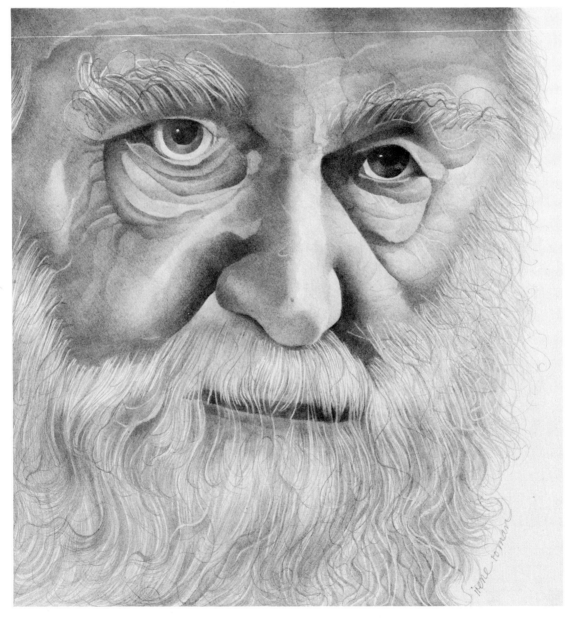

Chapter 1

THEORIES OF AGING

For more than a decade, the nursing profession has been seriously addressing itself to the task of developing theories for nursing practice. This effort is seen not only as "a way of discovering new knowledge, but also a way of looking at known facts and of organizing them into a system" (King 1978, p. 12). For nursing itself, such theory development is an attempt to establish the meaning of nursing, to improve its practice, and to help the profession achieve recognition as a science.

THEORY DEVELOPMENT

Theory development has many stages. One of the earliest is the formation of concepts and conceptual models—that is, conceptual representations of reality (Riehl and Roy 1974). According to Fawcett (1978), conceptual models are pretheoretic bases from which substantive theories may be derived. Nursing is now at the concept-building stage, and many conceptual models are being tested in both educational settings and actual practice.

Dorothy Johnson (1968), using a human behavioral system theory, has developed a conceptual model for nursing practice that considers human beings as many behavioral systems and subsystems that react with their environment. Nurses who use this model design their practice in such a way that their intervention works toward the optimum balance between system, subsystems, and environment.

Still another conceptual model developed to guide nursing practice is the adaptation model of Sister Callista Roy (1970). According to this model, the nurse practitioner focuses on assisting the client in efforts to satisfy four fundamental needs: (1) physiological, (2) psychological, (3) functional, and (4) social.

Examination and testing of conceptual models of nursing are critical as nursing attempts to develop its own theories. Nursing literature today is replete with such examinations and testing at the levels of education and practice. Nursing theories will emerge from these efforts—theories that will have internal consistency and will help give direction to the practice of nursing. However, as with all research, theory development requires a cadre of committed nurse scholars, time, and money.

In the meantime, since nursing is at present recognized as an applied science that draws upon knowledge from related disciplines, many of the theories within the psychosocial and biological sciences can be used to guide nursing in the development of conceptual models. Three psychosocial theories are particularly useful to nurses dedicated to delivering the best possible care to the elderly in our society. We will consider these before dealing with biological theories of aging.

THEORIES OF AGING

PSYCHOSOCIAL THEORIES OF AGING

A discussion of the psychosocial theories of aging might well begin with Bernice Neugarten's excellent summary of aging research done at the University of Chicago during the past several decades. In her Kleemier Award lecture delivered at the 1971 meeting of the Gerontological Society, she stated:

To sum up these findings then: in studying the same individuals we found asynchronous trends: in the covert or "inner" life—the eye of the mind—increased interiority and other changes which we interpreted as develop-

mental, occurring as early as in the 50s; on the adaptational side, no age related changes; and in social interaction, decrease occurring not until the late 60s and 70s. [Neugarten 1972, p. 11]*

These findings were based on a study of more than seven hundred relatively healthy subjects, age 40 to 70, interviewed at Kansas City. Three hundred of these subjects were seen over a six-year period and thus provided a longitudinal sample.

The first finding noted by Neugarten was the gradual tendency of aging subjects to move "inward"—that is, to become more concerned with their own life and its meaning and less concerned with passing affairs. Neugarten called this a movement to *interiority*. Other researchers (Erikson 1976; Clark and Anderson 1967) have suggested that with advancing years there comes a tendency, or better, a capacity, to enter more deeply into the self to creatively assess and reevaluate one's experiences, successes, and failures and to come at last to a more adequate acceptance of life and one's place in the scheme of things. Actually, this task is one that should occupy us throughout the life course. Stopping the rush and taking time to contemplate, to gather, and to integrate events of the preceding day or days should be a task for the young as well as the old. The research suggests that as we age, we are more likely to take the time to reflect on the real self and to become less concerned with passing things.

Neugarten also indicated that this trend toward "interiority" seems to be accompa-

*This quotation and the two that follow by Bernice Neugarten are from "Personality and the Aging Process," *The Gerontologist* (Spring 1972). © 1972 *The Gerontologist*. Reprinted by permission.

nied by an age-related change in the way people relate to the world around them. Forty-year-olds in her Kansas City study saw their environment as challenging and manageable; 60-year-olds saw it as complex, dangerous, and difficult to control. She noted that Gutman called the changing attitudes a move from active to *passive mastery*. This change may well be related to interiority in that it represents a realistic awareness that the world and human affairs in general are complex and not easily managed or controlled. For example, a 55-year-old man related that his 26-year-old son became involved in a dispute with a bank teller over what he regarded as an unjust business practice. While appreciating his son's frustration with the bank, the older man said with a smile, "I'd rather live to be 80 and put up with a few things that I don't like, than die at 60 worn out from fighting the world." The father seemed to be relating to the world from a different perspective than his son. This difference may be the result of aging and is probably a development of passive mastery.

Finally, Neugarten noted that the Kansas City study did find a gradual decrease in social activities beginning as early as in the sixties and continuing through the seventies. This gradual withdrawal, together with the tendency to inwapdneqs and passive mastery, led to the formulation of the now famous *disengagement theory,* first proposed by Cumming and Henry in 1961.

Disengagement Theory

Disengagement theory maintains that with advancing age individualq eradually withdraw their involvement in their social world, while at approximately the same time society encourages and affirms this withdrawal—in effect, it withdraws from them. Successful aging individuals, therefore, are those who withdraw "on time," when both they and society are ready. Retirement, for example, may be a societal "permission" to disengage; it provides older people with the time to develop in new ways and provides society with an organized way to keep the work force young and vigorous. The theory has provided a rather neat hypothesis that does, in fact, contain a good deal of truth about human ✓ aging as we know it. However, like most new and provocative theories, its chief value has been as a catalyst for a long and fruitful public discussion that has fostered a holistic appreciation of aging and aging persons. Its publication created a storm of controversy that has stimulated students of aging for a decade or more and has led to several other theories of aging, among them the *activity* and *continuity theories.*

Activity Theory

The most obvious objection to the notion that disengagement leads to successful aging and contentment with life is that it contradicts the commonsense dictum suggesting that successful aging individuals are those who are active and engaged. Proponents of this position developed a theory in response to the disengagement hypothesis, which appropriately has come to be known as the activity theory. This theory holds that people will remain content and satisfied in later years if they can maintain their activities and stay involved in the life around them. Therefore, as we lose roles and tasks, we must learn to substitute other things, such as hobbies, volunteer work, clubs and associations, and the like. The central point in this commonsense theory is exemplified by the comment of a 90-year-old man who told his audience that the secret of a long and happy life is to "keep busy."

Continuity Theory

Because neither the disengagement nor the activity theory was sufficient to explain the process of successful aging, a third theory developed, combining elements of the first two but emphasizing a dimension that brings them both into proper focus. In her summary Neugarten wrote:

> As we gathered more data . . . we did not find the consistent patterns that were predicted from the disengagement theory . . . . We found that high life satisfaction was more often present in persons who were socially active and involved than in persons who were inactive and uninvolved . . . . More important we found diversity. [Neugarten 1972, p. 11]

She continued:

> Certain personality types, as they age slough off various role responsibilities with relative comfort and remain highly content with life. Other personalities show a drop in role and in social interaction and show a drop in life satisfaction. Still others have long shown low levels of activity accompanied by high satisfaction and show relatively little change as they age . . . . We have concluded from this line of studies that personality organization or personality type is the pivotal factor in predicting which individuals will age successfully . . . . [Neugarten 1972, p. 12]

Continuity theory thus accepts the intrapsychic developmental changes expressed in disengagement, as well as the commonsense observation that keeping busy is important to many of today's elderly. It adds the notion that each person ages in a unique and personal way and does so according to the personality characteristics and the lifestyle developed throughout the greater part of the life course.

Lest this discussion seem merely academic, note that some clinicians and practitioners have taken the theories at face value and have tried to implement them in the lives of some of their older clients. A nursing home director who was an "activist" tried, for example, to encourage a 90-year-old man to come to activities because, she said, he spent so much time alone in his room. However, several days later at a discussion-group meeting, the old man described to the others how much he resented people's efforts to get him "involved." He explained that he needed this time alone in his room, where he was really very busy and very content, just thinking. He later said he liked to think and rethink about "all the things I've ever done." He seemed perfectly content to be disengaged"; and, in fact, this activity was appropriate for him. On the other hand, clinicians should not take the disengagement theory too literally and leave truly isolated and lonely clients alone when, in fact, they need to be invited and encouraged to join in social activities.

This brief discussion of three psychosocial theories of aging is offered to open the subject to you and to suggest a direction for individual practice. Older people, like everyone else, are poorly described by stereotypes. To understand an aging person, we must see him or her as an individual with a lifetime of unique and personal experiences, each of which contributes to a special way of dealing with old age.

6

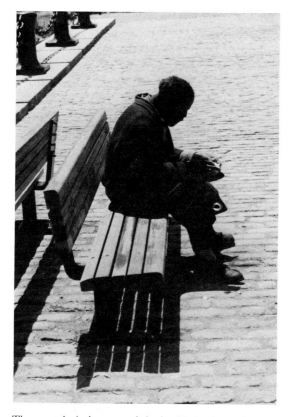

The gerontological nurse can help the elderly adapt to the aging process by recognizing that aging involves a movement to interiority; elderly clients need support and understanding as they spend more time reminiscing and reflecting on the self and become less concerned with the world around them.

BIOLOGICAL THEORIES OF AGING

As with most fields of scientific investigation, early reports on the biology of aging were mainly descriptive of gross organ changes. More recently, however, the cell itself has become the focus for study. Scientists have been examining cellular and molecular mechanisms in an effort to identify changes that lead to the organismic decline in efficiency and functioning that is associated with aging and, ultimately, death.

Understandably, much of the research has been conducted on lower animals.

In the mid-sixties Leonard Hayflick (1965) refuted the then current belief that cellular life, maintained in an optimal environment outside the body, could go on infinitely. Hayflick found that normal human fibroblasts from aborted fetuses divided vigorously for a time, then slowed down, stopped multiplying, and died soon after their fiftieth population doubling. Subsequent studies by many investigators have all supported the finding that somatic cells have a maximum division limit that precedes cellular death. (Abnormal tumerous HeLa cells, however, appear to be "immortal.") Further, recent research activities indicate that different species have characteristic and inheritable life spans.

While the early studies spoke to the duration of life, more recent investigations have addressed the decline of cellular efficiency and functioning. Hayflick himself attributes senescence to losses of cell function that occur before cells reach their maximum division limit. Many researchers who are currently studying the biology of aging appear to agree with this thesis. Their work involves primary aging, which depends on heredity, rather than secondary aging, which involves trauma and the chronic diseases that affect human beings.

The many attempts to link observed age changes in the whole organism to the cellular level have resulted in many theories of primary biological aging. To increase your awareness of current scientific investigations designed to answer the question "What is aging?" we will briefly discuss three of these theories: the error catastrophe theory, the redundant message theory, and the immunologic theory.

Error Catastrophe Theory

The *error catastrophe theory* was proposed in 1963 by Leslie Orgel of the Salk Institute in La Jolla, California. He suggested that biological aging was due to an accumulation of errors in amino acid sequence in proteins, especially errors that affect the specificity of enzymes needed for protein synthesis, which would result in further mistakes in protein synthesis and consequently lead to cell deterioration and death.

Evidence to support Orgel's hypothesis showed that abnormal forms of enzymes isolated from old human fibroblasts were more sensitive to heat than were normal enzymes isolated from young fibroblasts. Further supporting evidence revealed that the level of activity in enzyme proteins isolated from aged invertebrates (nematodes, or round worms) was lower than the level of enzymatic activity exhibited in young specimens.

Redundant Message Theory

The *redundant message theory* was proposed by the Russian geneticist and gerontologist Zhores A. Medvedev (1972). Earlier studies had noted that cells of higher organisms (eukaryocytes: cells with a true nucleus) have an excessive amount of DNA. The major portion of this extra DNA was found to contain repetitive or redundant sequences. According to Medvedev's theory, these repetitive or redundant sequences are called in to replace errors that accumulate in functioning genes. Since these sequences contain the same information, they take over until the redundancy in the system is exhausted and senescence results.

The Immunologic Theory

While many investigators continue their search for the biological cloci at the molecular level within cells, others are examining entire body systems. The immune system has been a particularly attractive system because, with the passage of time, the thymus lymphatic mass decreases in size. The thymus is where the lymphocytic "T" cells of the immune system develop. "T" cells are responsible for cell-mediated responses to antigens. A second type of response, the humoral response, is the property of the lymphocytic "B" cell. These cells produce immunoglobulin.

Investigators have further noted that with age there is a decline in the protective ability of the immune system and an impaired surveillance function, as well as a distortion of the system's protective mechanism, which results in a self-destructive autoaggressive phenomenon.

A relationship is apparent between longevity and at least two types of serum immunoglobulin concentrate—that is, death can come earlier to older individuals who have relatively low levels of immunoglobulin G (IgG) and immunoglobulin M (IgM). Dr. Roy Walford, an immunologist at U.C.L.A., believes that with age there is a breakdown in the surveillance function—the regulatory function that commences soon after birth when the body begins to catalog its native components. The end result is that in later life the body is unable to distinguish its own parts from intruders. With the breakdown of the surveillance function, the immune system fails to recognize cells of its own body and produces antibodies against them. This autoimmune reaction, according to Dr. Walford, plays an important role in aging. He also points out that autoimmune diseases appear to increase with age.

The biological explanation for aging may take years to develop; however, many scientists are devoted to the search for such a key to the nature of aging. The work of some of these investigators is briefly discussed by Kimmel (1974, pp. 343–356).

In addition to the three psychosocial and three biological theories we have briefly discussed, many other theories have been advanced and may also be particularly relevant to the care and treatment of elderly clients. We have presented these theories to help you appreciate the relationship between theory and nursing practice. Note, however, that although such theories provide useful guidelines for practice, the overriding considerations should always be the individuality of the client and nurse and the uniqueness of their situation.

REFERENCES

CLARK, M., and B. G. ANDERSON. 1967. *Culture and Aging.* Springfield, Ill.: Charles C. Thomas.

CUMMING, E. and W. E. HENRY. 1961. *Growing Old: The Process of Disengagement.* New York: Basic Books.

ERIKSON, E. 1976. "Reflections on Dr. Borg's Life Cycle." *Daedalus* 105:1–28.

FAWCETT, J. 1978. "The 'What' of Theory Development." *Theory Development: What, Why, How?* National League for Nursing, Publication No. 15–1708. New York.

HAYFLICK, L. 1965. "The Limited *in vitro* Lifetime of Human Diploid Cell Strains." *Experimental Cell Research* 37:614–36.

JOHNSON, D. 1968. "One Conceptual Model for Nursing." Unpublished paper presented at Vanderbilt University, Nashville, Tenn., April 25.

KIMMEL, D. C. 1974. *Adulthood and Aging.* New York: John Wiley.

KING, L. 1978. "The 'Why' of Theory Development." *Theory Development: What, Why, How?* National League for Nursing, Publication No. 15–1708. New York.

MEDVEDEV, Z. 1972. "Repetition of Molecular-Genetic Information as a Possible Factor in Evolutionary Changes of Lifespan." *Experimental Gerontology.* 7:227–38.

NEUGARTEN, B. 1972. "Personality and the Aging Process." *The Gerontologist* (Spring).

ORGEL, L. E. 1963. "The Maintenance of the Accuracy of Protein Synthesis and Its Relevance to Aging." *Proceedings of the National Academy of Sciences* 49(4):517–21.

RIEHL, J. and C. ROY. 1974. *Conceptual Models for Nursing Practice.* New York: Appleton-Century-Crofts.

ROY, C. 1970. "Adaptation: A Conceptual Framework for Nursing." *Nursing Outlook* 18(3)42–45.

WALFORD, R. 1969. *The Immunologic Theory of Aging.* Baltimore: Williams and Wilkins.

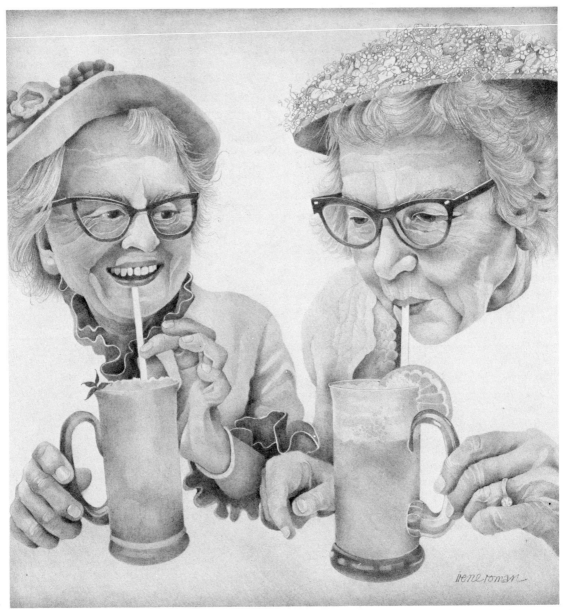

Chapter 2

AGING IN AMERICA

America is aging. By the year 2000, 30.6 million people will be age 65 or over (National Council on the Aging 1978, p. 6). This number represents a 35 percent increase over the current older population of 22 million (U.S. Bureau of the Census 1976). The demography and social profile of this growing segment of the population, as well as health care concerns and policies for the elderly, will be discussed in this chapter. To provide a foundation for our study of aging and the aged, we will begin by defining certain basic terms.

BASIC DEFINITIONS

GERONTOLOGY

Gerontology, the scientific study of the processes of growing old, is a complex field that crosses many disciplinary lines. Its basic concern is with older persons and with the processes of physical and social aging that begin with conception and end with death. The term is derived from the Greek *geron, -ontos,* meaning old man.

In contrast, *geriatrics,* derived from the Greek *geras* meaning old age and *iātros* meaning physician, refers to medical care of the aged. Geriatrics today is concerned primarily with medical intervention in the treatment of diseases of the elderly. When discussing the aging process, then, a distinction must be made between changes brought about over time—gerontology—and changes that occur as a result of diseases—geriatrics.

Research is making important contributions to a fuller understanding of the aging process. Investigations have shifted away from limited ". . . study of the sick and institutionalized to a broader inquiry into normal physiological changes occurring with age, the behavioral constitution of the

11

aged, and the social, cultural, and economic environment in which the elderly live" (Butler and Martin 1977, p. 71).

AGING

The study of aging has four separate but related aspects: biological, psychological, behavioral, and sociological (Atchley 1977, p. 5). The biological aspect deals with physical aging; the psychological aspect deals with sensory processes, perceptions, motor skills, intelligence, drives, and emotions; the behavioral aspect focuses on the social environment of the person and deals with biologically and psychologically induced changes in attitudes, motives, self-image, personality, social roles, and adjustment to aging; and the sociological aspect deals with matters related to society's influence on aging individuals and their influence on society, such as health, income, work, leisure, families, friends, the community, and government.

Biological aging is called *senescence.* Comfort describes it as a "deteriorative process":

> What is being measured, when we measure it, is a decrease in viability and an increase in vulnerability. . . . Senescence shows itself as an increasing probability of death with increasing chronological age: the study of senescence is the study of the group of processes, different in different organisms, which lead to this increase in vulnerability. [Comfort 1964, p. 22]

We should not confuse this term with *senility.* Senility is an outdated, abused term used to describe mental infirmities thought to be associated with aging. Research has shown that some so-called aging symptoms are specific treatable diseases. Such diseases and their management will be discussed in part III of this book.

A more useful definition of aging is given by Atchley (1977, p. 330): "A general term used for various biological, psychological and social processes whereby an individual acquires the socially defined characteristics of old age." Indeed, aging is difficult to define. To determine whether a person is aged, aging, or elderly, chronological age must also be considered with the biological, behavioral, and sociological aspects, for people can be "aged" at 40 or "aging" at 65, depending on the indicator used to define the word.

The Stages of Later Life

The definition of aging based on chronological age has in recent years undergone some refinement:

> It has been customary to assume that old age sets in somewhere during the seventh decade of life, and, until recently, much of the research and the majority of action programs have focused on the period beginning at or near age 65. It is now recognized, however, that the real turning point comes much earlier. On the basis of present knowledge, it seems possible to identify three stages of advanced adulthood: middle age, later maturity and old age. [Tibbitts 1960, p. 9]

Middle age is the time of life when the individual first becomes aware that energy levels are lower and health begins to fail. This period is also the one when children leave home. Middle age often marks a fresh assessment of a marriage, job, or the individual. It is a time when one seriously thinks about the future. These events normally occur during the forties and fifties.

Later maturity should be a period that includes freedom from earlier responsibilities and time to do things one wishes to do when one wishes to do them. However, in this period of the sixties and seventies several predictable crises occur, such as retirement, reduction of income, poor health, and loss of spouse.

Old age finds the individual cognizant of the fact that the end is approaching. Past 80, the likelihood of becoming more frail and disabled increases significantly.

These last two stages are at present being further divided into *young-old* (55–70) and *old-old* (85–100+) by chronological age. Because the elderly segment of the population is so diverse, care should be taken when describing the aged chronologically. They, like all people, should never be rigidly categorized.

The chronological age 65 was first used by Bismarck in Germany to denote the beginning of "old age" in social policy legislation during the 1880s. America adopted the same age indicator to determine eligibility for retirement and social services for its Social Security legislation in 1935. But "age 65" is clearly a tool for policy making and does not accurately reflect the refinements described above in the stages of later life.

DEMOGRAPHIC FACTS ABOUT THE ELDERLY

NUMBER AND PROPORTION

Approximately 10.5 percent of the total U.S. population, or more than 22 million persons, were over 65 years of age in 1976 (U.S. Bureau of the Census 1976). The rate of increase for the elderly population was greater between 1960 and 1970 than that for the general population (Kart, Metress, and Metress 1978, p. 2). The 75-and-over age group has grown more rapidly since

1900 than has the 65-to-74 age group (NCOA 1978, p. 3). This rapid increase in both number and proportion of the elderly has created a new phenomenon in our society.

The growth in the over-65 population can be attributed to three factors: the high birth rate of the late nineteenth and twentieth centuries, the high immigration rate prior to World War I, and the dramatic increase in life expectancy rates. This higher life expectancy rate reflects increased life expectancy at birth rather than at upper age levels. While the rates of infant and childhood mortality have decreased, the diseases of old age have not yet been conquered.

Recent life-expectancy projections (U.S. Dept. of Health, Education, and Welfare 1975) show that a white male reaching age 60 is likely to live until age 77 and a white woman until age 82. Blacks and other nonwhites who formerly had less favorable prospects for longevity are closing the gap: a nonwhite male at age 60 is likely to live until 76, a female until about 81. Women will continue to live longer than men, and the difference between male and female life expectancy is likely to increase.

The proportion of the very old (over 85) among the elderly is also increasing (see table 2.1). This particular growth pattern is predominately due to the improvements in health care and nutrition that have increased survival rates. Despite these improvements, different categories of elderly still have varying life expectancies. As stated above, men have shorter life expectancies than women and blacks have shorter life expectancies than whites.

Demographic projections show that the growth rate of the U.S. population over age

TABLE 2.1
Percentage of Older Persons by Age Group in Total U.S. Elderly Population, 1900–2000

Age	1900	1950	1975	2000
65–74	71	68	62	53
75–84	25	27	30	34
85+	4	5	8	11

Source: *National Council on the Aging,* Fact Book on Aging: A Profile of America's Older Population *(Washington, D.C.: NCOA, 1978), p. 7.*

65 will decline around 1990 (NCOA 1978, p. 11). This drop reflects the aging of individuals born during the depression and World War II years when birth rates were down. However, a dramatic increase in older persons will again be evident around 2010 because the postwar ("baby-boom") babies will be reaching age 65. Much will depend on fertility and mortality rates, but after 2030 the figure is expected to peak at 17 percent and decline thereafter (see table 2.2).

Demographers now are analyzing other factors—social, economic, psychological, and physiological—that have implications for gerontology. This multidimensional approach is useful in anticipating the needs of the elderly. For instance, family composition, and rates of institutionalization or disability among the older population can aid social planners when projecting personnel and space needs.

SEX AND MARITAL STATUS

Today, women outnumber men in America. Despite the fact that more male than female babies were born in 1974, male

TABLE 2.2
Percentage of Persons Age 65 and Over in Total U.S. Population, 1900–2050

Year	Percentage	Year	Percentage
1900	4.1	1980	11.0
1910	4.3	1990	11.7
1920	4.6	2000	11.7
1930	5.4	2010	11.9
1940	6.8	2020	14.6
1950	8.1	2030	17.0
1960	9.2	2040	16.1
1970	9.8	2050	16.1
1975	10.5		

Source: *U.S. Bureau of the Census,* Demographic Aspects of Aging and the Older Population in the United States, *Current Population Reports, Special Studies, Series P–23, no. 59, Washington, D.C., 1976, p. 9.*

death rates still remain higher beginning at birth, so that by age 20 women outnumber men. The sex differential in the older population, shown in table 2.3, is attributable to differing trends in mortality rates for males and females.

The U.S. population includes many widows, who at present outnumber widowers five to one. Approximately five of ten older white females are widows, while six of ten older black females are widows (NCOA 1978, p. 19). The difference reflects the higher mortality rate of the blacks and the greater age difference between black husbands and wives. In 1974 the number of married men age 65 and over was twice the number of married women age 65 and over (NCOA 1978, p. 19).

RACE AND ETHNICITY

In 1970, 15 percent of the elderly U.S. population was foreign born (Kart, Metress, and Metress 1978, p. 8), whereas blacks made up 7 percent of the elderly population. The foreign-born elderly are predominately in the Northeast; the black elderly, in the South.

Of the 11.2 million Spanish-Americans, approximately 6 to 7 million are of Mexican extraction and about 80 percent of the latter live in urban areas primarily in Arizona, California, Colorado, New Mexico, and Texas (Butler and Lewis 1977, p. 13). Overall, the elderly make up approximately 4 percent of the Spanish-American population.

Little is known about the American Indian elderly. Butler and Lewis (1977) state that they are the poorest segment of the U.S. population and suffer many disadvantages, such as minimal health care and education.

Hawaii and California have a large number of East Asian–American elderly. Statistics here are unreliable because of illegal immigration status but about 95 percent of these elderly live in cities such as San Francisco (Kart, Metress, and Metress 1978). They, too, are poor, disadvantaged, and many have language difficulties.

LIVING ARRANGEMENTS

Most older persons in the United States continue to reside in family settings, the most prevalent arrangement being a husband and wife living as a two-member family (NCOA 1978). A higher percentage of older men (81%) than of older women (58%) live in family settings (U.S. Bureau of the Census 1976).

TABLE 2.3
Proportion of Men to Women in the Age 65 and Over U.S. Population, 1975

Age	Men	Women
65–74	76.8	100
75 +	61.5	100
85 +	48.5	100

Source: *U.S. Bureau of the Census*, Demographic Aspects of Aging and the Older Population in the United States, *Current Population Reports, Special Studies, Series P–23, no. 59, Washington, D.C., 1976, p. 13.*

The proportion of elderly living alone, however, has increased in recent years mainly because of the growing number of widows and because more of the elderly can now afford to live alone (Kart, Metress, and Metress 1978, p. 18).

While many elderly do live alone, the percentage of those living in institutional settings increases after age 75 (see table 2.4). Even so, according to the 1970 census fewer than 5 percent of the elderly are institutionalized. Relationships with a "significant other"—someone who takes an interest in and maintains a positive relationship with the elderly person—contributes to deterring early institutionalization.

EDUCATION

According to the 1970 census, the elderly have completed a median of 8.7 years of school, compared with 12 years for the general population. Elderly blacks have completed a median of 5.6 years of school. However, educational attainment is improving steadily for persons 65 and over: by 1990 nearly one-half of the elderly population will be high school graduates (U.S. Bureau of the Census 1976).

GEOGRAPHIC DISTRIBUTION

Seventy-three percent of the older population resides in urban areas (Atchley 1977, p. 14). The geographic concentration of the elderly has not changed much over the last decade: in 1960 9 percent of the rural population was elderly; in 1970 the proportion was 10 percent (Kart, Metress, and Metress 1978). Of the 40 percent of the elderly who live in nonmetropolitan areas, only 5 percent actually live on farms and the remaining 35 percent reside in small towns (Butler and Lewis 1977, p. 15). Although fresh air, sunshine, and freedom from urban congestion abound in rural and semirural settings, unfavorable features such as lack of transportation, poor health facilities, low income levels, and rising property taxes also prevail and thus leave the elderly with few resources.

According to 1975 data approximately 45 percent of the over-65 age group lives in the six largest states (New York, California, Pennsylvania, Illinois, Texas, Ohio) and in Florida. Kart, Metress, and Metress (1978, p. 13) have found that "although relatively few elderly individuals show a propensity to be residentially mobile, some pattern is emerging with regard to which regions of

TABLE 2.4
Living Arrangements of Elderly Men and Women, 1975

	Men			Women		
Age	Family	Alone	Institution	Family	Alone	Institution
65–74	85.0%	12.1%	2.9%	64.6%	32.9%	2.5%
75+	74.5%	18.2%	7.4%	49.4%	40.6%	10.0%

Source: *U.S. Bureau of the Census,* Demographic Aspects of Aging and the Older Population in the United States. *Current Population Reports Special Studies, Series P–23, no. 59, Washington, D.C., 1976, p. 48.*

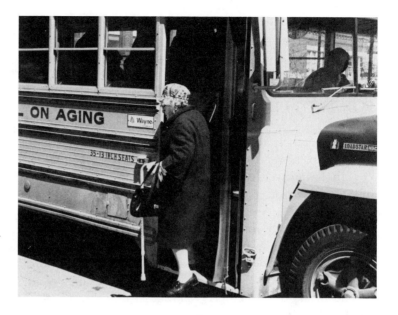

The gerontological nurse can help the elderly adapt to the aging process by encouraging them to be functionally independent; elderly clients need to be made aware of appropriate services, programs, and activities available to them in the community.

the country the elderly are mobile to and mobile from." Florida and Arizona show high in-migration rates, as do Nevada and New Mexico. The northeastern and midwestern states show high out-migration rates, particularly New York, Massachusetts, and South Dakota.

INCOME

The elderly have lower incomes than most younger people do. Many elderly persons have always had low incomes, but old age compounds the problem for them. Other elderly persons become poor only upon retirement. Statistics also show that a greater proportion of the elderly (15%) than of the total U.S. population (12%) are poor; older persons living alone or with nonrelatives are more likely to be poor than those living in families, regardless of race (NCOA 1978, p. 43).

In 1975 Social Security represented 90 percent or more of total income for one out of four single elderly persons and one out of twelve older couples (U.S. Senate 1976, p. 77). Originally conceived as a supplementary source of income, Social Security—along with Supplemental Security Income (SSI), a welfare program that provides for the aged, blind, and disabled—is proving to be the major source of income for most older aged. These two social programs are described in chapter 19. Earnings, private pensions, and assets are an additional source of income for some elderly.

The tendency for persons to continue to work after age 65 has declined since the turn of the century (NCOA 1978, p. 71). This trend is expected to continue: projections are that only one out of six older adults will be employed in 1990. Mandatory retirement policies are a major factor in the decline of employment for the eld-

17

erly, but the trend will probably shift as retirement policies allow work after age 65.

HEALTH CARE CONCERNS FOR THE ELDERLY

The Social Security Administration indicated in a report published in 1976 ". . . that the average annual health care bill for a person 65 years or older was $1,360 in 1975, almost six and one-half times the average annual health care expense of persons under age 19 and three times that of people age 19 to 64" (Zarit 1977, p. 113).

The needs of the elderly change from short- to long-term health care as a result of chronic diseases and disabling conditions or impairments and thus further reduce their incomes. Medicare is oriented toward short-term acute illnesses and accidents and removes some of the insecurity caused by medical bills for short-term illnesses. For example, in 1974 Medicare covered 60 percent of hospital care and 50 percent of physicians' services. However, it paid for only 3 percent of nursing-home–care expenses because dental care, prescription drugs, and chronic care for long-term illnesses were not covered (Schulz 1976, p. 162).

The funding of health care and related human services is a current major social policy issue. At present most programs and health care services for the elderly are inadequate. Problems include insufficient facilities, personnel, and funding; funding of services that do not include health services; lack of training programs for care-taking personnel and lack of educational programs for the public; and fragmented, poorly coordinated services and agencies for the elderly.

Contrary to popular belief, the majority of the elderly are not in poor health. Although about 86 percent of people over 65 have one or more chronic conditions (NCOA 1978, p. 98), most are functionally independent and are not institutionalized. Ninety-five percent of these elderly live at home in the community; only 5 percent are confined to institutions.

PHYSICAL HEALTH

The major health care problem of the older population is treatment of chronic conditions. Such conditions many times are a result of one's lifestyle, including patterns of alcoholic consumption, smoking, nutrition, and exposure to pollution. Thus, improving the health care system is only one solution to a complex problem. Throughout their lives individuals must be taught to practice preventive health measures and to seek early treatment for health problems in order to deter disabling effects.

The five most prevalent chronic conditions affecting the physical health of the aged, according to the National Council on Aging (1978, p. 109), are arthritis (38%), hearing impairments (29%), vision impairments (20%), hypertension (20%), and heart conditions (20%). Two surveys conducted by the National Center for Health Statistics (1973) found that arthritis, hypertension, and heart conditions, as well as diabetes, are more prevalent in women than in men, and that hypertension and heart disease are more prevalent among blacks than among whites. (Persons living in institutions were excluded from the surveys.) Visual and auditory dysfunctions increase dramatically with age. After age 45 the defective vision-acuity prevalence rate steadily increases until only 15 percent of the 75-to-79 age group has 20/20 vision even with correction (NCOA 1978, p. 111). After age 30 sharp increases in prevalence rates for hearing problems occur. Nineteen percent of the 45-to-54 age group has some hearing difficulties, while about 75 percent of the 75-to-79 age group has hearing impairment (DHEW 1975, p. 250).

Periodontal disease and tooth loss increase steadily with age. For persons over age 65, tooth loss caused by periodontal disease is the most prevalent dental problem (NCOA 1978, p. 111).

Major causes of death for persons 65 years and over are diseases of the heart, malignant neoplasms, cerebrovascular diseases, influenza, and pneumonia (DHEW 1975). Diseases of the heart far outrank the other causes of mortality.

MENTAL HEALTH

Old age represents a period of changing life circumstances. The ability to adapt to such changes has important consequences for the emotional and mental health of the elderly. Mental health status can be divided into three categories: (1) life-crises reactions—common emotional reactions such as anxiety, depression, and grief following the death of loved ones; (2) functional disturbances—psychiatric disturbances that may affect day-to-day functioning, but cause no impairment of brain function; and (3) organic disorders—impaired or permanently damaged brain cells.

Little is known about the extent of life-crises reactions and of organic disorders in the elderly. Most elderly presumably pass through life crises without developing severe emotional or functional disabilities. More is known about functional disturb-

ances. In 1971 the American Psychological Association estimated that 15 percent of the elderly required mental health services (Butler and Lewis 1977, p. 51). One percent of persons age 65 and over are in mental institutions; an additional 2 to 3 percent reside in nursing homes and related settings (NCOA 1978, p. 148).

We will give special consideration here to the statistics regarding suicide, depressive reaction, alcoholism, and drug abuse because these problems place the elderly in immediate need of mental health services.

Suicide

Suicide rates increase with age. The highest rate of suicide occurs in white males in their eighties. The elderly account for 25 percent of the reported suicides—about 5,000 to 8,000 yearly in the United States (Resnik and Cantor 1970, p. 153). Although suicide rates for women of all ages have been increasing, they peak in middle age (Butler and Lewis 1977, p. 67), as do rates for black men and women.

Depressive Reactions

Evidence indicates that the incidence and prevalence of depression rise through the life span and that the majority of people who commit suicide have shown previous signs of depression (Pfeiffer and Busse 1973, pp. 124 and 125). Early diagnosis and intervention may prevent serious mental illness later.

Alcoholism

Data indicate that alcohol problems among older people have been underestimated and hidden. The problem is greater among older males than females, but evidence suggests that the incidence of problem drinking among older females is likely to increase (NCOA 1978, p. 161). Elderly widows show the highest rate of alcoholism among all groups in a study by Bailey, Haberman, and Alksne (1965).

Drug Abuse

Little research has been done on the extent and nature of drug abuse among the elderly. Some of the abuse is intentional but much of it may be unintentional (NCOA 1978, p. 163). Mixing drugs, taking too much, not taking prescribed medicine, and saving or taking old drugs are some forms of abuse. Overuse of tranquilizers is one form of abuse that can create serious brain damage. Tardive dyskinesia is an irreversible syndrome that appears as a side effect of phenothiazine therapy or from withdrawal after being on moderate dosages and is most common in the brain damaged (Butler and Lewis 1977, p. 54).

HEALTH CARE POLICIES FOR THE ELDERLY

POLITICAL POWER

The potential political strength of the elderly may surprise political watchers in the future. "Almost 90 percent are registered to vote and two-thirds vote regularly," according to Butler and Lewis (1977, p. 13). Older individuals must *organize* themselves, however, in order to influence policy. A desire for "senior power" does seem to exist, and as Butler and Lewis further comment, "along with political strength can come a new sense of self-respect and a respect from others that will not be dependent on solicitude but will be a sober recognition of power at the ballot box on public issues." Binstock (1972), in con-

trast, takes the opposite view and doubts that older people as a group can mobilize themselves and exert political pressure by bloc voting.

Nevertheless, one example of elderly organization is the "Gray Panthers," a group promoting alternative lifestyles for older people. The strength of this organization led by Margaret Kuhn derives from an alliance of both young and old. Although such groups of elderly have not yet effectively made drastic power moves for equality, they have helped bring about current programs benefiting the elderly. What role the elderly will play in future politics remains to be seen.

SOCIAL POLICY AND THE AGING SOCIETY

The increasing number of older persons in the population necessitates comprehensive planning for them. However, investigations into U.S. social policy patterns on old age show many different programs but no coherent overall plan. For example, according to Gold, Kutza, and Marmor (1976, p. 9), "If aging policy means an intentional, coherent, overall plan about what the United States should do about aged citizens, then the United States does not have a social policy on old age." Their contention is that the unsystematic development of programs is due to the committee structure of Congress, which does not lend itself to program integration. Therefore, new programs do not necessarily build on their forerunners.

Although policy should set the goals that programs are intended to implement, many times the programs do not meet any goals, and sometimes the goals that are met are contrary to those set by policy makers. In addition, and perhaps more importantly, the art of understanding the impact of programs is not well developed (Gold et al. 1976, p. 9).

Not only are questions of impact important, but the ethical implications of policies and programs must be considered. "Our policies may be said to reflect ethical underpinnings of Western culture in general, and those of U.S. society in particular, but an awareness of the particular values implicit in particular policies may lead, not only to identification of value conflicts, but also to the re-examination of value priorities in a changing society" (Gold et al. 1976, p. 9).

Indeed, governmental influence on people's lives has become immense as federal expenditures for human services have grown. Much of the outlay has been through increased grants to state and local governments or direct cash transfers to individuals. Cash transfer programs include Social Security benefits; federal contributions to the aged, blind, and disabled (SSI); and civil service and railroad retirement benefits. Prior to the 1930s care for the aged and infirmed was the responsibility of the state or local municipality or was left to private charitable organizations. The depression led to a new type of federal policy regarding income redistribution. An example of a program under the new policy is the Social Security Act.

The Social Security Act of 1935 significantly affected the incomes of the elderly. The elderly also benefited from public housing under the Housing Act of 1956. But the Medicare law of 1965, which provides a national health insurance system for older persons, has had the greatest impact on the elderly.

Since the passage of the Medicare law, several smaller programs have developed, such as senior service centers, homemaker services, transportation services, and nutrition programs, but their impact on the 22 million aged has not yet been determined. Social Security and Medicare remain the two key programs for the elderly and will help shape future policy on old age.

Policy Issues

An analysis of social programs that affect the elderly and of programs developed specifically for the elderly is presented in chapter 19. Here let us consider issues that may influence future policy. At present, economic, political, psychosociological, and ethical-philosophical rationales have directed public investment in older persons (Gold et al. 1976). Statements that reflect these considerations range from "The elderly are economically disadvantaged" to "The elderly deserve special measures because of their past contribution." Whatever the reason for increased aid, redistribution of funds to the elderly will almost certainly continue. Social Security and Medicare will be the major programs; programs funded under the Older Americans Act will have little impact because of limited and restrictive funding; and Medicaid will continue to help the elderly who need nursing home care.

Issues that must be resolved in future policy making are:

1. The need for a reevaluation of the Social Security welfare function and its relationship to the Supplemental Security Income (SSI) program;
2. The question of spreading benefits such as health insurance to all the people or allocating them to a constituency group with a problem;

3. The high costs associated with policy decisions, including tax implications for citizens and political costs for policy makers;

4. The responsibility of the government versus that of individuals and their families for supporting older persons.

Problems in Health Services. Inadequate health care and retirement income are probably the two most critical problems affecting the well-being of the older population. The two are closely interrelated. Medicare is at present providing, along with Medicaid, the major portion of payments for health services. These programs are described in chapter 19. Evaluation and redirection of these two programs are badly needed, for they do not cover necessities such as out-of-hospital drugs, convalescent and custodial care, dental service, and hearing and vision services and devices.

The health care system needs changes that will benefit the entire adult population. Medical and technological advances have increased longevity to the point where national health policies are being made to counter the social, economic, and health problems of the elderly. At the present time health care in this country tends to follow a medical model that is designed for cure rather than for prevention of disease or for maintenance care. Some health workers are concerned essentially, if not solely, with acute diseases for which there are recognized treatments or palliative measures. They are interested in chronic diseases only if they promise, with more investigation, to yield better understanding and curative treatment.

Caring for the elderly has been left to the nonprofessional nurse for the most part. Duff and Hollingshead concluded in *Sickness and Society* (1968, p. 368) that care depends on the class structure of individuals and on their ability to pay. This study showed that patients who have insurance plans or who are classified as upper or middle class by the admissions officer receive attention from professional workers (doctors and nurses); patients designated as lower class and economically indigent are rendered care by nonprofessionals and by interns. Because many of the aged are economically disadvantaged, they fall into the group receiving care from the nonprofessional caregiver and intern. Duff and Hollingshead cited case studies that demonstrated care to be minimal and haphazardly given in wards where most patients were elderly.

The response of paraprofessionals to the care of the elderly has been judged inadequate because of their lack of knowledge of how to assess the health needs of the elderly. Utilization of the nursing profession to a greater degree in primary and long-term health care facilities and in the community at large is suggested. The degree of confusion surrounding the roles of the helping professions must be recognized. Change in the roles of the helping professions is necessitated not only by the need to broaden the base of skilled workers in critically needed services, but to give these workers the fullest satisfactions and benefits of contributing to the public well-being.

REFERENCES

ATCHLEY, R. 1977. *The Social Forces in Later Life,* 2d ed. Belmont, Calif.: Wadsworth.

BAILEY, N., P. HABERMAN, and H. ALKSNE. 1965. "The Epidemiology of Alcoholism in an Urban Residential Area." *Quarterly Journal Studies of Alcohol* 26:13–15.

BINSTOCK, R. 1972. "Interest-Group Liberalism and the Politics of Aging." *Gerontologist* 12:265–80.

BOUVIER, L., E. ATLEE, and F. McVEIGH. 1975. "The Elderly in America." *Population Bulletin.* Population Reference Bureau. Washington, D.C.: U.S. Government Printing Office.

BROTMAN, H. 1970. *The Older Population: Some Facts We Should Know.* Administration on Aging Publication #SRS–AOA–164–1971. Washington, D.C.: U.S. Government Printing Office, April.

———. 1975. *Every Tenth American.* Prepared for U.S. Senate Special Committee on Aging. Washington, D.C.: U.S. Government Printing Office, June.

BUTLER, R. 1975. *Why Survive? Being Old in America.* New York: Harper and Row.

——— and M. LEWIS. 1977. *Aging and Mental Health,* 2d ed. St. Louis: C. V. Mosby.

——— and A. MARTIN. 1977. "What You Should Know about Aging." *Pharmacy Times,* September.

CLARK, M., and B. ANDERSON. 1967. *Culture and Aging.* Springfield, Ill.: Charles C. Thomas.

COMFORT, A. 1964. *The Process of Aging.* New York: New American Library.

DUFF, R., and A. HOLLINGSHEAD. 1968. *Sickness and Society.* New York: Harper and Row.

GOLD, B., E. KUTZA, and T. MARMOR. 1976. "United States Social Policy on Old Age: Present Patterns and Predictions." In B. Neugarten and R. Havighurst, eds., *Social Policy, Social Ethics, and the Aging Society.* Washington, D.C.: National Science Foundation.

KART, C., E. METRESS, and J. METRESS. 1978. *Aging and Health: Biologic and Social Perspectives.* Menlo Park, Calif.: Addison-Wesley.

KIMMEL, D. 1974. *Adulthood and Aging.* New York: John Wiley.

LEAF, A. 1973. "Getting Old." *Scientific American* 229(3):45–52.

National Center for Health Statistics. 1973. *Current Estimates from Health Interview Survey (1972).* P. H. Service Publication No. 1000, series 10, no. 52. Washington, D.C.: U.S. Government Printing Office.

National Council on the Aging. 1978. *Fact Book on Aging: A Profile of America's Older Population.* Washington, D.C.: NCOA.

NEUGARTEN, B., and R. HAVIGHURST, eds. 1976. *Social Policy, Social Ethics, and the Aging Society.* Washington, D.C., National Science Foundation.

———, eds. 1977. *Extending the Human Life Span: Social Policy and Social Ethics.* Washington, D.C.: National Science Foundation.

OSTFELD, A., and D. GIBSON, eds. 1975. *Epidemiology of Aging.* U.S. Department of Health, Education, and Welfare, National Institutes of Health, DHEW Publication No. (NIH) 77–711.

PFEIFFER, E., and E. BUSSE, eds. 1973. *Mental Illness in Later Life.* Washington, D.C: American Psychiatric Association.

RESNIK, H. L., and J. M. CANTOR. 1970. "Suicide and Aging." *Journal of the American Geriatrics Society* 18:152–58.

SCHULZ, J. 1976. *The Economics of Aging.* Belmont, Calif.: Wadsworth.

TIBBITTS, C., ed. 1960. *Handbook of Social Gerontology.* Chicago: University of Chicago Press.

U.S. Bureau of the Census. 1973. *Some Demographic Aspects of Aging in the United States.* Current Population Reports, series P–23, no. 43. Washington, D.C.: U.S. Government Printing Office.

———. 1976. *Demographic Aspects of Aging and the Older Population in the United States.* Current Population Reports Special Studies, series P–23, no. 59. Washington, D.C.: U.S. Government Printing Office.

U.S. Department of Health, Education, and Welfare. 1975. *Health United States 1975.* Washington, D.C.: Public Health Service, Health Resources Administration, National Center for Health Statistics.

U.S. Senate. 1976. *A Report of the Special Committee on Aging.* Washington, D.C.: U.S. Government Printing Office.

ZARIT, S., ed. 1977. *Readings in Aging and Death: Contemporary Perspectives.* New York: Harper and Row.

23

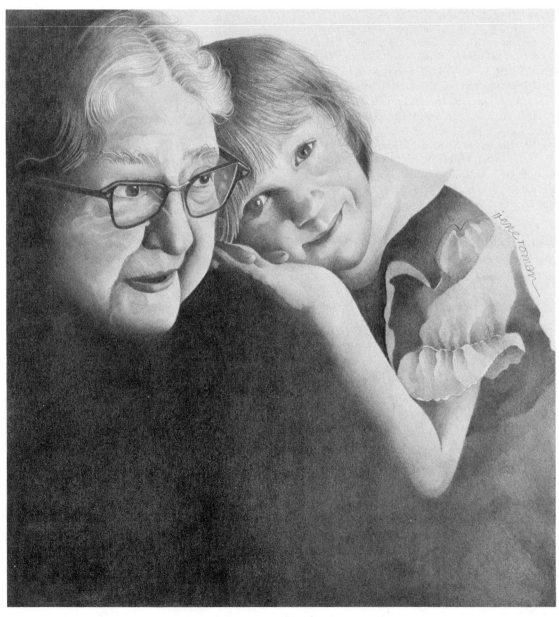

Dorothy Karpowich

Chapter 3

NEEDS OF THE ELDERLY AND HEALTH PROMOTION

Most gerontological nurse practitioners/ clinical nurse specialists are likely to be employed in a variety of primary care settings—for example, ambulatory care centers, clinics for the aged, doctors' offices, or health maintenance organizations. Regardless of the setting, their role responsibilities to their elderly clients will require that they: (1) strengthen the ability of the "normal, healthy, and walking" to maintain and promote their own health; (2) supervise and coordinate the care of common health problems and chronic illnesses; (3) evaluate and plan the treatment of illnesses; (4) evaluate the need for referral to appropriate medical personnel for acute illnesses or deterioration of conditions; and (5) work in collaboration with other health care providers and agencies to provide and coordinate services for the aged and their families. The gerontological nurse will stress education for health maintenance

and promotion and will teach relevant self-care measures to the elderly.

In the past, preventive health programs for the elderly have not been commonplace. But medical advances and an increase in living standards for most Americans have prolonged life to the extent that more and more individuals are now concerned with the quality of their increased longevity.

Many of the elderly have chronic, noncurable illnesses that require continuous and long-term health care services. The present American health care delivery system is geared toward "repair," and cure of acute illness. If the values of our pluralistic society dictate comprehensive health services for all individuals, then certain changes must occur. The health care delivery system must be organized in such a way that it becomes a health promotion system. Such a system would provide necessary health information, care, and services from the very beginning to the end of the life span.

The American Association of Colleges of Nursing's definition of primary care strongly supports the view that *illness prevention and health maintenance must be viable and integral components of primary care* within the total health care system (A.A.C.N. 1976). Their definition of primary care is both timely and appropriate for gerontological nurse practitioners and is in agreement with the definition of primary care contained in the Nurse Practitioner Act (Federal Register, Nov. 1977).

The A.A.C.N. definition goes beyond first-contact, on-going, and coordinated care of common health problems and chronic illnesses to emphasize illness prevention and health maintenance. It recognizes the importance of care over time and across specialty and agency boundaries as well as the importance of teaching all individuals about health and self-care.

Accessible and comprehensive health services suited to the needs of our elderly population and health promotion efforts should help reduce the necessity for short-term hospitalization and long-term institutionalization. The gerontological nurse, by virtue of seeing an aged client on a regular, continuous basis, will be able to identify changing levels of wellness and by so doing intervene before serious illness occurs.

The elderly require accessible and comprehensive health service; they also need health workers who care. They want not so much a diagnosis as an affirmation of their self-worth. Health care, then, should be delivered and given in an atmosphere that increases the self-respect of the elderly person. It is imperative that in any primary care setting the gerontological nurse will make time for the development of a trusting and mutually satisfying relationship between nurse and client. One of the major needs of the aged person is meaningful relationships with others. Only within a satisfying nurse-client relationship will true needs and problems of the elderly be revealed and effective solutions planned and implemented.

Often aged persons find themselves in care settings that are both busy and complex. The elderly become frustrated and confused by a large number of short, superficial contacts with a wide variety of health personnel as well as by long, tiring sojourns in waiting rooms. Whenever possible, therefore, reducing the number of "helpers" and scheduling the same nurse to see the same client on a continuous basis are sensible measures. True collaborative relationships built on trust and sharing among professionals will obviate the need for everyone to see and interview the client. Certainly, however, if the therapeutic process demands interventions by a variety of personnel and services, explanations and advocate services are desirable.

The aged face multiple and diverse problems. A humanistic and holistic view of the aged and of those closest to them is essential in efforts to help them maintain health and cope with various levels of wellness.

NEEDS OF THE ELDERLY

Many professionals in the behavioral and health sciences have written of the needs of the elderly and their special problems brought on by physical decline, role adjustment, societal attitudes, and decreased income. As all the needs of humanity in general and of the aged in particular are more or less related to the promotion and maintenance of physical and mental health, we will take a brief look at some of the universal needs of humanity and the special needs of the aged.

UNIVERSAL HUMAN NEEDS

Certain human needs are generally accepted as universal. Many lists of these needs may be found in the literature (Murray 1938; Maslow 1943, 1970; Alderfer 1969). Most contain a category of physical needs (hunger, thirst, activity, rest, sex, temperature regulation, elimination, oxygen, and avoidance of pain, injury, and illness) and a category of psychosocial needs (security, status, affection, esteem, affiliation, independence-dependence, and achievement). Such needs are viewed as motivating forces that initiate behavior. When a need exists and is unsatisfied, the individual is anxious, restless, and tense. When the need is satisfied, a temporary state of equilibrium is established and the individual ceases activity directed toward the fulfillment of the need. Behavior is then directed toward the meeting of other needs.

Maslow's hierarchical classification of needs seems to be well known among health personnel because of its organismic point of view. According to Maslow the following five levels of needs must be satisfied in order to achieve and maintain physiological and psychological homeostasis: (1) physiological needs; (2) the need for safety, security, stability, and freedom from pain, threat, or illness; (3) the need to belong and to be loved; (4) the need for recognition or respect from others and self-esteem, and (5) the need for self-actualization, sometimes described as the need to grow and develop or the need to realize one's potential.

Maslow theorizes that the strength of any need is determined by its position in the hierarchy (physiological needs being most important) and by the degree to which lower order needs have been satisfied. While Maslow states that the hierarchy of needs is not a rigidly fixed order—that is, it is not the same for all individuals—he does contend that physiological needs, because they are most crucial to survival, are the most prepotent and that self-actualization needs are the least. Furthermore, in contrast to the other levels of needs, motivation based on the need to grow and develop (self-actualize) does not decrease as the need becomes satisfied, but creates a desire for more growth.

Some evidence suggests that unless physiological and safety-security needs are satisfied, behavior will not be directed toward satisfaction of high order needs (Keys et al. 1950; Lawler and Suttle 1972). Thus needs for social acceptance, self-esteem, and self-actualization will appear only when the first two levels of needs are satisfied. Little evidence has been found to support the existence of a hierarchy above the physiological and safety-security levels. Therefore, the acceptance of a two-level hierarchy with physiological and safety-security needs at the first or fundamental level and the others at the second level seems to be a safer course, as no one can predict what higher order needs will come into play once the first level has been satisfied (Lawler 1973).

Many who care for the elderly would take issue with Maslow's hierarchical classification theory and even with the latter two levels suggested. They would point out that many of the elderly who have adequate funds to meet basic physiological and safety-security needs commit suicide, many die of loneliness, and others simply do not have "the will to live."

On the other hand, most observers of our elderly "well" population would agree that meeting basic survival needs is most important to the majority of the elderly. Poverty poses a formidable barrier to many elderly attempting to meet basic survival needs, associated as it is with inadequate nutrition, poor housing, and minimal health care. Estimates are that while persons over 65 make up 10.5 percent of the general population, they constitute 20 percent of the poor, or one out of every three elderly Americans.

The aged, many of whom live in high-crime areas of cities, also have difficulty meeting safety-security needs. Fear of bodily harm and material loss prevents many from venturing outside their homes. This deplorable situation is described almost daily in our newspapers.

In caring for the elderly who cannot meet certain physiological and safety-security needs, the gerontological nurse may have to go beyond the health care system and contact other appropriate community systems (social welfare, housing councils, public health, councils for the aging, etc.) if social workers are not available. Only when living conditions improve in some environments can basic needs of many of our aged be met and their quality of life improved.

SPECIFIC NEEDS OF THE ELDERLY

The White House Conference on Aging (1971) identified nine areas in which the needs of the elderly are directly or indirectly related to health promotion: nutrition, retirement roles and activities, spiritual well-being, transportation, education, employment-retirement, physical and mental health, housing, and income.

Goldfarb (1967) has summarized the specific needs of the elderly as the need to be physically and socially independent and to have a sense of purpose, self-confidence, and self-esteem. Because of problems in later life, many find it hard to satisfy these needs. Thus Goldfarb argues that it is more important for health workers to give the elderly a feeling of self-worth than to give them routine physical care.

From the experiences of community health nurses working with the elderly, Austin (1959) has summarized six basic needs of the elderly person: (1) an income and economic security gained through socially useful and personally satisfying means, (2) a sense of maximum personal effectiveness, (3) a suitable place in which to live, (4) opportunities to spend leisure time constructively, (5) a sense of positive and well-integrated social relationships within the family and community, and (6) a sense of achieving and maintaining spiritual values and goals.

In his interesting study done in England, Skelton (1977) found that the following problems of the elderly were overlooked by health and welfare services: depression, visual defects, hearing impairment, obesity, inadequate foot care, symptomatic anemia, inappropriate use of drugs, loneliness, prolonged bereavement, poor housing, and financial difficulties. This particular study identified nearly two (statistically 1.8) previously unrecognized problems for every one problem known to the health and welfare services. Comparative data from Shanas (1969) relating to unreported needs of the aged also point out the need for more comprehensive health services and better methods of case finding for this group. Both researchers point out, however, that such case finding is questionable practice if the system is unable to provide for these needs.

Gerontological nurses will be working primarily with the ambulant elderly who live in their own homes. In caring for such clients, the following list of needs of the elderly will be helpful. It has been taken from many sources, including those mentioned above, with no attempt to rank items in order of importance.

Needs of the Elderly

Adequate income

Adequate nutrition

Adequate housing

Convenient transportation

A meaningful and purposeful life

Spiritual belief, guidance, and growth

Accessible, coordinated, and comprehensive health services

Opportunities for companionship and recreation

Good personal health habits

Privacy and personal space

Opportunities to voice consumer complaints

Control over life situations to the degree possible

Life with integrity

Death with dignity

Opportunities to learn and practice new skills

One-to-one relationships with caring, loving people

Maintenance of a good physical appearance

Solitude if so desired

Physical intimacy and sexual expression

Counseling and advice regarding role loss, retirement, legal problems, and money management

Physical and psychological independence to the degree possible

Maintenance of family and peer roles

Health insurance coverage

A caring attitude, attentive listening, and careful assessment of each unique elderly client will help gerontological nurses identify their clients' specific needs. Working cooperatively and collaboratively with other health workers in the social and health systems, they will be in a position not only to assess changing levels of wellness, but also to work with others in the community to initiate, develop, and evaluate health and social programs required by the elderly. For only with a full awareness, appreciation, and understanding of the total needs—physical, mental, and spiritual—of the elderly can gerontological nurses promote health and prevent illness in the elderly. The physical health needs of the elderly are discussed in this chapter and in chapter 6; various aspects of the elderly's mental health and spiritual needs will be discussed in chapter 7.

CONCEPTS OF HEALTH AND HEALTH PROMOTION

With more people living longer, American society needs to become more concerned with the health and quality of life of its older citizens. An emphasis on health promotion throughout the life cycle, including old age, would reduce disability and chronic illness in later life. One of the most logical ways to decrease ever-rising medical and institutionalization costs is to emphasize positive health attitudes and habits by stressing prevention of disease and encouraging people to take more responsibility for their own health maintenance.

DEFINITIONS OF HEALTH AND ILLNESS

Many definitions of health and illness exist. For example, the World Health Organization defines health as a state of complete physical, mental, and social well-being, not merely the absence of disease. According to an even more flexible and dynamic definition by Murray and Zentner (1975), health is the purposeful, adaptive response (physically, mentally, emotionally, and socially) to internal and external stimuli to maintain stability and comfort. Illness, then, is defined as a disturbed adaptive response to internal and external stimuli, resulting in disequilibrium and inability to utilize the usual health-promoting resources.

In caring for the elderly, a useful definition of health and illness is one formulated by Dunn (1959). Dunn conceives of health and illness in terms of a graduated scale or continuum that ranges from high-level wellness to extreme poor health. High-level wellness is a state in which the individual's physical, mental, emotional, and social functioning is oriented toward maximizing his or her potential within a given environment. Thus in Dunn's view the individual is an integrated bio-psycho-social being whose level of wellness is dynamic and ever changing. This concept of high-level wellness, which focuses on maximizing potential and recognizes the influence of environment, helps health workers to focus on the elderly's assets and resources rather than on their liabilities when planning for their care.

PREVENTIVE HEALTH MEASURES

Health promotion for the elderly, then, may be defined as the promotion of all those factors that help them achieve the maximum level of wellness or functioning of which they are capable. Among the factors are preventive health measures. These measures vary according to the elderly's level of wellness.

Phases of Prevention

1. *Primary prevention:* measures aimed at averting the occurrence of disease
2. *Secondary prevention:* Measures aimed at minimizing the progress of disease and its complications through early diagnosis and prompt treatment
3. *Tertiary prevention:* measures aimed at avoiding further progress of sequelae from disease

Leavell and Clark (1965) have developed a comprehensive model showing levels of application of preventive health measures (see figure 3.1). Most health workers are familiar with this model, which covers a span of time and events from prepathogenesis through rehabilitation. Leavell and Clark stress that the phases of prevention and levels of application are not

FIGURE 3.1   Levels of Application of Preventive Health Measures.
Source: H. R. Leavell and E. G. Clark, Preventive Medicine for the Doctor in His Community, *3rd ed. (New York: McGraw-Hill Book Co., 1965). Reprinted by permission.*

THE NATURAL HISTORY OF ANY DISEASE OF HUMANS

Prepathogenesis Period	Period of Pathogenesis
Interrelations of Agent, Host, and Environmental Factors → Production of STIMULUS →	Reaction of the HOST to the STIMULUS Early Pathogenesis → Discernible early lesions → Advanced disease → Convalescence

HEALTH PROMOTION

Health education

Good standard of nutrition adjusted to developmental phases of life

Attention to personality development

Provision of adequate housing, recreation, and agreeable working conditions

Marriage counseling and sex education

Genetics

Periodic selective examinations

SPECIFIC PROTECTION

Use of specific immunizations

Attention to personal hygiene

Use of environmental sanitation

Protection against occupational hazards

Protection from accidents

Use of specific nutrients

Protection from carcinogens

Avoidance of allergens

EARLY DIAGNOSIS & PROMPT TREATMENT

Case-finding measures, individual and mass

Screening surveys

Selective examinations

Objectives:

To cure and prevent disease processes

To prevent the spread of communicable diseases

To prevent complications and sequelae

To shorten period of disability

DISABILITY LIMITATION

Adequate treatment to arrest the disease process and to prevent further complications and sequelae

Provision of facilities to limit disability and to prevent death

REHABILITATION

Provision of hospital and community facilities for retraining and education for maximum use of remaining capacities

Education of the public and industry to utilize the rehabilitated

As full employment as possible

Selective placement

Work therapy in hospitals

Use of sheltered colony

Primary Prevention	Secondary Prevention	Tertiary Prevention

isolated but overlap and form a continuum.

In working with the aged more than with any other age group, the gerontological nurse will be applying preventive health measures in all phases of prevention. In caring for an elderly client, the nurse may be teaching the client what an adequate diet consists of for a given age, amount of activity, and budget *(primary prevention)*; performing a physical examination and providing a health evaluation and management plan *(secondary prevention)*; and referring the client to appropriate facilities in the community for job retraining *(tertiary prevention)*. See Dr. Giorgi's "Considerations in Health Promotion of the Aged," at the end of the chapter for numerous examples of primary, secondary, and tertiary prevention.

INDIVIDUAL RESPONSIBILITY AND HEALTH PROMOTION

Increasingly in health literature authorities are recognizing that people have the capacity to determine their own health potentials and are emphasizing the need for individuals to assume basic responsibility for their own well-being. Recent research (Belloc and Breslow 1972; Belloc 1973; Somers and Breslow 1977) has shown that basic health habits, lifestyle, and environment have an effect on life expectancy and health. For example, Belloc and Breslow (1972) studied 7,000 adults for five and a half years and found that longevity and better health were significantly related to the practice of seven basic health habits.

Basic Health Habits

1. Three meals a day at regular times instead of snacking
2. Breakfast every day
3. Moderate exercise
4. Seven or eight hours of sleep at night
5. No smoking
6. Moderate weight
7. No alcohol or moderate consumption

Individuals practicing many of these good health habits exhibited better physical health than those who practiced only a few. Mortality rates were more directly related to poor health habits than to physical health status or income levels. Many other lists of factors promoting personal health have been formulated. Most include regular physical examinations and selective checkups; learning the warning signals of disease and the predisposing factors of illness; personal hygiene; cholesterol control; avoidance of extreme stress, fatigue, or exhaustion; avoiding substances injurious to health; and adequate nutrition.

According to Spector and Spector (1977), however, many of these preventive measures simply ignore the realities of the daily existence of many elderly people as well as of ethnic minorities and others who live in poverty. Such measures are frequently alien to their cultural patterns. Spector and Spector conclude that if prevention is not to be a myth for the groups mentioned above, living conditions must improve and preventive health programs and services must be accessible and available to nonpaying clients as well as to those with health insurance. Preventive programs must also be geared to the cultural traditions of different groups.

Certainly the elderly population that the gerontological nurse will be caring for has profited from the better health care and living standards of the last half century. But the particular socioeconomic backgrounds and ethic origins of the elderly have been important determinants of their environment, lifestyles, and ability to practice good basic health habits. The elderly in our pluralistic society represent diverse ethnic origins, cultural patterns, religions, social classes, and socioeconomic means. An awareness of and sensitivity to this diversity will enable the gerontological nurse to give meaningful and effective care to elderly clients and to determine the degree of responsibility that they are ready and willing to accept in promoting their own health.

THE "BIG THREE" IN HEALTH PROMOTION: DIET, EXERCISE, AND THE HAZARDS OF SMOKING

Health education in diet, exercise, and the hazards of smoking should be communicated to clients in a way that is acceptable to them. Inadequate diet, lack of exercise, and smoking can play important roles in predisposing the elderly to coronary heart disease, cancer, and cerebrovascular disease. These diseases rank first, second, and third, respectively, as causes of death in the United States today.

If elderly clients have an existing or newly diagnosed disease, they may be even more receptive to health education in the "big three" than those with no evidence of disease. Teaching people about their illnesses and how to manage them is usually easier than teaching preventive measures aimed at avoiding problems before they occur. The information seems more relevant to the individual afflicted with the condition.

However, diet, exercise, and the hazards of smoking need to be stressed even to persons without these aforementioned condi-

tions, as many other chronic conditions of the aged (respiratory problems, diabetes, hypertension, arthritis, etc.) are affected by one or more of the "big three." For example, smoking is a predisposing or high-risk factor in cancer of the lung and emphysema; obesity is a high-risk factor in diabetes and coronary heart disease and certainly interferes with the coping power of the elderly arthritic client.

Diet

Nutritional Requirements. The elderly need carbohydrates, fat, protein, vitamins, minerals, and water as part of their daily dietary intake. These nutritional requirements vary according to individual differences in body structure, metabolism, and, possibly, different past or current disease processes.

Most elderly require fewer calories than younger people do because of reduced basal energy requirement caused by loss of functioning cells and by lessened physical activity. Probably the simplest criterion for determining adequate calorie intake is the maintenance of desired and proper weight.

In planning specific nutrient intakes with the elderly, the gerontological nurse can use the recommended dietary allowances provided by the National Research Council (1974) (see table 3.1). By comparing the older adult's food intake (kinds and amounts of solids and liquids) ingested over three days with the recommended daily allowances, the nurse can better evaluate the client's nutritional status. Essentially the National Research Council states that caloric intake for persons over age 50 should be reduced to 90 percent of the allowance for mature adults. However, allowances in the intake of other nutrients, 33

TABLE 3.1
Recommended Dietary Allowances for Persons Over Age 50

Nutrients	Women	Men
Calories (kcal)	1,800.0	2,400.0
Protein (g)	46.0	56.0
Vitamin A (I.U.)	4,000.0	5,000.0
Vitamin E (I.U.)	12.0	15.0
Ascorbic Acid (mg)	45.0	45.0
Niacin (mg)	12.0	16.0
Riboflavin (mg)	1.1	1.5
Thiamin (mg)	1.0	1.2
Calcium (mg)	800.0	800.0
Iron (mg)	10.0	10.0

Source: *National Research Council,* Recommended Dietary Allowances, *8th rev. ed. (Washington, D.C.: National Academy of Science, 1974). Reprinted by permission.*

such as protein, vitamins, and minerals, do not call for any reduction.

Nutritional Problems. Some of the most common nutritional problems of the elderly are overnutrition, undernutrition, dehydration, and iron-deficiency anemia. In a ten-state nutrition survey taken between 1968 and 1970 on a population sample of men and women over 60 years of age, the most prevalent nutritional deficits were iron in both sexes, vitamin A in Spanish-American men and women, riboflavin in black and Spanish-Americans of both sexes, and vitamin C in males of all racial and ethnic origins. This sample consisted of those in the lowest quartile of income at the time of the 1960 census (Center for Disease Control 1972). In a similar survey on a sample representative of the U.S. civilian population (ages 1–74 years), the most frequent deficits in the age group over 60 years were those of dietary iron, vitamin A, vitamin C, and calcium (Abraham et al. 1974).

Overnutrition, especially in carbohydrates, coupled with decreased physical activity, causes many of the aged to become overweight or obese. Statistics indicate that obesity reduces life expectancy in the middle-aged and aged population; and clearly many conditions known to decrease longevity are less severe when uncomplicated by obesity.

The elderly tend to buy carbohydrate foods in abundance because they are easy to store and eat, are generally less expensive than other foods, and require little, if any, cooking. Many are snack foods that "taste good" (crackers, pies, cakes, potato chips, etc.). Such foods satisfy hunger but meet few nutritional requirements. Some of the elderly supplement such a diet by taking vitamins and minerals, but protein deficiency commonly results.

Undernutrition among the elderly is also common partly because budgetary restraints often force them to skimp on food purchases. Other factors that may contribute to undernutrition are reduced perception of smell and taste and limiting enjoyment of eating, depression, chronic illness, and drug therapy. The aged often eat alone, and grocery shopping and meal preparation can be difficult, especially if sensory deprivation or other physical limitations exist.

While dental condition is frequently cited in the literature as a factor contributing to undernutrition, Mikelson (1976) reports evidence from a number of sources suggesting that the nutrient intake of older people is not influenced by their dental condition. The nurse should be aware of the availability of Meals on Wheels and other sponsored meal programs in the community. Such programs have been successful in providing nourishing meals for the elderly in their homes and in central locations that also offer an opportunity for socialization. Sometimes an older person's principal need is to help others; meal programs frequently fulfill this need by welcoming volunteers of any age.

Dehydration is seen frequently in the elderly; they need to be continually reminded that adequate hydration is necessary for proper body functioning. Dehydration and lack of fiber in the diet of the aged frequently cause and aggravate constipation, hemorrhoids, and colitis. Helping the elderly person write out a definite schedule of fluid intake is one way to encourage adequate hydration.

Both nutritional surveys mentioned previously pointed to the prevalence of *dietary iron deficiency* in older age groups (see chapter 18 for symptomatology and treatment of nutritional anemia). Usually an iron supplement or a diet high in iron is prescribed after a complete and thorough health assessment. Foods high in iron include liver and other organ meats, lean meats, egg yolks, seafood, whole wheat bread, green vegetables, apricots, raisins, nuts, and legumes.

Vitamin and mineral supplements may be necessary if nutritional requirements cannot be met by food intake. A food consumption survey taken in the mid-1960s indicated that 26 percent of men and women age 65 to 74 use vitamin or mineral supplements, as do 35 percent of those over 74 (U.S. Dept. of Agriculture 1972). These findings may indicate that older people are interested in diet and health and/or have difficulty meeting nutritional requirements by diet alone. Research suggests that increased intake of calcium and certain vitamins such as C and E might have beneficial health effects for the aged, but further research is needed before definitive statements can be made.

Although changing the dietary patterns of the elderly is very difficult, gerontological nurses will have a better chance of being effective if they develop a good relationship with their clients and teach them on a one-to-one basis. Therapeutic diets may be prescribed for some clients, and nutritionists may be available to help plan and teach these diets to the elderly. Increasingly, modified low-cholesterol diets are prescribed to reduce elevated serum lipid levels. Clients on such diets should restrict their intake of saturated fat—cholesterol—and substitute polyunsaturated fats for saturated fats whenever possible. Cholesterol-rich foods include egg yolk, organ meats, shellfish, and dairy fat.

In summary, adequate hydration and the need for all nutrients must be stressed to the elderly. Fresh fruits and vegetables, whole grain bread, lean meats, fish, and legumes should be encouraged if obtainable, economically feasible, and culturally acceptable. Nurses working with many different cultural groups should know the food preferences and staples of their clients. Clients are more likely to comply with needed dietary changes if sample menus include culturally preferred foods.

Exercise

Physical activity improves overall health, reduces susceptibility to many diseases, and promotes longevity. Although environment and climate may limit the ways one can exercise, more and more opportunities for exercise are becoming available. Some elderly are joining health clubs or signing up for exercise or dancing classes at the local "Y," community college, or other adult-education–oriented organizations. The elderly should be encouraged to exercise daily within the limits of their tolerance. Previously sedentary persons who want to begin an exercise regimen should be cautioned to begin slowly, build up gradually, and take rests between exercises. Exercise programs should have physician approval if the elderly client has any kind of illness or chronic condition. Exercise can help aged individuals lose weight, maintain cardiovascular fitness, prevent the formation of cellulite, and improve their self-image by improving their appearance. While exercise does not alter the rate of aging, scientific studies demonstrate that it can reduce the incidence of disease. More and more elderly will be reaping the rewards of safe and appropriate exercise through such means as walking; swimming; jogging; flexibility exercises; disco, ballroom, and square dancing; and using basic exercise equipment. The nurse should review with the elderly the exercise options available to them. Most people who exercise say it makes them feel better. The nurse should encourage the elderly to give exercise in any form a "test run."

The Hazards of Smoking

Estimates are that 54 million Americans smoke in spite of the fact that smoking was proved harmful to health more than fourteen years ago. Research has shown that smoking can initiate and promote disease processes (cardiovascular and respiratory diseases and some types of cancer) and is also one of the most important negative predictors of longevity. Analyses of disease patterns from the National Cancer Institute indicate that 30 to 35 percent of all cancer-related deaths in this country are the direct result of cigarette smoking. Although smoking is a habit difficult to give up once established, some elderly will be motivated to quit because of the seriousness of their symptoms or the discomfort brought on by smoking. Smokers Anonymous and other programs frequently available at health centers can help the aged client to quit.

IMPORTANT AREAS IN HEALTH PROMOTION OF THE ELDERLY

Promoting the Safe Use of Drugs

The elderly, who constitute roughly 10 percent of the U.S. population, account for 25 percent of the drugs used in this country (Kayne 1976). They are probably the largest purchasers of over-the-counter drugs, which they use for self-treatment. Susceptible to advertising on television (watching television is one of their favorite pastimes), they are prone to use many remedies for their various ailments.

Because many of the elderly need prescribed drugs, tend to self-medicate, and increasingly use multiple drugs in one vehicle, gerontological nurses must devote adequate time for taking an accurate drug history. Many times the elderly do not know the names of the drugs they are taking and are not taking their prescribed drugs in the right dosage or at the right times for optimum effectiveness. Research (Schwartz 1962; Neely and Patrick 1968) indicates that the incidence of drug errors among the aged is high. By taking an accurate drug history, nurses will be able to learn the extent of their clients' knowledge about the drugs being taken and to identify areas that require teaching and/or review.

The elderly ambulatory client, while receiving many benefits from the necessary medications, must be closely monitored by the gerontological nurse for possible adverse drug reactions. The importance of such monitoring is highlighted by the fact that 3 to 5 percent of all hospital admissions are a consequence of adverse drug reactions (Miller 1973; Caranasos et al. 1974). Furthermore, proportionately more clients over 61 years of age than under 61 require hospitalization for drug-induced illnesses. Therefore, the nurse should keep in mind that changes in the client's physical and/or mental condition might be drug induced. Too frequently, symptoms brought on by adverse drug reactions are attributed to disease or to the age of the client. Some of the most common of the serious drug-induced diseases are digitalis toxicity and dehydration and electrolyte disturbances caused by diuretic therapy.

To avoid problems, the elderly need counseling about the drugs they are taking. If many drugs are to be taken, the names of the drugs and the times they are to be taken should be written down and given to clients. Important side effects should also be written down. If elderly persons have difficulty remembering what time they should take a drug or whether they have taken a certain drug, a clock can be made out of a paper plate, and small baking cups can be glued at hours when medication is to be taken. In the morning, the client or another person can put the designated allotment of pills for the day into the proper time cups. In this way, if clients forget whether they took their 10 A.M. drug, they can look at the 10 A.M. cup to see if the pill is there. Some elderly have found this method very helpful. Those responsible for the older person can also use this method to check whether the daily drug allotment has been taken. Some elderly individuals rely on alarm clocks to remind them to take necessary drugs.

The creative and imaginative nurse will be able to identify methods that work with individual clients. Drug taking by the elderly in the home can be a safe procedure when proper instruction is given initially, followed by regular monitoring and review when necessary.

Promoting Foot Care

Foot care is a very important aspect of health promotion in caring for the elderly. Arteriosclerosis, diabetes, and other circulatory problems commonly found in the aged frequently cause small cuts, hangnails, calluses, and ulcers to become major handicaps that cannot only restrict social-

37

ization and independence, but eventually lead to hospitalization. Feet, nails, shoes, canes, crutches, and prosthetics should be examined by the nurse. Shoes should fit properly, presence of skin breakdown or redness should be noted, and walking aids should be of proper height and used correctly to promote safety and comfort. The elderly should be taught the basics of good foot care if they are not practicing preventive care and should be encouraged to seek proper care at the first sign of a foot problem. Podiatric services should be recommended whenever necessary.

Maximizing Dental Function

The condition of the teeth or dentures, gums, and mouth may have an effect on the nutritional intake and physical appearance of the elderly. Therefore, gerontological nurses should assess this area carefully and make recommendations whenever appropriate. Referral may be difficult, as economical and accessible services are not always available.

The goal in this area is to prevent further decay and to maximize whatever dental function is left. Unfortunately, many dental problems (loss of teeth, periodontal disease) are irreversible, but efforts can be made to take advantage of whatever function is left and to promote good oral hygiene. Dentures should be obtained when indicated, and ill-fitting dentures should be replaced. Sugars, snacks, and soft, sticky foods should be eliminated or reduced in the diet. A well-balanced diet, an adequate water intake, and the chewing of firm solids will help the elderly maintain dental health.

Identifying Sensory Deficits

Vision and hearing deficits are common in the elderly and frequently act as a deterrent to adequate socialization and the development of satisfying relationships. Safety problems are also multiplied for those with failing eyesight and hearing loss. A careful home assessment is usually indicated for those elderly with one or more sensory deficits. Safety hazards can be identified and procedures instituted to give the elderly person with a sensory loss a greater feeling of security when living alone.

Vision Deficits. One of the most common causes of vision deficit in the elderly is glaucoma. Estimates are that 2 out of every 100 persons over age 40 may have glaucoma. Glaucoma is an insidious disease and can lead to blindness. The disease and loss of sight are irreversible, so it is important to identify the condition in its early stages. Case finding of glaucoma depends on eye tonometry, as the disease is asymptomatic in its early stages. Therefore, some physicians recommend that eye tonometry measurements be included with every examination on persons age 40 and above, particularly those with a family history of the disease.

Hearing Deficits. Hearing losses are fairly common in the elderly; deficits usually begin around the late forties and early fifties, when many lose the ability to hear high-frequency sounds. A nurse can easily discover if cerumen is causing the hearing deficit. If this is the case, an ear irrigation will solve the hearing problem.

In cases of obvious hearing loss, referral should be made to an otologist who can properly diagnose the condition and initiate proper treatment if the loss is not due to irreversible nerve damage. The loss of hearing can have devastating effects on some individuals, particularly those whose work requires good hearing or who are highly involved in the community and/or in social activities.

Interestingly, only 35 percent of persons over age 65 who have a hearing loss have had their condition checked by a doctor. Frequently individuals try to conceal their hearing loss. Elderly persons whose hearing can be improved by hearing aids will need psychological preparation and instruction about the particular instrument they will be using.

Promoting Safety and Preventing Injury

Accidental injuries account for approximately 20 percent of acute conditions in the aged, and more than half of such injuries occur in the home. The most common accidents among the aged are falls, many of which are related to sensory deprivation or loss of functional capacity. Of persons age 65 and over, 43 percent have limitation in activity and 16 percent are unable to carry out major activities. Hip fractures and other musculoskeletal injuries often result from dropping or lifting heavy objects; slipping on wet floors or bathtubs; tripping over rugs, pets, or cords; and falling when getting out of bed.

Many factors predispose the aged to injuries. The aged may be poorly coordinated, have slow reflexes, and walk with difficulty. They may also have illnesses, such as cerebral ischemia, arthritis, or osteoporosis, or neurological disorders that affect locomotion and the senses. For these reasons the home environment must be made as safe as possible and the elderly must become accustomed to taking certain precautions, depending on their particular deficits. The elderly should be advised not to rise from a horizontal position too rapidly after rest: dizziness caused by postural hypotension or rapid head movement may make the elderly fall and injure themselves. Dr. Giorgi has made a detailed outline listing steps that can be taken to prevent injury in the aged—see "Considerations in Health Promotion in the Aged" at the end of this chapter. Gerontological nurses and others can use this outline as a checklist in teaching the aged about preventive measures or during a home safety evaluation. The list is presented in its entirety because it is both comprehensive and succinct.

LEARNING AND THE AGED

Today's society is making greater demands upon people to adapt and change. Because changes are occurring rapidly in all spheres of life and because people are living longer, the need for continuous learning throughout the life span is imperative. The elderly are attending classes in record numbers and taking many diverse courses. Long-held but inaccurate beliefs that old people cannot learn or do not want to learn are slowly disappearing. Increasingly education is providing the elderly with an opportunity to "broaden their world" and/or increase their skills in areas of their choice. Health educators can take advantage of this emphasis on lifelong

39

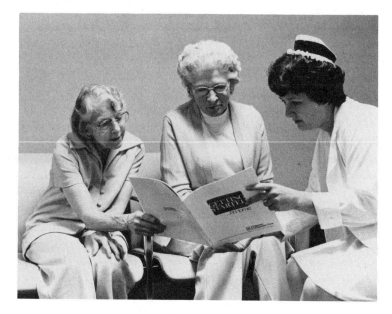

The gerontological nurse can help the elderly adapt to the aging process by promoting preventive health measures through the teaching process; elderly clients need to understand their own roles and responsibilities in maintaining their health.

learning to promote health among the elderly.

LEARNING CAPACITY

Some studies have been done to determine the learning capacity of individuals as they age. Conclusions have been difficult, as the studies have differed in methodology (cross-sectional, longitudinal, time-lag) and subjects (healthy, unhealthy).

According to Chown (1972), results from some studies of aging and intelligence exaggerate somewhat the deleterious effects of "pure age." Convenience sampling, tests taken under the stress of time limitations, and the elderly's lack of motivation in performing tasks that seem meaningless may account for some of the negative results. The risk-taking behavior of the aged may also play a role: many older persons are reluctant to take action in any risk-taking situation if the effects are uncertain. The elderly tend to be anxious in learning and testing situations because society has convinced them that they will fail. Furthermore, if the elderly have sensory losses, their perception of test material and grasp of instructions may be deficient, resulting in lower test scores.

Several studies show that in teacher-made tests, virtually no sign of decline appears in the intelligence of normal, healthy individuals past 60. What studies have shown to decline is speed in performance. However, individuals with such health problems as cardiovascular conditions, hypertension, and other active diseases of the brain or blood supply apparently do less well on intelligence tests than healthy individuals (Birren and Spieth 1962; Spieth 1964).

Birren (1964) has stated that with advancing age decrease in the primary capacity to learn is minor. The differences between learning capacities of younger and of older people are due to physiological state, perception, set, attention, and motivation. He concludes that older people can learn as well as younger people if they are given adequate time to learn.

Educational psychologists have identified many factors that influence learning performance. Among these factors are intelligence, previous learning, socioeconomic status, personality, interests, health status, methodology, climate, readiness, attentional variables, perseverance, goals, fatigue, and motivation. Gerontological nurses must remember that the elderly are a heterogeneous group as far as intellectual functioning is concerned, and few generalizations apply. Nurses should rely on their own knowledge and assessment of their clients. If the intellectual functioning of a particular client appears to be on the wane, the nurse should consider such causes as depression, social isolation, disease processes, adverse drug reactions, and malnutrition.

The assets of the aged should be recognized: aging helps with learning because growing old involves experience, and experience helps to organize input. The nurse can preserve the self-esteem of the elderly by acknowledging their intelligence and/ or skills. If possible, the elderly should be allowed to get involved in teaching their peers if they have the interest, knowledge, and skills necessary.

MEMORY

Some studies indicate that short-term memory (1 second to 10 minutes) and long-term memory (10 to 20 minutes) decline with age. But old memory (recall of events in the distant past) shows little decline, provided the individual is in good health.

Other studies have demonstrated that older people do not remember as well as younger people under the following conditions: (1) when the task or procedure is not meaningful, (2) when the pace is not the client's own, and (3) when the learning situation includes a constant switching of attention or requires a change of set.

Evidence exists that older people are able to "store" information but may have difficulty retrieving it. They have difficulty remembering tasks or events upon free recall, but if they are provided with "cues" or recognition tasks, little or no deficit is observed. Therefore, the elderly tend to do better on multiple-choice questions in tests than on completion questions.

The general public presumes that learning capacity and memory decline with age. The gerontological nurse can help dispel this myth by sharing the knowledge that "normal" older persons can maintain the quality of their intellectual functioning if they are in good health, are motivated, and have a stimulating environment.

PRACTICAL CONSIDERATIONS IN TEACHING THE AGED

About a half dozen major theories of learning and more than a score of theories applicable to learning behavior exist. These theories have produced many definitions of learning. For our purposes learning will be defined as a process involving a modification or change in behavior, not attributable to growth, that helps individuals adapt to circumstances of their lives.

We do not intend to identify comprehensively all teaching-learning principles, types of learning, or conditions of learning and relate them to the teaching of elderly.

But because health teaching is such an important component of health promotion, a brief practical treatment follows.

After the nurse has prepared a thorough, written assessment of the aged client, the planning stage of the nursing process begins. The nurse and client may concur that some of the client's health care needs can be met through health teaching. At this stage the nurse must remember that change in health-related behavior is seldom brought about by new knowledge alone. Only if clients see the health information or self-care procedure as a direct solution to a felt need will they change their behavior. Human motivation, or what people feel they want or need, is one of the most important determinants of behavioral change. When planning care with the elderly, listening carefully to what they see as their problems or needs is therefore crucial.

Success in teaching the elderly depends a great deal on this initial assessment and mutual planning with the client. Unless aged persons can appreciate the difference this new knowledge will make in their lives, little change in behavior will take place.

In some cases an individual client may have multiple health problems, and seemingly an overwhelming amount of information must be communicated to the client. In such a situation the following questions may help the nurse and client to determine priorities.

Criteria for Determining Priorities in Teaching the Elderly

What knowledge is of most worth to the client at this time?

What lack of knowledge will contribute to the rapid deterioration of physical and/or mental health?

What information could be given during the next visit?

What teaching could best be done by a community health nurse in the home?

What does the client perceive as the most important problem or need?

What written information would help the client or those who care for the client?

The gerontological nurse must become aware of cultural differences among clients. Attitudes toward health care, diet, learning, body image, self-care, grief, death and dying, male-female roles, and drug-taking practices may all be explained by cultural differences. Some of these attitudes may provide clues on how to proceed more successfully in teaching the elderly. In addition, the following factors are most conducive to providing an effective learning situation for the aged.

Guidelines for Teaching the Elderly

Identify both short- and long-range objectives; change as necessary according to needs, progress, and additional information.

Consider the motivation, intellectual and emotional readiness, and previously acquired capabilities of the elderly.

Consider the self-esteem and personal adjustment of the individual.

Consider the impaired sensory perception of many elderly before choosing methodology.

When using visual aids, keep in mind the poorer peripheral vision of many aged.

Provide a well-lighted and quiet environment, particularly for the aged with visual-hearing impairments.

Allow the elderly to set their own pace when learning.

Keep the teaching-learning sessions short; the elderly have a shorter concentration time than younger people and tire more easily.

Give one message at a time and teach slowly.

When teaching procedures of self-care or how to use equipment, use the same materials and/or equipment that the client will use at home.

Require frequent, active response from the client.

Positively reinforce the aged whenever appropriate and immediately after a successful response.

Give immediate and specific feedback to correct errors during task performance.

Provide the client with cues at each step of the task if necessary; do not allow the older person to become disappointed or embarrassed if unable to remember.

If possible, simplify the demands of the procedure to be learned; leave out meaningless steps and irrelevant information.

Be sure of the client's physical ability to perform procedures requiring fine-muscle movement and coordination.

Avoid classroom lectures in teaching older persons; small informal groups are more effective.

Do not encourage note taking unless clients believe they will profit from them.

When designing health information pamphlets or procedures, keep them simple, require large print, and avoid complex illustrations or diagrams.

Capitalize on the older person's experience, if possible.

Allow the client to repeat the task as many times as necessary to acquire mastery and self-confidence; avoid fatigue.

If written information is given to the client and family, go over the material with them to be sure they can read and understand it.

Avoid medical, nursing, and educational jargon.

Forgetting may necessitate frequent review; provide for evaluation and review at next visit.

Review and apply principles to increase retention (e.g., apply Basic Four in nutrition to cultural diet and set up appropriate daily menus).

Frequently lack of communication between the health provider and elderly client leads to noncompliance with the health regimen. We hope that gerontological nurses will be able to communicate with their elderly clients and will make a real difference in the lives of many because of the nurses' understanding of the total health needs of the elderly, their efforts in helping the elderly maintain their own health, and their ability "to reach and to teach" the elderly.

Considerations in Health Promotion in the Aged

1. *Prevention of injury (Primary prevention)*
   a. Good lighting, especially on landings and stairwells.
   b. Handrails on both sides of staircases and halls or at least on one side, designed to show when top and bottom steps have been reached.

43

c. Top and bottom steps and risers should be painted in easily seen colors, and nonskid treads should be used.

d. Eliminate loose extension cords, small mats, sliding rugs, slippery linoleum.

e. Use rubber-backed nonskid rugs and nonskid floor waxes.

f. Tack down edges of rugs or use wall-to-wall carpeting.

g. Advise use of corrugated soles on shoes.

h. Adequate lighting from the bedside tables to the bathroom with baseboard light. Easily available switches and flashlight at bedside.

i. Levers rather than doorknobs.

j. Telephone at bedside. (Aged; health educator; telephone company; builders)

k. Eliminate casters on chairs, rickety tables, sharp-cornered furniture, and high beds.

l. Advise against looking up when climbing stairs or sudden movement of the head to the side, since this may interfere with the blood supply to the brain and cause fainting.

m. Avoid sedation.

n. Distinct and complete labeling of medications, including large letters indicating if it is for internal or external use, and good illumination of the medicine cabinet in order to avoid errors in self-administered medicine.

o. Avoid smoking in bed.

p. Distinct markings of dials on stoves.

q. Use of controls outside the tubs and showers.

r. Complete instructions on accident prevention to all personnel in hospitals and other institutions.

s. Use of grab rails and nonskid mats or emery strips in the tub.

t. Use of high sinks, high toilet seats, and high refrigerators to prevent undue bending of the head, which may cause dizziness and falls.

u. Careful training in use of wheelchairs.

v. Careful feeding of aged people in institutions to prevent aspiration and asphyxiation in presence of poor gag reflex.

w. Avoidance of large bowls of food for same reason as above.

x. Frequent reevaluation of capability for driving a motor vehicle. To be checked are such things as type of medication being used, type of underlying chronic illness, understanding of new rules and new signs. Curtailment of driving at night and in bad weather or on high-speed routes.

y. Pedestrian escort in bad weather or even in good weather, depending on the person's physical and mental capabilities.

z. Frequent testing of vision and hearing and immediate treatment of eye, ear, and foot abnormalities to prevent stumbling, etc.

2. *Specific prevention of disease and early disease detection (Secondary prevention)*

a. Instruction (if possible) concern-

44

ing familial incidence (genetically and unknown genetically induced) of disease in premarital education in order to promote healthier underlying constitutional factors.

b. Periodic checkups to discover and effectively treat the conditions which may lead to chronic illness (e.g., chronic draining ears to deafness, chronic bronchitis to respiratory insufficiency, etc.).

c. More frequent periodic health examinations in the aging person because of constant breakdown of tissue. Close attention to all symptoms and signs. Avoid thinking in terms of "not expecting to feel well" when one becomes older.

d. Awareness of the fact that the aging person can mask the usual signs and manifestations of severe illness, especially infection such as fever, acute abdominal disease, etc. A high degree of suspicion is very essential.

e. Immediate repair and treatment of defects while motivation is still present—e.g., foot, eye, and hearing trouble, arthritic changes, sustained and intermittent high blood pressure, early congestive heart failure, etc.—rather than procrastination because of the person's chronological age.

f. Continuation of immunizations required in that age group (e.g., tetanus, influenza).

g. Avoid exposure to communicable disease insofar as possible.

h. Periodic screening tests for early detection of occult disease in order to arrest it before the damage is severe or irreversible; at least annually in young and mature and biannually in aging or chronically ill. These should include the following: hemogram; sedimentation rate; urinalysis; electroencephalogram; stool specimen after being meat-free for four days; two-hour postprandial blood sugar; x-ray of heart and lungs; cancer detection tests such as sigmoidoscopy, Papanicolaou vaginal smear, acid phosphorous, sputum if a smoker of cigarettes.

i. Thorough and complete evaluation of specific body system if any tests show deviation from normal, no matter how slight.

j. Hormone replacement as indicated (early) rather than attributing fatigue, etc., to "old age."

k. Prevention of pressure point erosion and ulceration (especially in bed-bound or partially bed-bound patients) by frequent turning of patient and padding such areas.

3. *Personal health habits (Primary prevention)*

a. Stress the need for maintenance of optimal weight.

b. Instruct in the value of good nutrition and the harmful effects of certain foods such as polyunsaturated fats, high calorie foods, etc.

c. Motivation towards optimum body care (cleanliness, good dental repair, adequate attention to feet, etc.).

45

d. Stress the need for initiation and continuation of an adequate exercise program.

4. *Social habits and mental health (Tertiary prevention)*

a. Constant motivation towards optimal fulfillment in all spheres of living rather than just work and family.

b. Preparation for period of loss of family and work roles by discussing these possibilities frequently in the mature years.

c. Motivation for substitution for work, community, and family roles by specific and general interests along other lines, such as hobbies, volunteer works, clubs, visiting friends, going on trips, etc.

d. Provide easy availability of proper substitute interests. The Mount Sinai Hospital-based Geriatric Day Center is an example of this. Here a small group (20 persons) is engaged in recreation and discussion sessions which closely resemble group psycho-social therapy in connection with a select group of patients motivated towards illness and isolation rather than health and community and environmental interests. This plan is now being considered on a wider scale by other community groups. These will be school- and church-based, etc. The basic plan is to keep the groups small so that they are given closer, more individual attention which motivates them to resume their lost community role.

e. Family instruction on the adverse effects of overprotectiveness of senior citizens. It is just as important to know how to intervene as it is to know when to intervene. They should be allowed and encouraged to do as much as possible for themselves. The latter applies to institutional settings also. Families should be instructed in avoidance of poor communication or misunderstanding based on guilt feelings which ultimately lead to irreversible disruption of families.

5. *How to get health care and prepayment for health care (Primary prevention)*

a. Free selection of physician should without question remain the prerogative of each person. It is fair, however, to acquaint him with the criteria which usually (though not always) apply to the selection of a well-trained, well-motivated physician such as type of hospital he is associated with, type of training necessary for specialization, etc.

b. All, especially the aging, should be made aware of the resources available to them in their particular community to serve their health needs. If they are medically or socially indigent, they should be informed as to how they may secure the proper assistance.

c. Prepaid health insurance should be encouraged. However, it is good to secure authoritative advice as to which plan best covers the individual needs of the person. [Adapted from Giorgi 1971]*

REFERENCES

ABRAHAM, S., F. W. LOWENSTEIN, and C. L. JOHNSON. 1974. *Preliminary Findings of the First Health and Nutrition Examination Survey, U.S. 1971–1972: Dietary Intake and Biochemical Findings.* DHEW Publication No. (HRA)74–1219–1. Rockville, Md.

ALDERFER, C. P. 1969. "An Empirical Test of a New Theory of Human Needs." *Organizational Behavior and Human Performance* 4:142–75.

American Association of Colleges of Nursing. 1976. "Prevention in Primary Care." Position paper.

AUSTIN, C. L. 1959. "The Basic Six Needs of the Aging." *Nursing Outlook* 7:138.

BELLOC, N. B. 1973. "Relationship of Health Practices and Morality." *Preventive Medicine* 2:67–81.

——— and L. BRESLOW. 1972. "Relationship of Physical Health Status and Health Practices." *Preventive Medicine* 1(3):409–21.

BIRREN, J. E. 1964. *The Psychology of Aging.* Englewood Cliffs, N.J.: Prentice-Hall.

——— and W. SPIETH. 1962. "Age, Response Speed and Cardiovascular Functions." *Journal of Gerontology* 17:390–91.

BOTWINICK, J. 1973. *Aging and Behavior.* New York: Springer.

CARANASOS, G. J., R. B. STEWART, and L. E. CLUFF. 1974. "Drug-Induced Illness Leading to Hospitalization." *Journal of the American Medical Association* 228:713–17.

CARLSON, S. 1972. "Communication and Social Interaction in the Aged." *Nursing Clinics of North America* 7(2):269–73.

CASTER, W. O. 1976. "The Role of Nutrition in Human Aging." In M. Rockstein and M. L. Sussman, *Nutrition, Longevity, and Aging.* New York: Academic Press.

Center for Disease Control. 1972. *Ten-State Nutrition Survey, 1968–70.* DHEW Publication No. (HSM) 72–8130. Washington, D.C.: U.S. Government Printing Office.

CHOWN, S. M. 1972. "Intelligence in Adulthood and Old Age." In W. D. Wall and V. P. Varma, eds., *Advances in Educational Psychology.* Vol. 1. New York: Barnes and Noble Books.

DUNN, H. L. 1959. "What High-Level Wellness Means." *Canadian Journal of Public Health* 50:447–57.

———. *High-Level Wellness.* 1971. Arlington, Va.: Beatty.

GIORGI, E. A. February 1971. "Aging and Mental Health." Workshop paper. University of Southern California, Los Angeles, 6.

GOLDFARB, A. I. 1967. "Psychiatry in Geriatrics." *Medical Clinics of North America* 51:1515–27.

"Health, Education, and Welfare Secretary Califano Initiates Anti-Smoking Campaign." 1978. *Los Angeles Times,* January 23.

KAYNE, R. C. 1976. "Drugs and the Aged." In I. M. Burnside, *Nursing and the Aged.* New York: McGraw-Hill.

KEYS, A., et al. 1950. *The Biology of Human Starvation.* Minneapolis: University of Minnesota Press.

LAWLER, E. E., 1973. *Motivation in Work Organization.* Monterey, Calif.: Brooks/Cole.

LAWLER, E. E., and J. L. SUTTLE. 1972. "A Causal Correlation Test of the Need Hierarchy Concept. *Organizational Behavior and Human Performance* 7:265–87.

LEAVELL, H. R., and E. G. CLARK. 1965. *Preventive Medicine for the Doctor in His Community.* New York: McGraw-Hill.

MANN, G. V. 1973. "Relationship of Age to Nutrient Requirements." *The American Journal of Clinical Nutrition* 26:1096–97.

MASLOW, A. 1943. "A Theory of Human Motivation." *Psychological Review* 50:370–96.

———. 1970. *Motivation and Personality.* New York: Harper and Row.

MIKELSON, O. 1976. "The Possible Role of Vitamins in the Aging Process." In M. Rockstein and M. L. Sussman, *Nutrition, Longevity, and Aging.* New York: Academic Press.

MILLER, R. R. 1973. "Hospital Admissions Due to Adverse Drug Reaction: A Report from the Boston Collaborative Drug Surveillance Program." *Clinical Pharmacology and Therapeutics* 14:142–43.

MURRAY, H. A. 1938. *Explorations in Personality.* New York: Oxford University Press.

MURRAY, R., and J. ZENTNER. 1975. *Nursing Concepts for Health Promotion.* Englewood Cliffs, N.J.: Prentice-Hall.

---

* Elsie Giorgi, "Aging and Mental Health," paper distributed to USC gerontology students, Los Angeles, February 6, 1971. Reprinted by permission of the author.

National Research Council. 1974. *Recommended Dietary Allowances*, 8th rev. ed. Washington, D.C.: National Academy of Science.

NEELY, E. and M. L. PATRICK. 1968. "Problems of Aged Persons Taking Medications at Home." *Nursing Research* 17:52–55.

ROCKSTEIN, M., and M. L. SUSSMAN. 1976. *Nutrition, Longevity, and Aging.* New York: Academic Press.

SCHWARTZ, D. 1962. "Medication Errors Made by Elderly, Chronically Ill Patients." *American Journal of Public Health* 52:2018–29.

SHANAS, E. 1969. "Measuring the Home Health Needs of the Aged in Five Countries." *Proceedings of the 8th International Congress of Gerontology* 1:260. Washington, D.C.: Federated American Society for Experimental Biology.

SHARK, R. E. 1976. "Nutritional Charcteristics of the Elderly." In M. Rockstein and M. L. Sussman, *Nutrition, Longevity, and Aging.* New York: Academic Press.

SKELTON, D. 1977. "The Future of Health Care for the Elderly." *Journal of the American Geriatric Society* 25(1):39–46.

SOMERS, A., and L. BRESLOW. 1977. "Lifetime Health Monitoring Program." *New England Journal of Medicine* 296:601–08.

SPECTOR, M., and R. E. SPECTOR. 1977. "Is Prevention Myth or Reality?" *Health Education* 4:23–25.

SPIETH, W. 1964. "Cardiovascular Health Status, Age and Psychological Performance." *Journal of Gerontology* 19:277–84.

U.S. Dept. of Agriculture. 1972. *Household Food Consumption Survey, 1965–66.* Report no. 11.

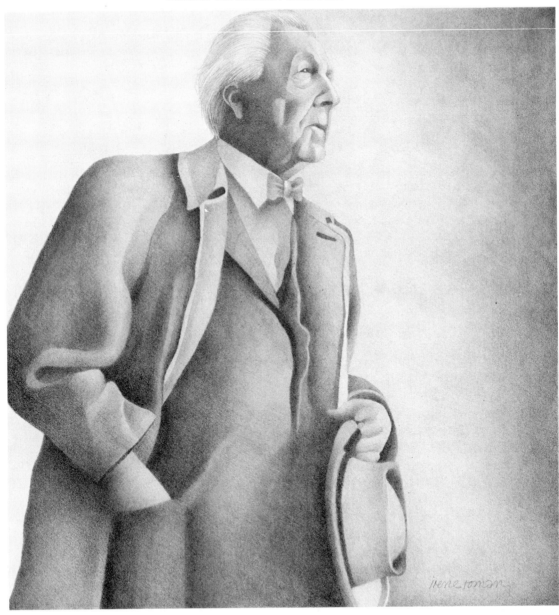

Chapter 4

THE EXPANDED ROLE OF THE GERONTOLOGICAL NURSE

For more than a decade nursing has played a major role in the delivery of primary health care. This commitment has necessitated expanding the unique nursing practice role. It has also required more communication and collaboration with other health professionals. This chapter discusses primary health care, the American Nurses Association definition of and scope of practice for the nurse practitioner/clinician and clinical specialist, and the expanded role of the gerontological nurse in primary care of the older adult.

PRIMARY HEALTH CARE FUNCTIONS

Nurses have expanded their roles and increased the level of their functions in order to keep pace with changes in the health care delivery system. With the change from traditional roles to the expanded role has come confusion in terminology, credentials, education, and relationships among health professionals. In order to clarify this confusion, the secretary of the U.S. Department of Health, Education, and Welfare appointed a committee in 1971 to determine the responsibilities of nurses in expanded roles. The committee published a report, "Extending the Scope of Nursing Practice," in November 1971. The following excerpts from that report elaborate nurses' functions in delivering primary health care as defined elsewhere in this book.

Primary Care

One of the most important opportunities for change in the current system of health care involves altering the practice of nurses and physicians so that nurses assume considerably greater responsibility for delivering pri-

51

mary health care services. The term Primary Care as used in this paper has two dimensions: (a) a person's first contact in any given episode of illness with the health care system that leads to a decision of what must be done to help resolve his problem; and (b) the responsibility for the continuum of care, i.e., maintenance of health, evaluation and management of symptoms, and appropriate referrals. . . .

The nurse's primary care functions include:

Routine assessment of the health status of individuals and families.

Institution of care during normal pregnancies and normal deliveries, provision of family planning services, and supervision of health care of normal children.

Management of care for selected patients within protocols mutually agreed upon by nursing and medical personnel, including prescribing and providing care and making referrals as appropriate.

Screening patients having problems requiring differential medical diagnosis and medical therapy. The recommendation resulting from such screening activities is based on data gathered and evaluated jointly by physicians and nurses.

Consultation and collaboration with physicians, other health professionals, and the public in planning and instituting health care programs. [Secretary's Committee to Study Extended Roles for Nurses 1971, pp. 11–12 and 14–15]

ROLE DEFINITIONS

The 1971 DHEW report was followed by a proliferation of educational programs to prepare nurses for their expanded role.

There was no agreement on the title that would describe the nurse prepared for such a role. In an attempt to help nurses, employers, and consumers, the Congress for Nursing Practice sponsored by the American Nurses' Association in 1974 defined nurse practitioners, nurse clinicians, and clinical nurse specialists. These definitions are provided here to show the three nursing "roles" for a historical perspective.

Nurse Practitioners

Nurse practitioners have advanced skills in the assessment of the physical and psychosocial health-illness status of individuals, families or groups in a variety of settings through health and development history taking and physical examination. They are prepared for these special skills by formal continuing education which adheres to ANA approved guidelines, or in a baccalaureate nursing program.

Nurse Clinicians

Nurse clinicians have well-developed competencies in utilizing a board range of cues. These cues are used for prescribing and implementing both direct and indirect nursing care and for articulating nursing therapies with other planned therapies. Nurse clinicians demonstrate expertise through clinical experience and continuing education. Generally, minimal preparation for this role is the baccalaureate degree.

Clinical Nurse Specialists

Clinical nurse specialists are primarily clinicians with a high degree of knowledge, skill, and competence in a specialized area of nursing. These are made directly available to the public through the provision of nursing care to clients and indirectly available through guidance and planning of care with other nursing personnel. Clinical nurse specialists hold a master's degree in nursing preferably with an emphasis in clinical nursing. [American Nurses' Association]*

The ANA Congress for Nursing Practice updated the definitions in May 1976. The current definitions are found in a document entitled "The Scope of Nursing Practice, Description of Practice, Nurse Practitioner/Clinician, Clinical Nurse Specialist," May 1976, which can be acquired from the American Nurses' Association. A brief presentation of these new definitions is included here and encompasses the definition of and scope of practice for the gerontological nurse practitioner.

Nurse Practitioner/Clinician

Operational Definition

A nurse practitioner/clinician† is a registered nurse with preparation in a specialized educational program. This preparation at present may be in the context of a formal continuing education program, a baccalaureate nursing program, or an advanced degree nursing program. It is envisioned that in the future a nurse practitioner/clinician will be academically prepared at the baccalaureate or higher degree level. This preparation enables the nurse practitioner to provide nursing care as a primary health care provider in a variety of settings. Primary care provides health care to individual clients or groups of clients in order to maintain the

clients' health status and to prevent serious illness or disability. In any health care setting the focus is mainly on the maintenance of wellness, the prevention of illness, and dealing with acute or chronic health problems.

Scope of Practice

At present the nurse practitioner/clinician as a primary care provider, assesses the physical and psychosocial status of clients by means of interview, health history, physical examination and diagnostic tests. The nurse practitioner/clinician interprets the data, develops and implements therapeutic plans, and follows through on the continuum of care of the client. The practitioner/clinician implements these plans through independent action, appropriate referrals, health counseling, and collaboration with other health care providers. All aspects of the therapeutic plan and the continuum of care are documented in the client's records. The nurse practitioner/clinician accepts the responsibilities and the obligations to practice in accordance with accepted standards of nursing as defined by the profession and adhere to similar standards of ethical practice exemplified in the ANA Code for Nurses. The nurse practitioner/clinician accepts accountability for these professional and ethical activities.

Clinical Nurse Specialist

Operational Definition

The Clinical Nurse Specialist (CNS) is a practitioner holding a Master's degree with a concentration in specific areas of clinical nursing. The role of the CNS is defined by the needs of a select client‡ population, the

---

* Definitions of the ANA, Congress for Nursing Practice, Kansas City, May 1974. Reprinted by permission.

† The Congress for Nursing Practice approved the recommendation of the ad hoc committee, Nurse Clinician, that since consistent and significant differences in education, practice, or place of practice could not be identified, the term *practitioner/clinician* be used and the description of practice apply to both roles.

‡ The word "client" is intended to mean patient, family, and/or community.

expectations of the larger society, and the clinical expertise of the nurse. By exercising judgement and demonstrating leadership ability, the CNS functions within a field of practice that focuses on the needs of client system and encompasses interaction with others in the nursing and health care systems serving the client. The CNS role includes participation in activities designed to continue self-development, advance the goals of the nursing profession, and promote effective collaborative relationships with members of other health care disciplines.

The function of the CNS is unique with respect to the particular use of clinical judgement and skills regarding client care, service as an advocate when the client is unable to cope with a particular situation, and influence for change as necessary in the nursing care and in the health care delivery system.

The CNS is obligated to operate within and to affect nursing care delivery systems and the total health care delivery system. While roles may change by circumstances for a certain period of time, this practitioner ceases to be recognized as a CNS when the patient-client-family ceases to be the basis of practice.

Fields of Practice as a Practitioner

As a practitioner, the clinical nurse specialist operates within three separate fields which remain in a state of dynamic change. These fields represent the health status of the client, the nursing care delivery system, and the health care delivery system. Each of these fields is so interrelated as to continuously affect the other. [American Nurses' Association]*

---

* Updated definitions of the ANA, Congress for Nursing Practice, Kansas City, May 1976. Reprinted by permission.

O. Marie Henry (1978, p. 4) states that "approximately 12,000 nurses have been formally prepared for the expanded role with over 72 percent of these graduates working as nurse practitioners providing primary health care. Other graduates are employed in areas such as teaching, consultation and administration." She points out that because 50 percent of the nurse practitioners are working in inner city or rural areas, they have been a factor in the improvement of accessibility of health services.

The federal government's initiative and financial support have stimulated growth of the nurse practitioner movement. The 1975 Nurse Training Act provided a separate program of grants and contracts for nurse practitioner programs. The gerontological/geriatric nurse practitioner movement was given a boost in 1975 when the federal government sent out a "request for proposals" for educational programs. Six programs were funded: University of Lowell, University of Miami, University of North Carolina, University of Wisconsin, Rush University, and State University of New York at Buffalo. Five of the programs were at the certificate level; the University of Lowell's program was at the master's level. The latter program meets with ANA expectations of future preparation for the nurse practitioner/clinician.

GERONTOLOGICAL NURSING

According to Stone (1976), gerontological nursing offers many role opportunities to nurses. They are: (1) primary-care provider, (2) health assessor, (3) high-level patient-care manager in nursing homes, (4)

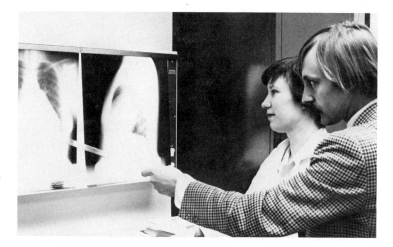

The gerontological nurse can help the elderly adapt to the aging process by facilitating the integration of health interventions, health education, and supportive counseling; elderly clients have multidimensional problems that require coordination and collaboration by all members of the health care team.

independent practitioner, (5) researcher, and (6) teacher. The role opportunities proposed by Stone make possible the delineation of numerous roles for the gerontological nurse.

Gerontological Nursing Roles

Direct provider of health services

Independent practitioner

Educator of clients, families, community, and self

Researcher

Consultant in gerontological nursing to community agencies, long-term care facilities, day and ambulatory centers

Collaborator with other health professionals and community agencies

Role model for other nurses and initiator of innovative health care modes

Advocate for aged individuals and the aging population

Health planner and potential social policy maker for services and resources needed by the elderly

Administrator of health agencies rendering service to the elderly

Counselor

Nurses prepared at the master's level are capable of assuming these roles when they specialize in gerontological nursing.

The specialty of gerontological nursing includes the "well" aged as well as the "sick" aged. Persons in both categories require nursing care. At the present time the number of qualified gerontological nurses is insufficient. This shortage may be due to cultural attitudes. Although some studies have revealed that nurses show more positive attitudes than do other professionals toward the elderly and toward working with the elderly (Futrell 1977), many studies indicate that nurses do have negative attitudes toward the aged. Much research has indicated that age, education, cultural attitudes, and one's personal feelings toward aging may influence these negative attitudes.

The educational system must promote ways for nursing students to examine their present attitudes and values with respect to aging. At the same time, students must be involved in collaborative ventures with other professionals in order to learn how to promote and maintain health for the eld-

55

erly. Thus, there is a need to produce nurses who can teach the specialty and thus prepare a cadre of qualified nurses.

Gerontological nursing is not geriatric nursing; geriatric nursing primarily involves meeting the needs of the *ill* elderly. Gerontological nursing is broader in concept. It is concerned with assessment of health care needs of the elderly, planning and implementing health care to meet the needs, and evaluating the effectiveness of the care. Emphasis is placed on preventing illness and promoting, maintaining, and restoring health.

ADVOCACY

Gerontological nurses need to serve as advocates for the elderly and at the same time teach the elderly how to be advocates for themselves. Advocacy is action by or for the powerless to restore to them a measure of control (power) over their own destiny. The advocate has three aims: (1) to provide access to community resources, (2) to assist the elderly in the exercise of their rights and privileges, and (3) to secure benefits and services to improve the quality of life for the client (Pennsylvania Department of Public Welfare 1977).

MULTIDIMENSIONAL ASSESSMENT

The elderly have unique needs and problems; consequently nurses must be involved in obtaining services that address their needs and problems. One of the major needs of the elderly is for health assessment. This assessment must be multidimensional and include physical, psychological, and social components. In order to make such an assessment, the nurse must develop appropriate attitudes and skills.

Nursing Requirements for Assessing the Elderly

Free oneself of biases toward aging and the old

Identify pathologies and latent strengths of the elderly individual through multidimensional assessment tools

Perform periodic assessments to determine response to interventions

Help families and communities overcome hostilities toward the elderly

Challenge constructively the self-destructive behavior of the elderly toward themselves

The gerontological nurse must consider the past and present identity and lifestyle of individual clients when planning care. How have they adapted? What are their strengths? Another area of concern should be the clients' understanding of their illnesses and their expectations. Can they manage, or do family members need to help? And lastly, old people in today's society expect and need companionship and warm relationships with people around them.

Educational programs in gerontological nursing must focus on the need to:

1. Know the literature about midlife change and aging,
2. Understand what older widowed women experience,
3. Understand ethnic backgrounds of clients,
4. Understand "time" concepts and clients' feelings of "not having much time left to live,"
5. Know what one is doing and why one is doing it,
6. Make contracts with clients,
7. Help clients integrate past life with present,

8. Know that elderly clients need more structure and thus more input from their nurses,
9. Utilize research findings.

The gerontological nurse needs to become involved in research that focuses on aging. In order for nursing to help improve the delivery of health care to the elderly, nurses must gather data that can be used in social policy decisions and in altering attitudes of the population toward the elderly. Gerontological nursing research is in the embryonic stage and offers opportunities to nurses for the addition of new knowledge to the field of aging.

The future holds many challenges for gerontological nursing. The major challenge is to provide a cadre of nurses with specialized skills that will enable more elderly individuals to remain healthy. Utilization of professional nurses in the health care of the elderly promises to improve the quality of life for both the elderly and the nurse if both educate each other about health, living, and longevity.

REFERENCES

AIKEN, L. 1977. "Primary Care: The Challenge for Nursing." *American Journal of Nursing* 77(11): 1828–32.

American Hospital Association. 1975. *Hospital Statistics.* Chicago.

BRUNETTO, R. A., and P. BIRK. 1972. "The Primary Care Nurse: The Generalist in a Structured Health Care Team." *American Journal of Public Health* 62:785–94.

DONABEDIAN, A., et al. 1972. *Medical Care Chart Book,* 5th ed. Ann Arbor: University of Michigan.

DRAYE, M. A., and L. A. STETSON. 1975. "The Nurse Practitioner as an Economic Reality: Everett Clinic—A Private Medical Clinic, Seattle, Washington." *Nurse Practitioner* 1:60–63.

FARRAND, L. L., and M. COBB. 1975. "Perceptions of Activities Performed in Ambulatory Care Settings." *Nurse Practitioner* 1:60–72.

FLYNN, B. C. 1974. "The Effectiveness of Nurse Clinicians' Service Delivery." *American Journal of Public Health* 64:604–11.

FUTRELL, M., and W. JONES. 1977. "Attitudes of Physicians, Nurses, and Social Workers toward the Elderly and Health Maintenance Services for the Aged: Implication for Health Manpower Policy." *Journal of Gerontological Nursing* 3(3):42–46.

GARDNER, H. H., and R. OUIMETTE. 1974. "A Nurse–Physician Team Approach in a Private Internal Medicine Practice." *Archives of Internal Medicine* 134:956–59.

HENRIQUES, C. D., V. G. VIRGADAMO, and M. D. KAHANE. 1974. "Performance of Adult Health Appraisal Examinations Utilizing Nurse Practitioner–Physician Teams and Paramedical Personnel." *American Journal of Public Health* 64:47–53.

HENRY, O. M. 1978. "Progress of the Nurse Practitioner Research." *The Nurse Practitioner* 3(3):4.

KIRK, F. H., et al. 1971. "Family Nurse Practitioners in Eastern Kentucky." *Medical Care* 9:160–68.

LEVINE, D. M., et al. 1976. "The Role of New Health Practitioners in a Prepaid Group Practice: Provider Differences in Process and Outcomes of Medical Care." *Medical Care* 14:326–47.

LEVINE, E. 1977. "What Do We Know about Nurse Practitioners?" *American Journal of Nursing* 77(11):1799–1803.

LEWIS, C. E., and B. A. RESNICK. 1967. "Nurse Clinics and Progressive Ambulatory Patient Care." *New England Journal of Medicine* 277:765–69.

————, et al. 1969. "Activities, Events, and Outcomes in Ambulatory Patient Care." *New England Journal of Medicine* 280:645–49.

————, and T. K. CHEYOVICK. 1976. "Who Is a Nurse Practitioner? Process of Care and Patients' and Physicians' Perceptions." *Medical Care* 14:365–71.

————, and L. LINN. 1977. "The Content of Care Provided by Family Nurse Practitioners." *Journal of Community Health* 2:259–67.

MERESTEIN, J. H., H. WOLFE, and K. M. BARKER. 1974. "The Use of Nurse Practitioners in a General Practice." *Medical Care* 12:445–52.

MILIO, N. 1975. *The Care of Health in Communities.* New York: Macmillin.

Pennsylvania Department of Public Welfare, Office
for the Aging. 1977. *The New Older Citizens' Guide:
Advocacy and Action.* May.

RICHARDS, S. J., and F. J. DECASTRO. 1973.
"Communication with Patients: A Parameter in
Evaluating Nurse Practitioners." *Missouri Medi-
cine* 70:719–20.

RUNYON, J. 1975. "The Memphis Chronic Disease
Program: Comparisons in Outcome and the
Nurses' Expanded Role." *Journal of the American
Medical Association* 213:264–67.

Secretary's Committee to Study Extended Roles for
Nurses. 1971. *Extending the Scope of Nursing Practice:
A Report of the Secretary's Committee to Study Extended
Roles for Nurses.* DHEW Publication No.
(HSM)73–2037. Washington, D.C.: U.S. Gov-
ernment Printing Office.

SIBLEY, J. C., et al. 1975. "Quality of Care Appraisal in Primary Care: A Quantitative
Method." *Annals of Internal Medicine* 83:46–52.

STEIN, G. H. 1974. "The Use of a Nurse Practitioner in the Management of Patients with Diabetes Mellitus." *Medical Care* 12:885–90.

STEINWACHS, D. M., et al. 1976. "The Role of
New Health Practitioners in a Prepaid Group
Practice: Changes in the Distribution of Ambula-
tory Care between Physician and Nonphysician
Providers of Care." *Medical Care* 14:95–120.

STONE, V. 1976. "The Nurse and the Aged." *R.N.*,
February.

II

GERONTOLOGICAL NURSING PROCESS

Overview

GERONTOLOGICAL NURSING PROCESS
HEALTH APPRAISAL OF THE OLDER ADULT

Health appraisal is a goal-oriented process in which the primary concern is the resolution of health-related problems. As with any other problem-solving process, ultimate success depends on adequate data collection and the establishment of a data base that can be used for diagnostic decision making.

The nursing process is a system of problem solving. It consists of four parts: assessment, planning, intervention, and evaluation. According to Campbell (1978, p. 41) the process can be subdivided as follows:

Assessment
    Subjective data (symptoms)
    Objective data (signs)
    Related data
Possible Etiology
Nursing Diagnosis
Nursing Plan
    Patient needs
    Primary nurse–patient goals

Nursing Interventions
    Nursing treatments
    Nursing observations
    Health teaching
    Medical treatments performed by
      nurses
Evaluation

It is with this concept of nursing process in mind that parts II and III are written. Part II discusses methods of assessment and planning, and part III will describe management and evaluation of common health problems of the elderly.

Preventive health care requires thorough assessment of the client's health status. Planning for promotion of health in the individual and/or family comes only from a complete data base. Therefore, part II describes the specifics of history taking, physical assessment, mental health assessment, and recording of the data. Formal physical assessment is an essential part of

61

the data base. It not only expands the available information but also serves as a control on the diagnostic hypotheses formulated during history taking.

Because the primary health care provider's major concern is with wellness, the term *client* rather than *patient* is used throughout this text. The client participates in the plans for health care. "Client," according to Malasanos et al. (1977, p. VII), "is a term that implies the ability of a person to contract for health care, whether well or sick, as a responsible participant with the providers of health care."

Using the nursing process, nurses gather information by means of the health history, physical examination, and laboratory findings. The data (physiological, behavioral, sociological, spiritual, and environmental) are analyzed in order to identify the client's functional abilities and the etiology of the client's problem(s). This step leads to the nursing diagnosis, which is the recognition of those problem(s) the nurse can treat.

The nursing plan identifies a client's needs and sets the health care goals with the client. These goals are listed in the problem-oriented record. They serve as guideposts for therapy. Nursing interventions follow from nursing diagnosis and planning and differ from medical diagnosis in that they reduce, or prevent problems, aid in the restoration of normal independent function and "maintain optimum health and independent patient functioning" (Campbell 1978, p. 46). Medical diagnosis is primarily concerned with responding to illness or injury.

Periodic reassessment of problems permits evaluation of progress in terms of these goals or may lead to modification of the goals into more realistic terms. Thus reassessment serves as a control of the total process. It is important to include the family during all phases of the nursing process.

Nursing process is used to develop a framework for primary health care rendered by a gerontological nurse. It is essential that physicians and nurses share their skill and knowledge in a common goal of wellness for the elderly client.

REFERENCES

CAMPBELL, C. 1978. *Nursing Diagnosis and Intervention in Nursing Practice.* New York: Wiley.

DUNN, H. L. 1976. *High-Level Wellness.* Arlington, Va.: Beatty.

HURST, J. W., and H. K. WALKER. 1972. *The Problem-Oriented System.* New York: Medcom Press.

LAMONICA, E. 1979. *The Nursing Process: A Humanistic Approach.* Menlo Park, Calif.: Addison-Wesley.

MALASANOS, L., et al. 1977. *Health Assessment.* St. Louis: C. V. Mosby.

MITCHELL, P. H. 1973. *Concepts Basic to Nursing.* New York: McGraw-Hill.

WEED, L. L. 1970. *Medical Records, Medical Education, and Patient Care.* Chicago: Yearbook Medical Publishers.

YURA, H. and M. WALSH. 1973. *The Nursing Process.* New York: Appleton-Century-Crofts.

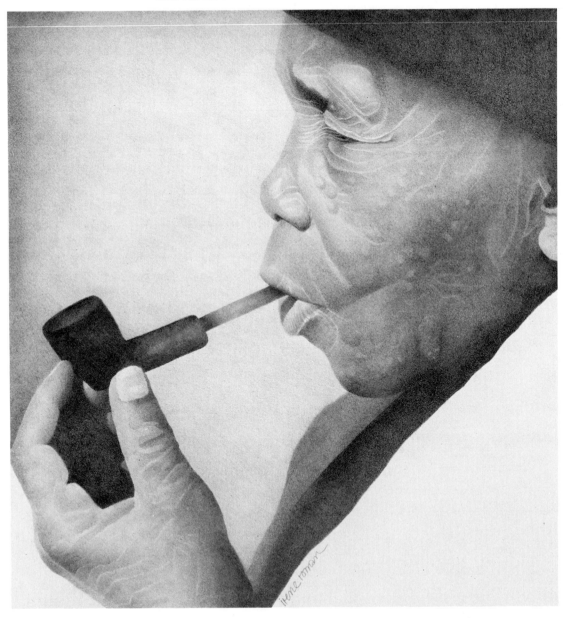

D. L. Anderson

Chapter 5

THE HISTORY

Nursing assessment is dependent upon the collection of pertinent data obtained in the health history. Its importance lies in the fact that "... the nurse observes and interprets minimal as well as gross signs and symptoms associated with both normal aging and pathological changes and institutes appropriate nursing measures" (ANA 1973). The health history is the initial component of the comprehensive health assessment. The mental health assessment (chapter 7), which will help establish the reliability of the client, can be obtained concurrently with, or independent of, the health history. The other components of the comprehensive assessment include the physical examination and diagnostic testing (chapter 6) and the problem list and the therapeutic plan (chapter 8).

The history is a goal-oriented interviewing process. Its purpose is to obtain information related to the elderly client's current and past health status, family role, and socialization level. Information gathered in initial visits is used to establish the data base, to which information obtained in following visits is added. Immediate decisions regarding intervention are made from the base line data gathered during the initial visits. The data base changes as problems are identified and resolved in subsequent visits.

The data gathered from the health history is subjective, and the information supplied by the client or significant other alerts the nurse to focus on key areas of investigation during the objective data gathering portion of the comprehensive health assessment—namely, the physical examination and the diagnostic testing.

INTERVIEWING PROCESS

The interviewing process allows for the establishment of a relationship with the elderly client, which is essential to the collection of useful, significant data. "The greatest desire of older people is for relationships with others" (Mezey 1977, p. 47). The development of relationships may be impeded by fear resulting from the elderly's experiences of coping with multiple losses. Multiple losses of spouse, relatives, and friends, as well as of bodily functions can contribute to their feelings of helplessness and hopelessness. Under these circumstances, the elderly may be fearful of establishing new relationships that could again lead to feelings of loss. Recognizing this fact, the nurse should attempt to establish the relationship slowly. Although it may take several visits before rapport is accomplished, the relationship must be built on trust because the nurse often becomes the "significant other" in a client's life.

The person-to-person contact in the interview situation provides an initial opportunity for the nurse to convey a caring attitude to the older person. Sincere interest in the individual is easily transmitted when the nurse utilizes a nonjudgmental, open, empathetic approach during the interview. The credibility of the gerontological nurse is established through consistency, honesty, and a caring attitude.

TECHNIQUES

With the exception of clients who have considerable health care experience, the average client does not readily provide the nurse with a detailed health history. The data must be obtained through a skillful, goal-directed interviewing process. The use of both directive and nondirective techniques will guide the interview.

Statements such as "You seem to be having difficulty answering this question . . ."

or "Perhaps you can tell more about it . . ." are nondirective and allow clients to express themselves verbally rather than answering yes or no. Open-ended questions such as "How do you feel?" as well as restatements of clients' own words and encouraging remarks such as "continue" or "go on" all assist client expression. When elderly clients move away from the focus of the question, the reason may be that they have misunderstood the question. Rewording of questions often helps, but if clients still seem unable to focus on questions, they may be trying to avoid answering. In this situation, an attempt should be made to obtain the information in a nonthreatening manner.

During the interview the nurse should use terminology appropriate to the client's educational level. The nurse must also be sure to avoid talking down to an elderly client, particularly one who may be timorous in seeking clarification of confusing or unknown terms. Some elderly immigrants to the United States may be unable to speak and/or understand the English language, and the use of an interpreter is essential if the nurse cannot speak such a client's native language. The use of short sentences will help to eliminate misunderstanding and misinterpretation among the interpreter, nurse, and client. The interpreter must be instructed to translate questions and answers word for word, as failure to do so may significantly alter the meaning and context of both questions and responses.

THE SETTING

The setting for the interview is important when trying to establish a nurse-client relationship of trust. Hospitals, emergency rooms, clinics, and waiting rooms are a familiar and comfortable habitat for health care professionals. Yet, to the elderly client, these areas are sources of anxiety, confusion, and uncertainty. Examining rooms that are harshly lit and full of extraneous noises can heighten the anxiety level of an elderly client.

The first major responsibility of the gerontological nurse, then, is to minimize environmental stimuli that can contribute to clients' confusion and anxiety. The use of a paging system in the waiting room to call clients can be distracting to them. Personal greeting of each individual and escorting the client to the examining room takes little extra time and contributes to an atmosphere of reassurance.

Once in the examining room the nurse should eliminate all interruptions. They only serve to increase anxiety and distract the client. The reassuring milieu that should be created during the interview is considerably weakened by the nurse's leaving the room for even short periods. Clients often report that nurses appear "so busy" as they answer phone calls or move from one examining room to another. The hidden message, "so busy," can be translated to mean "too busy" to care enough about them as individuals.

Burnside (1976, p. 385) proposes a number of suggestions that will assist the sensorially impaired elderly in adapting to their environment. These techniques can be used to decrease anxiety and facilitate communication during the interview with the visually and/or hearing-impaired client (Mummah 1975; Burnside 1976).

Interviewing Elderly Clients with Visual and/or Hearing Acuity Impairments

Make sure adequate lighting is present.

Avoid seating the client in bright glare; for example, near highly polished floors, enamel walls, or windows without curtains or shades.

Face the person when speaking.

Speak slowly and in low tones to accentuate both vowels and consonants.

The gerontological nurse can help the elderly adapt to the aging process by allowing them to discuss their personal concerns as well as their health problems in an atmosphere of trust; elderly clients need to perceive open, empathetic, and nonjudgmental attitudes in order to communicate all of the information necessary for appropriate and comprehensive interventions.

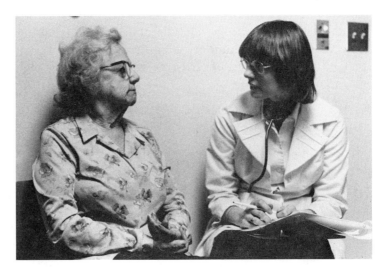

Sit close to and at the same level as the client.

For men, trim mustache and beards well to avoid covering the lips to facilitate lip reading.

For women, wear bright red lipstick to facilitate lip reading.

Do not cover mouth while speaking.

Do not smoke or chew gum while speaking.

CONTENT OF THE HEALTH HISTORY

A comprehensive health history consists of seven parts: the identification or biographical data; chief complaint (CC), history of present illness (HPI), past history (PH), family history (FH), psychosocial history (PSH), and review of systems (ROS).

IDENTIFICATION OR BIOGRAPHICAL DATA

The client's preliminary identification data, often collected by a receptionist on a form such as shown in figure 5.1, provide a frame of reference for the history. The data should include at least the client's name, address, telephone number, significant other, ethnic origin, date of birth, sex, religion, and marital status.

CHIEF COMPLAINT (CC)

The chief complaint establishes the major reason for the client's seeking care. The reported complaint is often a symptom and is briefly recorded in the client's own words. The duration of the complaint should also be noted, as shown in figure 5.1.

Other examples of chief complaints and ways to record them include "chest pains for one hour," "headache for past two days," "shortness of breath since yesterday." The chief complaint should be recorded as stated by the client. A frequent mistake made by a beginning examiner is to change a chief complaint such as "shortness of breath" to "dyspnea," which is a more precise term with diagnostic implications.

Feinstein (1967) feels that the use of the term *chief complaint* during the interview may be misleading and recommends that the examiner look for the iatrotropic stimulus ("What is your reason for seeking help today?"). People seek help from health care providers for different reasons. Unlike Mr. Harris whose history is presented in the figures in this chapter and who clearly expressed a chief complaint, some clients' reasons may not be readily apparent. For example, upon appearing at a clinic, one 68-year-old man stated that his health was perfect but that his wife had encouraged him to have a checkup. The iatrotropic stimulus ultimately came to light during questioning on the psychosocial history portion of the interview when he reported that his alcohol consumption had steadily increased in the past three years to eight beers each evening and that he felt the desire to drink more. Concern over alcohol consumption was his actual reason for the "checkup," and he expressed fear that his increased drinking was endangering his health and family relationships. Determination of the client's real reason for seeking

FIGURE 5.1 Health History of William Harris: Biographical Data. ▶

Identification or Biographical Data   Date _4/25/79_

Name _William Harris_   Sex M _✓_ F ___

Address _47 Hale Road_   Date of Birth _Feb 2, 1901_
Boston   _Mass_   _02114_
Town   State   Zip   Social Security No. _—_

Telephone No. _444-3112_   Medicare No. _033-60-7593A_

Religion _Catholic_   Medicaid No. _8465552_

Marital Status _Widowed_   Other Assistance:

Nationality/Ethnicity _American/30 African Black_   Name _None_

Occupation _/Retired_   No. _____

Person to notify in case of emergency:

Name _James Harris_   Relationship _Son_

Address _32 Hoob St., Hartford, Ct._   Phone No. _632-453-8712_

Chief Complaint: _____

"Pain in my chest" (2 days' duration)

help during the interview assisted the nurse in assessing and evaluating the client's problems and in formulating a plan of care that included supportive counseling to help him deal with and overcome his alcohol problem.

HISTORY OF PRESENT ILLNESS (HPI)

Information obtained in the history of present illness (HPI) portion of the health history provides data to support and define the chief complaint. Written in abbreviated narrative format, it outlines the nature of the problem. The purpose of the HPI is to elicit information describing the chief complaint and its pattern since onset, along with predisposing factors, the ameliorating factors that reduce or alleviate the problem, the effects on daily living, the effects of any ongoing therapeutic intervention, and the preexistence of any related problems in the past. The problem, or symptom, must be fixed in time and reviewed chronologically from inception to the present. The HPI is, initially, the most important part of the comprehensive health history. As shown in figure 5.2, the examiner has noted relevant information about Mr. Harris's chief complaint (pain in precordial area), previous health problems, family history, and health-related habits.

Onset

The nurse must start with the onset of the first symptom. Eliciting specific information about the time period provides both the examiner and the elderly person with a starting frame of reference. Clients' statements such as "a few days" or "several weeks" are ambiguous, and the nurse may find "several weeks" may actually mean eight weeks upon further questioning. Fixing the time also helps other health care professionals examining the client six months later by providing a specific date of reference. Although chronic problems may be difficult to pinpoint exactly, every effort should be made to do so.

The mode of onset is also significant. For example, did the problem begin suddenly (the sudden onset of pain due to mesenteric infarction) or gradually (the onset of insomnia following the loss of a loved one)? Examination of predisposing factors may assist in the understanding of the chief complaint. What was the client doing when the symptom began? Another aspect contributing to predisposing factors includes life circumstances.

Character

The nurse must elicit information that provides a description of the symptom. For example, is the type of pain knifelike, sharp, dull, throbbing, aching, burning, or constricting? What is the degree of severity (excruciating, severe, moderate, mild)? A good indicator of the severity of the symptom is whether the elderly client had to alter activity at the time.

Pattern

Questions regarding the pattern of the symptom explore changes in the intensity and course of the chief complaint. Was the pain steady or intermittent? How has the

FIGURE 5.2 Health History of William Harris: History of Present Illness (HPI).

Name: _William Harris_   Date: _4/25/79_

HPI: 4/24/79 a. m. after raking leaves approx. 25 mins., noticed "intense, severe, stabbing" pain of abrupt onset in precordial area. Immediately ceased work and sat on ground until pain subsided (4 to 5 mins.). No radiation of pain to jaw, neck, arms or epigastric area. Denies shortness of breath, palpitations, or nausea prior, during, or after episode. For remainder of day, stayed in bed — after taking a "nerve pill".

No further episodes until following afternoon (4/25/79) While walking to store, again noticed precordial pain (sharp, intense, and continuous) — after walking 1 mile. Resting relieved the pain in 5 mins. Resumed walking after 10 mins. rest and was again stricken with some pain — after walking 3/4 to 1 mile. Got a taxi and proceeded to clinic without further episodes of pain.

In February 1975, had a "heart attack" requiring a month's hospital stay at St. Francis. Treated by Drs. Smith and Jones.

In March 1978, had pneumonia. Hospitalized at St. Francis for 2 weeks. Treated by Dr. Smith. Told he had a "heart murmur" at this time.

Two younger brothers died of heart attacks (ages 51 and 58).

Smokes 1½–2 packs of cigarettes per day for past 40 years.

pain changed since its onset? Was it initially mild and then severe, or vice versa? Each episode of the problem should also be explored by beginning with the first episode and moving forward in time. (How many episodes occurred? How long did each last? Was each episode the same or different?)

Location

When possible, information on the location of the symptom should be elicited by asking the client to point to the involved area. Questions on radiation, referred pain, and localization also help the client to define the location. When dealing with the symptom of pain, the nurse should inquire whether the pain remained localized or whether it spread or radiated to other areas.

Ameliorating and Exacerbating Factors

The nurse needs to determine whether the client has observed activities or maneuvers that relieve the symptom or make it worse. For example, the client with intermittent claudication may have noticed that leg cramps begin after walking a certain constant distance and disappear soon after walking is stopped. The client with a peptic ulcer may have noticed that the pain begins thirty minutes to one hour after meals and is relieved by eating.

Effect on Activities of Daily Living

Particularly where problems or complaints are severe, the nurse should elicit information on ways in which the client's lifestyle may be altered. For example, pain or breathlessness induced by exertion may cause an elderly client to become sedentary, while loss of visual or auditory acuity cause isolation, loneliness, and frustration. In older clients these changes can significantly modify their lives and relationships with family and friends and ultimately have implications for nursing management decisions and the client's compliance with these decisions.

Preexistent Factors

Other factors that may have importance on a client's response to treatment as well as the nature of that treatment need to be elicited during the HPI portion of the interview. For example, the complaint of progressive increasing breathlessness in a client with a history of hypertension is different from that of one with recurrent pulmonary infection and many years of cigarette smoking. The former may indicate congestive failure while the latter may represent chronic obstructive lung changes.

Often the elucidation of preexistent factors or past events may be obtained during a later period of the history—during the past history, social history, family history, or even systems review.

PAST HISTORY (PH)

A client's current life and health are affected by illnesses of the past, and even those in the remote past may have great significance in relation to the client's current health problems. For example, primary tuberculosis may have a long latent period with secondary disease appearing in old age, or a severe trauma in the twenties may cause articular degeneration many years later. The past history (PH) portion of the client's health history thus allows the examiner to gain an understanding of and appreciation for the natural history of a disease and its effects on the client.

The PH helps the nurse identify and establish dates of the client's long-standing problems, hospitalizations, illnesses, injuries, and their sequelae. As figure 5.3 shows, the PH entails recording childhood diseases, immunizations, allergies, a statement of general health, and use of medications.

When asked about past problems, elderly clients may be unable to remember exactly when the problems first occurred. In such a case, the nurse can help obtain specificity of dates of onset through the use of historical landmarks that could have made an impression on their lives. The use of world events is important in helping clients reach into the past because of the large number of people who have immigrated to this country in the past hundred years. To assist elderly clients remember personal dates, the nurse can mention such world events as the following:

1898	Spanish-American War
1906	San Francisco earthquake
1912	Sinking of the *Titanic*
1914–15	World War I
1918	Influenza epidemic ("Spanish flu")
1927	Lindbergh crosses the Atlantic in the *Spirit of St. Louis*
1929	The stock market crash
1937	*Hindenburg* is destroyed
1940–45	World War II
1950–53	Korean War
1960	Kennedy elected
1963	President Kennedy's assassination
1968	Nixon elected
1974	Watergate

In addition to using a list of world events, the nurse might consider a client group's geographic origin and formulate a list of cultural events of possible importance to the particular clients being served. In other cases, the nurse might formulate a list based on an awareness of the fact that many elderly clients maintain deep religious ties and may be more in tune to religious events than historical events. Recognition of historical events that are worldwide, religious, and cultural can thus provide the nurse with an opportunity to gain specific time frames for past problems that affect clients' current health.

Medications

During the PH portion of the history, the medications used by the client is an important area of the client's history that must be examined in greater depth. Client compliance and adverse drug reactions are two critical aspects to be explored. Numerous studies have documented that errors in self-administration of medications by clients are frequent. Examples of common errors are overmedication, undermedication, nonuse of medication, wrong medication, or any combination of these errors. Studies (Donabedian and Rosenfield 1964; Hecht 1974) have also shown that the rate of compliance in self-administration of medicines for chronic diseases decreases with time. Visual impairment in the elderly client adds another dimension. By being unable to read labels correctly, elderly persons may believe they are taking medications as prescribed, but are unknowingly administering lethal doses to themselves.

Name: _William Harris_   Date: 4/25/79

PH: <u>Childhood Illnesses</u>: Had measles, mumps, chicken pox as a young child. Denies german measles, diptheria, rheumatic fever.

<u>Immunizations</u>: Date of last tetanus toxide during World War II.

<u>Allergies</u>: Denies allergies to food, medicine, dust, or pollen.

<u>Hospitalizations</u>: Spring 1918 — "Spanish flu" — Boston Hospital for 1 wk. Physician unknown.

August 1952 — "constipation" (Ba enema reported neg.) — Boston Hospital for 2 days. Dr. Smith attending physician. No sequela.

February, 1975 — "heart attack" — see HPI

March 1978 — "pneumonia" — see HPI

<u>Surgery</u>: Denies any surgery.

<u>Injuries</u>: December 1934 — fractured (R) humerus (fell off streetcar in snow). Treated at Dr. Hanes' office, Beacon Road, Dorchester. No sequela.

<u>Medication</u>: Unable to recall names of drugs.

Current: 1. "nerve pill" — used for anxiety — taken 1-2 times wk. (2 yrs).
2. "heart pill" — taken once a day to help "heart beat stronger" (4 yrs).
3. "water pill" — taken once a day to "get rid of fluid" (4 yrs.)

Previous: 1. laxative for 2 yrs. (1952-54). Stopped taking because constipation resolved.

Feels general health, up to this point in life, has been "very good."

FIGURE 5.3 Health History of William Harris: Past History (PH).

In a study conducted by the Armed Forces Institute of Pathology in 1974 (Irey 1976, p. 578), of 827 autopsies, 3.0 percent died because of therapeutic errors, and 26.6 percent died from unexpected adverse drug reactions. The most frequently used drugs that can result in an adverse condition or death include: antibiotics, antihypertensive agents, anticholinergic agents, antiparkinsonian agents, antituberculosis agents, and phenothiazines. These medications are usually taken for prolonged periods of time and are often used to treat chronic health problems common in the elderly.

To assist nurses in evaluating drug actions and interactions, Bird (1976) has devised a record-keeping system for the collection and organization of the drug history of a client. A medication profile (see figure 5.4) is part of the PROVE (Problem Oriented Visually Enriched) medical record. This profile allows recording all drugs taken or being taken by the client and categorizing them in order to observe patterns and interactions. As can be seen in figure 5.4, drugs are classified in the following eight categories on the PROVE medication profile:

1. Drugs acting on the *nervous system,* including central nervous system agents, local anesthetics, drugs acting on synaptic and neuroeffector junctional sites, and antacids;
2. Drugs acting on *cardiovascular* function, *renal* function, and *electrolyte* balance, including water, ions and salts, heavy metals and antagonists, and drugs affecting uterine mobility;

FIGURE 5.4 Health History of William Harris: PROVE Medical Record.
Source: Kenneth T. Bird, M.D., Massachusetts General Hospital, Boston. Reprinted by permission of the author.

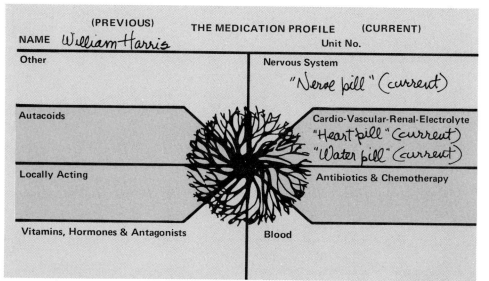

3. *Antibiotics and chemotherapy,* including drugs acting on parasitic diseases, microbial diseases, and neoplastic diseases;
4. Drugs acting on the *blood* and blood-forming organs;
5. *Vitamins, hormones,* and hormone *antagonists;*
6. *Locally acting* drugs, including antiseptics, disinfectants, and drugs used in the chemotherapy of infectious diseases;
7. *Autacoids* or vasoactive agents, histamines and antihistamines;
8. *Other*—drugs that do not fall under the specified categories.

The use of such a system in the collection of a medication history clearly facilitates the nurse's understanding of interactions and actions of drugs in each client. Since it is not unusual to discover that elderly clients are taking multiple medications that affect either a single system or many systems, the nurse must understand the possible interactions of these drugs in relation to each drug's specific action.

FAMILY HISTORY

Many disorders have a genetic or familial relationship, and a review of a client's family members during the family history (FH) portion of the health history allows the examiner to identify the client's particular health and risk patterns. The information elicited about the client's parents, grandparents, and siblings can be simply but explicitly diagramed as shown in figure 5.5 to help the examiner see possible risk patterns. For example, this family history documents that three people (maternal grandfather, mother, and father) died of heart attacks, two sisters have hypertension, one brother has had a heart attack, and one person (paternal grandfather) died of a cerebral vascular accident. Thus, the client should be made aware of the risk factors involved in cardiovascular disease and the management plan should include preventive intervention.

Because of the high incidence of risk factors, information about the incidence of the following diseases among family members should be elicited from the client: diabetes, tuberculosis, heart disease, hypertension, cancer, neurological or bone disorders, psychiatric conditions, kidney disease, arthritis, allergies, bleeding tendencies, gall bladder disease, thyroid disorders, and migraine headaches. In figure 5.6 Mr. Harris's family diagram shows a high-risk potential for cardiovascular problems.

PSYCHOSOCIAL HISTORY

As shown in figure 5.7, the psychosocial (PSH) portion of the health history provides a profile of the client's past and present life. To obtain a holistic view of the client's health, the nurse must explore the client's lifestyle, life satisfaction, interpersonal relationships, and support systems. Such factors as the home, economic level, supportive relationships, spiritual life, and neighborhood are all elements to consider. The individual's past coping mechanisms provide guidance for assisting the elderly in adapting to new stress.

In reviewing the elderly client's family relationships, the nurse should examine the level of satisfaction with family relationships and/or significant others. Loss of spouse, children, brothers, and sisters may

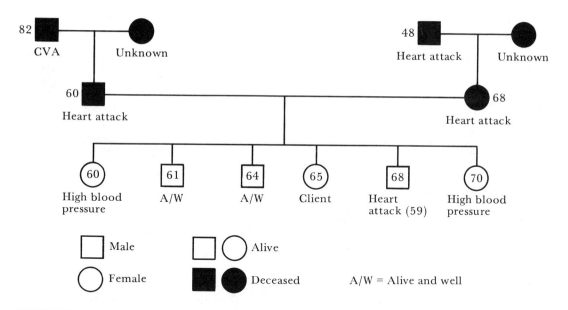

FIGURE 5.5   Diagrammatic Method of Recording a Client's Family History.

isolate the individual who has failed to establish new relationships.

Often, culture and heritage must be considered in order to understand the client's role within and relationship to both family and community. The United States has always prided itself on being the great melting pot of the world, and while immigrants have traditionally adopted cultural aspects of the American society, they have maintained an ethnicity that creates feelings of individuality and heritage. Consideration of such feelings is essential when serving clients from ethnic neighborhoods not only in large cities such as San Francisco (Chinatown), Boston (the North End), and New Orleans (the French Quarter) but in smaller communities throughout the country.

Religious attachments are important to many elderly clients. Thus the following significant areas should be considered during the PSH since they may aid the nurse

in understanding such clients' life relationships as well as their attitudes and activities:

Religious identification,
Church attendance,
Religious associations,
Personal religious observances,
Participation in religious rituals,
Religious faith,
Religious "experience,"
Religious beliefs,
Personal importance of religion,
Religious morality [Atchley 1977, p. 279].

Eliciting information about the manner in which a client spends the day may permit the evaluation of both the degree of socialization and the level of self-satisfaction. Note that the quantity of the client's activity does not equate with satisfaction derived from that activity. Some clients may be perfectly satisfied with sitting by the

77

Name: William Harris　　　　　　　　　Date: 4/25/79

FH:

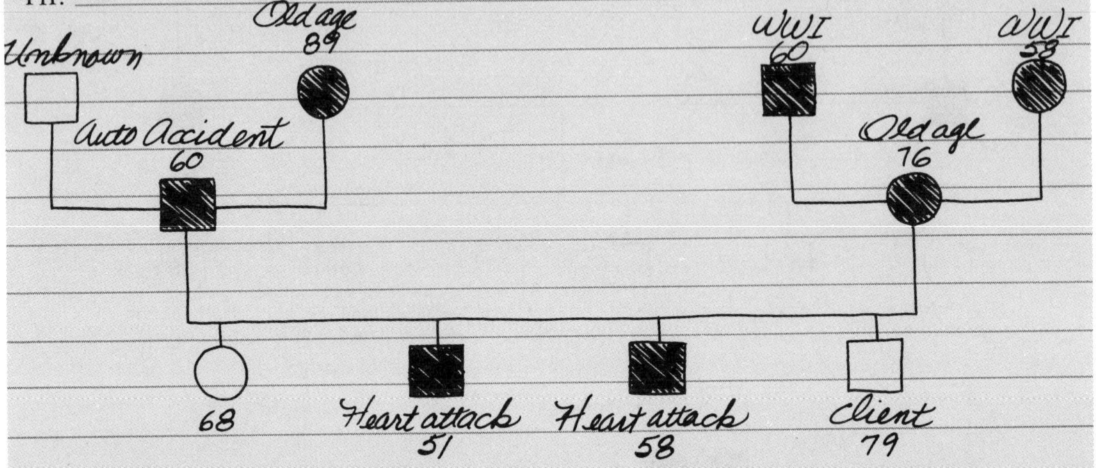

Denies family history of diabetes, tuberculosis, hypertension, cancer, allergies, gall bladder disease, bleeding tendencies, thyroid disorders, or migraines.

　　FIGURE 5.6　Health History of William Harris: Family History (FH).

Name: William Harris   Date: 4/25/79

PSH: Born in Boston, at home, oldest of four children. Recalls early life as "poor but happy". Quit school after graduating from 8th grade and worked on fishing trawler for several months before joining Army. Stayed in Army for 8 yrs. and reached rank of sergeant. Married at age 24 and discharged from Army following yr. Has since lived in same 3-family home in Boston with his family — 2 sons and 2 daughters, all now living out of state.

Worked at Penn's Printing Co. for 42 years. Retired 13 yrs. ago.

Loved wife very much and has been "very lonely" since her death 10 yrs. ago (she was 56 and he 69). Does not see friends much or go to church. Sees some children and grandchildren at Christmas time only.

Retirement income is #398/month. Budgets carefully. Description of typical day: "Days of week have lost their meaning — they're all the same." Arises 7:00 a.m. feeling tired and has breakfast. Spends morning watching television and doing yard work. Has lunch around 12:00 noon and then naps for 1–2 hrs. Afternoon is spent walking to store or park. Has dinner at 5:00 p.m. and then watches television until 10:00 p.m., at which time he retires. Never has difficulty getting to sleep; usually gets up once per night to void.

Smokes 1½–2 packs of cigarettes per day (×40 yrs. = 60–80 pack yrs.).

Denies use of marijuana, drugs, or any alcohol. Drinks 3–4 cups of tea per day (see ROS).

Denies any sexual activity since death of wife — unable to obtain erection.

FIGURE 5.7 Health History of William Harris: Psychosocial History (PSH).

window all day. An elderly client's impairment and independence may also be assessed by the degree and type of activity the person can carry out. Washing, combing hair, and cooking are examples of activities of daily living that should be considered.

Once a trust relationship is established between client and nurse and an uncritical, professional manner is communicated by the nurse, discussions regarding sexual activity will be easier. Many health professionals do not realize an 80-year-old male or female may experience an active sex life. When appropriate, clients should be asked such questions as when did they last have sexual intercourse and how frequently, how satisfactory was the sexual relationship; and, for males, questions concern ability to maintain erections in intercourse as well as obtaining early morning erections. Sexual activity is part of a healthy adult life, and the examiner needs to be aware of changes that may indicate problems of health and vigor.

Finally, knowledge of a client's economic status will help the nurse assess the individual's ability to pay for referral visits to community agencies. People who have "paid their own way" all of their lives may disregard health care recommendations, treatments, and return visits because they are unable to afford them. An inquiry into the client's knowledge and use of community resources will assist in identifying which resources may be indicated.

REVIEW OF SYSTEMS (ROS)

The review of systems (ROS) portion of the health history is a descriptive review of all the body systems in regard to any symptoms or past problems. Positive findings are explored and described in the same manner as in the HPI. The descriptive information provided in the ROS thus includes date of onset; manner, date, and frequency of recurrence; what, if anything, seems to affect the problem; and any information concerning previous diagnosis or treatment. While problems previously described in the client's history should not be included in the ROS, all pertinent negatives should be recorded as such.

Figures 5.8a, b, and c provide examples of the way in which the descriptive information is recorded for each system and region of the body. This type of useful descriptive information can only be gained by careful and systematic exploration of specific topics during the ROS. Following are examples of the specific topics for which descriptive information should be elicited for each body system.

Skin: Rashes, eruptions, dryness or sweating, pruritus (where and when), color change, texture, any contact or skin allergies (to what and how), hair loss, change of texture, nonhealing sores, lumps, sun sensitivity, characteristics of nails.

Head: Headaches, dizziness, masses, trauma (loss of consciousness, with or without amnesia, sequelae).

Eyes: Visual acuity defects (type, glasses, last exam, rapidity of deterioration), pain, double vision, blurring, inflammation, lacrimation, cataracts, infection.

Ears: Auditory deficits, infections, pain, discharge, tinnitus, vertigo.

Nose: Loss of sense of smell, strange odors, nose bleeds, discharge (color, fre-

FIGURE 5.8a   Health History of William Harris: Review of Systems (ROS–1).

Name: William Harris   Date: 4/25/79

ROS (1): ~~Skin~~: Denies rashes, eruptions, excessive dryness or perspiration, pruritus texture or color change, hair loss, nonhealing sores, lumps, or sun sensitivity. Nails considered healthy and unchanged.

Head: Denies headaches, loss of consciousness, trauma, or amnesia.

Eyes: States vision is good. Wears glasses for reading and watching television (for past 10 yrs.). Prescribed by Dr. Peterson, Allstate Road, Boston. Last eye exam, 1 yr. ago (May, 1978). Denies pain, diplopia, blurring, inflammation, infection, or cataracts.

Ears: Denies hearing loss, infections, tinnitus, pain, discharge, vertigo. Unable to recall last examination.

Nose: Denies loss of smell, strange odors, nose bleeds, discharges, or trauma.

Mouth: Able to taste all foods. Denies soreness or bleeding of tongue, mucosa, lips, or gums. Wears upper and lower complete dentures. Upper has three teeth missing. Last exam, 1972. Unable to recall dentist's name. Denies excessive or decreased salivation.

Throat: Denies frequent sore throats, strep infections, persistent hoarseness, painful swallowing, or lumps in throat.

Neck: Denies pain, stiffness limitation of movement, injury, thyroid problems, or masses.

Name: William Harris   Date: 4/25/79

ROS (2): <u>Respiratory</u>: Denies cough, dyspnea, painful respiration, night sweats. Last TB test, March 1978 — negative; Pneumonia, 1978; Spanish Flu, 1918 (see PH).

   <u>Cardiovascular</u>: Denies palpitations. Has had chest pain (see HPI). Denies vertigo, numbness, dyspnea, orthopnea. Sleeps with one thin pillow. Denies paroxysmal nocturnal dyspnea, history of hypertension, or varicose veins. Feels fatigued upon awakening (see PSH). Denies swelling of ankles, fainting, claudication, thrombophlebitis, or coolness or discoloration of extremities.

   <u>Gastrointestinal</u>: Yesterday's meals included:

Breakfast	Lunch	Supper
6 oz. tea and donut (plain)	8 oz. water and spaghetti	6 oz. tea and macaroni

Snacks included 2 cups of tea (8 oz.) and 1 bag (large) of potato chips.

Appetite is "good"; nutrition, poor.

Denies anorexia, weight loss, appetite change, nausea, indigestion, heartburn, water brash, sour regurgitation, nocturnal drool, dysphagia, odynophagia, vomiting, or pain.

Has bowel movement once a day after breakfast, denies changes. Constipation in 1952 — etiology unknown, spontaneously subsided in two yrs. with no sequelae (see PH). Stool is formed brown in color without any frank red blood. Denies rectal bleeding, use of laxatives or jaundice.

quency, uni- or bilateral, odor, consistency).

Mouth: Disturbance of sense of taste, soreness or bleeding (tongue, lips, or gums), dental problems, dentures, last dental exam, abnormalities of salivation.

Throat: Soreness, streptococcal infections, persistent hoarseness, painful swallowing, lump in throat.

Neck: Pain, stiffness, limitation of movement, injury, thyroid, masses.

Respiratory: Cough, when, how often, productive sputum (amount per day; color; consistency; odor; if bloody, describe color), shortness of breath, exercise tolerance, duration, pain with respiration, night sweats, skin testing and results.

Breasts: Nipple changes, discharge, tenderness, masses, deformity.

Cardiovascular: Palpitations (effort related, position related), pain (location, frequency, duration, character), radiation, ameliorating or exacerbating activities, effect of ambient temperature, dizziness (vertigo or not), numbness; dyspnea, orthopnea (number of pillows used), paroxysmal nocturnal dyspnea, hypertension, varicose veins, fatigue; swelling of ankles, fainting, claudication, thrombophlebitis, coolness and discoloration of extremities.

Gastrointestinal: Appetite, anorexia, weight loss, appetite change, nausea (when, time of day, relation to meals); digestion, indigestion (relation to meals); heartburn, waterbrash, sour regurgitation, nocturnal drool, dysphagia (liquids or solids), odynophagia (to citrus, carbonated, or solids); vomiting (type, color, quantity, relation to meals, whether awakening); pain (relation to meals or bowel movement); bowel habits, usual, changes in color, consistency; rectal bleeding; diarrhea (number of stools and amount, relation to meals, color, consistency, pus, mucus, blood); laxatives (type, frequency, period of time); jaundice.

Genitourinary: Urination (frequency, urgency), nocturia, dysuria (onset or terminal), incontinence (stress), urgency, overflow, enuresis, complete emptying, hesitancy, dribbling, straining, force of stream, thirst; hematuria (smoky urine), gravel, pain; vaginal or penile discharge (color, staining, treatment for V.D.); dyspareunia, postcoital bleeding, impotence, premature ejaculation, loss of libido (when, how long, any preceding events).

Menses: Menarche (date), menses (regularity), LMP (frequency/duration); dysmenorrhea (pattern), menorrhagia, metrorrhagia, menopause (any symptoms, any bleeding since), last pelvic exam, last Pap and result; pregnancies (gravida, para, abortions, stillbirths, Cesarean sections), complications (hypertension, toxemia, sugar, or TBC), sequelae.

Musculoskeletal: Arthritis, arthralgias (swelling, how long); stiffness; gout, rheumatism; redness or inflammation; deformities; limitation of activities; exercise, muscle strength or weakness; pain; cramps; back problems.

Hematopoietic: Anemia, bleeding disorders, bruising, blood dyscrasias.

Endocrine: Temperature intolerance; thyroid, history of growth and development; polyuria, polydypsia, polyphagia, hirsutism; changes in secondary sex characteristics.

Neurological: Weakness, numbness, changed or increased sensation; loss of posi-

FIGURE 5.8b   **Health History of William Harris:** Review of Systems (ROS–2).

Name: William Harris   Date: 4/25/79

ROS (3): <u>Genitourinary</u>: Denies frequency, urgency, dysuria, incontinence, hesitancy, dribbling, straining, hematuria, thirst, gravel, pain. Voids 3-4+ times and once during night. Denies penile discharge, VD. C/o of impotence since wife died. Has not had intercourse since then. Denies urge for intercourse. Denies nipple changes, discharge, tenderness, masses or deformity.

    <u>Muskuloskeletal</u>: Denies arthritis, arthralgias, stiffness, gout, rheumatism, inflamation, or limitation to activities. Fractured (R) humerus 1934 (see PH). Denies muscle weakness, pain, cramps, or back problems.

    <u>Hematopoietic</u>: Denies anemia, bleeding tendencies, bruising, or blood dyscrasias.

    <u>Endocrine</u>: Denies temperature intolerance, thyroid problems, polyuria, polydipsia, polyphagia change in secondary sex characteristics. Growth and development normal.

    <u>Neurological</u>: Denies weakness, numbness, loss of position sense, or changes in balance or coordination. Denies dizziness or lightheadedness, loss of vision, or seizure disorder.

◀ FIGURE 5.8c   Health History of William Harris: Review of Systems (ROS–3).

tion sense, balance, or coordination; dizziness (distinguish objective and subjective vertigo or simple lightheadedness); loss of vision (total or partial), blurring, double vision, difficulty following the printed page; seizures, loss of consciousness.

Since the ROS explores the regions and systems of the body, the nurse must understand the relationship of elicited symptoms to the physical findings and the pathophysiology of the body areas. Examples of subjective complaints are included in chapter 6 along with the objective findings of the physical assessment in order to help the nurse gain a better understanding of this relationship and thus develop the ability to explore the subjective complaints in greater depth during the health history interview.

REFERENCES

American Nurses Association. 1973. "Standards of Geriatric Nursing Practice." Kansas City, Mo.

ATCHLEY, R. C. 1977. *The Social Forces in Later Life.* Belmont, Calif.: Wadsworth.

BAER, E. 1977. "How to Take a Health History," *American Journal of Nursing* 77(7):1191–93.

BIRD, K. T. 1976. "The PROVE Medical Record." Unpublished paper. Massachusetts General Hospital, Boston.

BURNSIDE, I. M., ed. 1976. *Nursing and the Aged.* New York: McGraw-Hill.

BUTLER, R., and M. LEWIS. 1973. *Aging and Mental Health.* St. Louis: C. V. Mosby.

DONABEDIAN, A., and L. S. ROSENFIELD. 1964. "Follow-up Study of Chronically Ill Patients Discharged from a Hospital." *Journal of Chronic Diseases* 17:847.

FEINSTEIN, A. 1967. *Clinical Judgement.* Baltimore, Md.: Williams and Williams.

FOWKES, W., and V. HUNN. 1973. *Clinical Assessment for the Nurse Practitioner.* St. Louis: C.V. Mosby.

HECHT, A. B. 1974. "Improving Compliance by Teaching Outpatients." *Nursing Forum* 13(2):112–29.

IREY, N. S. 1976. "Adverse Drug Reactions and Death." *Journal of the American Medical Association.* 236(6):575–78.

KALISH, R., ed. 1977. *The Later Years.* Monterey, Calif.: Brooks Cole.

LEITCH, C., and R. TINKER, eds. 1978. *Primary Care.* Philadelphia: F.A. Davis.

MANSELL, E., et al. 1974. "Patient Assessment: Taking a Patient's History," *American Journal of Nursing* 74(2):293–324.

MEZEY, M., et al. 1977. "The Health History of the Aged Person." *Journal of Gerontological Nursing.* 77(3):47.

MUMMAH, H. 1975. "Group Work with the Aged Blind Japanese in the Nursing Home and in the Community." *The New Outlook for the Blind* 69(4):160–67.

MURRAY, R., and J. ZENTER. 1975. *Nursing Assessment and Health Promotion through the Life Span.* Englewood Cliffs, N.J.: Prentice-Hall.

PARKER, W. 1976. "Medication Histories," *American Journal of Nursing* 76(12):1969–71.

PRIOR, J., and J. SILBERSTEIN. 1973. *Physical Diagnosis.* St. Louis: C.V. Mosby.

ROBBINS, L., and J. HALL. 1974. *How to Practice Prospective Medicine.* Indianapolis: Methodist Hospital of Indiana.

STEINBERG, F. 1976. *Cowdry's The Care of the Geriatric Patient.* St. Louis: C.V. Mosby.

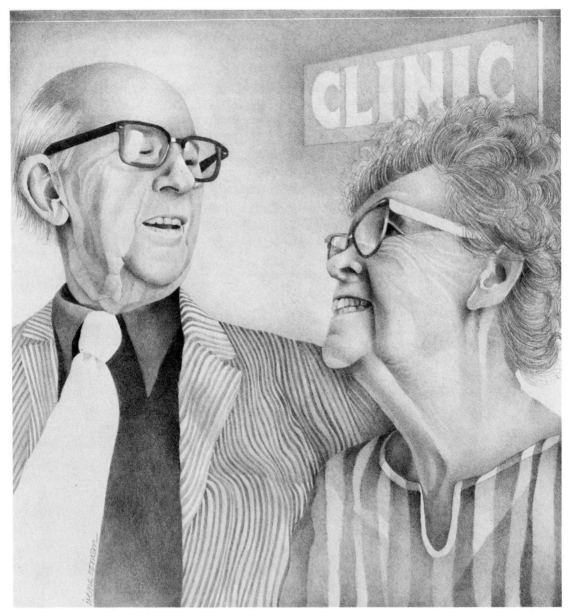

Chapter 6

THE PHYSICAL ASSESSMENT

The findings of a physical assessment provide the building blocks of objective data. Objective information that is acquired through evaluation becomes part of the data base utilized in diagnostic reasoning (Benbassat and Schiffman 1976) and helps to generate the practical decisions of management and care. Elstein and his colleagues (1972) demonstrated that the experienced clinician formed some diagnostic hypotheses very early in the encounter with a client, at the beginning of the health history. Diagnostic reasoning continues throughout the period of data collection and consists of the generation, testing, and acceptance or rejection of hypotheses.

A large part of a nurse's education is designed to promote sensitivity to the client's feelings and needs. This background in intuitive reasoning from subjective data frequently leads to remarkably correct decisions. However, when the nurse acts as the principal provider of primary care, the reasoning must be supported by objective fact. Diagnostic reasoning is not intuitive. It is the analysis of subjective data in the light of known pathophysiological mechanisms and is confirmed by the discovery of expected objective findings. Physical assessment is part of this search for objective data.

Thus the physical appraisal of the client is a vital component of a systematic nursing assessment. Once professional nursing had accepted McCain's (1965) concept of nursing process theory, as described in the overview to part II, the use of physical assessment skills by nurses was a logical development. Clinical decisions formed within the structure of modern nursing process require a complete and accurate data base. The enrichment of this base by the objective information gathered during a physical assessment allows nurses to render higher quality care (Lewis 1974) and prepares them to investigate and make appropriate decisions for a wider range of care and management problems (Lynaugh and Bates 1974). The objective data obtained from physical assessment permit nurses to measure their clients' disabilities and limitations and provide a baseline from which physiological change and the efficacy of nursing care can be measured.

The effective use of physical assessment skills requires that the nurse distinguish abnormal conditions from the wide range of normal variation that is even greater in elderly than in younger clients. This range is due to biological variation, the impact of pathology in one system on other systems, and the growth and development that occur over the life span (Rossman 1971; Timaris 1972; Linn 1975). Physical assessment skills are best learned under preceptorship and direct monitoring by skilled instructors (Butterworth and Reppert 1960; Feinstein 1967; Engel 1966; Anderson et al. 1974; Bates and Lynaugh 1975; Weiner and Nathanson 1976).

This chapter reviews some of the anatomical and physiological changes encountered in the healthy elderly, with particular attention given to age-related changes that affect the findings of the physical assessment. To facilitate the learning process and develop holistic thinking, each unit of this chapter begins with the subjective findings that point toward the particular system or region discussed in the unit. This section of the unit is followed by the objective findings that modify the examination. The unit concludes with some of the abnormal findings that commonly cause disability in older adults. Prerequisites for an effective use of this chapter are knowledge of anatomy and physiology and some experience in the examination of the normal adult. Nurses must be aware that biological aging is an irregular process occurring at different rates in different body systems. To find all of the described changes in one person would be unusual.

ASSESSING THE SYSTEMS AND REGIONS

TECHNIQUES OF EXAMINATION: SUBJECTIVE DATA COLLECTION

The interview is the most important part of the examination. It establishes rapport between the nurse and client and provides the precise information needed to guide diagnostic reasoning. This information determines the effectiveness of the entire health appraisal. The content of the health history was discussed in chapter 5; some useful techniques for obtaining the history are reemphasized here.

The anxiety that all examiners feel during a health encounter must not be communicated to the client. A warm, open, and interested attitude is essential. Sitting near the client will express concern and a desire to help; looking into the client's eyes will make the nurse appear unhurried and interested and thus permit the client to talk without worrying about taking up too much time. The elderly have long histories. The nurse should develop a personal style of interviewing that provides direction but does not interfere with communication. Techniques such as prompting and the use of open-ended questions are helpful and directive, but to elicit truly accurate information, the nurse must avoid leading with such questions as "Was the pain sharp?"

TECHNIQUES OF EXAMINATION: OBJECTIVE DATA COLLECTION

Physical appraisal is commonly performed after the history has been obtained. The physical appraisal broadens the data base and the nurse's perceptions of the client's problems (Bates and Lynaugh 1973). The appraisal is a deliberate, systematic, and thorough examination of the body, which permits an assessment of general health status and the identification of any abnormalities or limitations. Such an examination allows the nurse to assess functional ability, to test diagnostic hypotheses generated by the interview, and to discover physical data not previously known. If rapport is established during the interview, the transition into the examination should not pose any difficulty. If the client objects, the nurse has only to explain that the examination is necessary to evaluate the client's needs and to permit the formulation of an overall health care plan.

Each nurse must develop a personal approach to the routine of the examination. This order must be followed as closely as possible every time. Some flexibility is essential to allow for a client's limitations, but frequent changes in the routine cause disorganization and omissions in the examination (Weiner and Nathanson 1976). If the client appears fatigued and no apparent medical urgency exists, the nurse might well ask the client to come back and complete the examination at another session. Since the older client's energy levels are highest in the morning, the nurse might schedule the evaluations accordingly.

The skills needed for a complete examination are *inspection, palpation, percussion,* and *auscultation.* These techniques are reviewed in this section. Their specific application is described in the units of this chapter.

All observations are compared to a standard of normality that the nurse must acquire. This standard permits the nurse to distinguish conditions that are abnormal and in need of further evaluation from conditions in the broad range of normality. The client and the nurse must be in comfortable positions, as these may be held for a long time. The temperature of the room should be appropriate for the client's state of undress, and the client should be suitably covered to permit examination with minimum embarrassment and maximum relaxation. The examining area should insure privacy suitable for the intimate nature of the physical examination. Successful examination requires a knowledgeable nurse and a relaxed client.

Inspection

The detailed inspection of the client consists of a visual search for significant physical features. The nurse first notes the general appearance of the area examined and then its specific characteristics: color, size, texture, mobility, symmetry, comparison with the other side of the body, and presence or absence of normal or unusual landmarks and their location, appearance, and size.

This most important clinical skill is an art perfected by conscious, continuous practice. Inspection begins during the interview but is used more precisely during the actual examination. Experienced examiners will often couple it with palpation.

Palpation

Palpation is the evaluation of the tissues and organs of the body through the sense of

89

touch. First the client must be completely relaxed; then the nurse proceeds in an orderly manner to compare one side of the body with the other. Tender areas are always examined last. The tactile sense is used to evaluate all accessible areas of the body for texture and temperature; for appraisal of articular appearance and the presence of crepitus or grating in the joint; for fixation, mobility, and pulsation of blood vessels, glands, and tumors; for muscle tone or rigidity; for skin turgor and moisture content; and for the transmission of vocal or cardiac vibrations.

Palpation is performed with warm hands. The examination begins with light pressure and progresses to deeper palpation. Different parts of the hands are used. The *palmar surfaces of the fingertips* are the most sensitive and are used to evaluate vessels, small tumors, and the texture of the skin and organs. Sensitivity of the digital pads is enhanced if the examiner applies them with a slightly circular motion. Firm application of the *palmar surfaces of the metacarpophalangeal joints* is the most sensitive manner to assess vibrations. Temperature is best evaluated by applying *the dorsal surfaces of the hand and fingers.* The thinner skin of this area is most sensitive to temperature. Consistency and mobility are appreciated by *grasping with the fingers.* For deep palpation of the abdomen, a *bimanual technique* may be used. A passive sensing hand is placed on the abdomen and covered by the active hand. Pressure is applied by the active to the sensing hand. Palpation is performed by the digital cushions and palmar surface of the sensing hand. Any pressure exerted by the sensing hand diminishes its sensitivity. *Dipping* is a special form of bimanual palpation useful in the presence of ascites. The active hand applies a sudden, deep pressure and maintains it. Organs or tumors floating in the fluid are initially pushed away; as they return they are palpated by the sensing hand. By means of *ballottement* the nurse can evaluate rebound tenderness, the consistency of an organ, and the tension of an encapsulated fluid. In ballottement pressure is exerted on the organ and suddenly released; the sensing hand can then assess the impact on rebound.

Percussion

The technique of percussion consists of setting up vibrations by means of a sharp tap. This technique produces sounds that enable the examiner to assess the size, position, and density of an underlying structure. Percussion is particularly valuable for assessing the relative amounts of air and solid material in an underlying structure, the borders of organs or parts of the body of differing structural density, and changes from the normal density caused by the accumulation of fluid or the formation of a solid mass within a hollow organ.

Percussion may be either direct or indirect. *Direct, or immediate, percussion* is accomplished by striking the body surface directly with one or more partly bent fingers. If only one finger is used, it is usually the third or fourth finger. In *indirect, or mediate, percussion,* the nurse firmly places the distal phalanx of the middle finger of the left hand in contact with the tissues (see figure 6.1). Firm, close contact by the pleximeter finger is the secret of successful percussion. A sharp blow is then struck on the dorsum of the base of the distal phalanx of this finger by the tip of the middle (plexor) finger

90

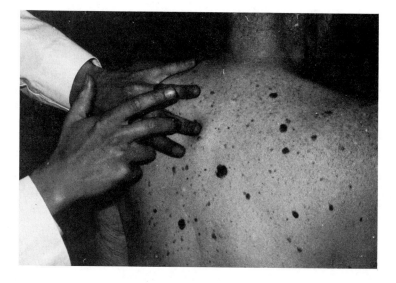

FIGURE 6.1 Mediate Percussion.
The distal phalanx of the pleximeter is held firmly against the chest wall and parallel to the ribs. The plexor finger is bent so that it is perpendicular to the pleximeter as it strikes. The blow is delivered from the wrist and not from the arm. Note the seborrheic keratoses typically distributed over the back (see also figure 6.4).

of the right hand. The blow is delivered by a movement of the wrist alone. The plexor finger is partially bent so that it falls and strikes the pleximeter at a right angle. If the organ or mass is close to the surface, percussion should be light; if it lies deeply, or if the mass is large, percussion should be heavy. The sounds of percussion may be intensified by using two plexor fingers or by using direct percussion. This skill is acquired by repeated practice. Common errors, causing a decreased percussion note, include incomplete and loose contact of the pleximeter with the skin and the absence of perpendicularity of the tip of the plexor as it strikes.

The sounds of percussion are classified according to the acoustical properties of the tones produced. *Resonance* is a sustained, low-pitched note. This sound is common in normal lungs and is caused by the mixture of air and tissue. If the pulmonary air spaces are overinflated, the resonance increases and a booming sound, called *hyperresonance,* is heard. Hollow organs filled with unloculated air, such as the large bowel or stomach, produce a drumlike sound. This extreme resonance is known as *tympany.* The absence of air in a solid organ such as the liver causes *dullness,* which is heard as a short, high-pitched note. Extreme dullness, called *flatness,* can be produced by percussion of the thigh. The sound is similar to that made by striking a container filled with water. The proficient examiner actually perceives as much of the percussion note through the finger as is heard by the ear. *Sonorous percussion* allows the nurse to distinguish the density of an organ, while *definitive percussion* may be used to outline the borders of organs of differing density.

Auscultation

Auscultation is the process of listening to sounds produced by various organs and tissues of the body in order to detect variations or deviations from sounds normally produced. Auscultation is an extremely

91

useful clinical tool and is most productive in the assessment of sounds produced by the lungs and heart. It is also used clinically to evaluate the neck and the abdomen. The complexity of the sounds and the difficulty of distinguishing abnormal from normal ones require that the nurse practice listening to normal sounds until familiar with them. Only then can the abnormal ones be appreciated.

Direct auscultation has rarely been performed since Laennec discovered, in the nineteenth century, that breath and heart sounds can be more comfortably heard through a roll of parchment. This mediate (or indirect) auscultation led to the development of the modern binaural stethoscope. This instrument consists of a bell or a diaphragm, or both, connected with rubber or plastic tubing to ear pieces. The tubing should be short, 18 to 20 cm long, with an internal diameter of 4 mm and a thick rubber or plastic wall. The double-tube stethoscope is acoustically superior to the single-tube type. The ear pieces must fit snugly and comfortably. If too small, they slip into the canal, causing discomfort and reducing sound transmission. The diaphragm best transmits high-pitched tones, such as the murmur of mitral regurgitation. The bell is distortion free and is best used for low-pitched tones, such as the murmur of mitral stenosis.

Sounds are evaluated as to pitch (frequency), intensity, quality, and duration. The *pitch* is a measure of the number of waves per second. The more waves per second, the higher the frequency and pitch; the fewer waves, the lower the pitch. The *intensity* is a measure of the energy or amplitude of the sound waves produced. High-intensity sound is loud, whereas low-intensity sound is soft. The *quality* of the sound is a measure of its timbre. Two sounds of equal intensity and pitch, coming from different sources, can be distinguished by their quality. *Duration* of sound is a measure of time. Evaluating duration means distinguishing the number of continuous vibrations. The duration of these vibrations is determined by the energy producing them and by the frictional resistance within the system, which absorbs the energy. This resistance is called *damping*. The vibrations produced by the internal organs are damped by the soft tissue overlying the organs.

To adequately perform auscultation, absolute quiet and concentration are essential. Many sounds are close to the limit of human hearing and only with practice and absolute concentration can they be discerned. To exclude extraneous sounds, the chest piece of the stethoscope is placed firmly against the skin. The pressure should leave a slightly blanched ring after a few seconds of application. Movements of the chest piece, clothing, or bandages between the skin and the chest piece; breathing on the tubing; or sliding one's fingers on the chest piece will produce extraneous sounds. Hair on the skin surface may cause crackling sounds if the chest piece is moved. If the skin surface is excessively hairy, wetting the hair or plastering it down with soap will help. The room must be warm and the client comfortable to prevent any audible involuntary muscle movement.

The key to successful auscultation lies in being systematic and in listening to one sound at a time. The nurse must listen to symmetrical points on each side of the body, one after the other. When examining the lungs, the nurse must proceed symmetrically from the top down. When listening to breath sounds, the nurse must ignore sounds produced by the heart; and when listening to the heart, the nurse must attend to each portion of the cardiac cycle separately while ignoring the rest. Only when the nurse has learned to recognize the normal sounds can the abnormal ones be appreciated. Once these sounds are distinguished, the nurse may begin the finer definition of the nature of the observed abnormality.

THE GENERAL EXAMINATION

The appraisal of the client's general condition is a constant feature of all health encounters.

The nurse continually notes the client's posture, color and texture of the skin and its appendages, facial appearance, and body movements. All of these attributes convey impressions about mental and physical health, limitations requiring further evaluation, as well as vigor, interest, intelligence, and the effects of aging.

HEALTH HISTORY AND SUBJECTIVE FINDINGS

During the interview the nurse concentrates on establishing rapport and appraising the client's vocabulary, intelligence, and general knowledge of body functions. In addition, the nurse observes the client's physical status and ease and spontaneity of movement and mimic. Subjective information of a general nature may be elicited. Loss of energy, fever, anxiety, blue feelings, and a change in sleeping habits may be spe-

cific complaints, or they may represent general manifestations of another specific disorder and are due to its impact on the body as a whole.

EXAMINATION AND OBJECTIVE FINDINGS

Upon completion of the interview, the nurse begins the examination of the client. The client's height and weight are recorded along with the vital signs—pulse, blood pressure, number of respirations per minute, and temperature. The techniques of measuring blood pressure and pulse are described in detail in unit 10 on the cardiovascular system. Other concepts beyond the simple measure of pulse and pressure are also outlined.

Aging is accompanied by modification in the significance of the vital signs. Changes occurring in the autonomic nervous system and nodal tissue lead to a diminution in the peripheral effects. The elderly client has a slower heart rate and an increased sensitivity to catacholamines, which causes an increased frequency of extrasystoles (Harris 1975). Thermoregulation is also modified. Not only are the elderly more sensitive to variations in ambient temperatures, but they are also unable to develop the fevers that may be found in younger persons (Timaris 1972). Frequently in the critically ill, the nurse will find temperatures below the usually accepted normal of 37°C (98.6°F) (Agate 1971).

After measuring the vital signs, the nurse assesses the general appearance of the client. Does the client appear healthy or can the nurse see evidence of a systemic disorder? For example, jaundice may indicate a liver or hemolytic problem; air forced

93

through pursed lips may indicate a respiratory or cardiac condition. Does the client show signs of acute or chronic ill health? What is the client's state of nutrition? The nurse must keep in mind that in the elderly the redistribution of body fat creates a boniness, a prominence of tendon insertions and joints, a loss of fat on the face, and an increase of fat around the hips and abdomen (Hejda 1963; Wesel et al. 1963). Is the client's physical development normal? Here the nurse must recognize that breasts sag and hair distribution changes markedly with advancing years, so clients may appear to suffer from endocrinopathies, which are actually nonexistent. Posture and stature are modified, so that the elderly have a dorsal kyphosis and stand with bent knees and hips in the absence of any pathological condition.

Changes of a local nature may indicate unusual exposure to sunlight or to a toxic environment or a particular genetic effect as in familial balding. General alterations of appearance due to aging are a good index of the individual's rate of biological aging. The elderly are often stooped because of decreased muscle mass and strength. People lose 1.2 cm in stature every twenty years after age 30 (Brown and Wigzell 1964). With age, hair often turns gray or white and becomes thinner in both men and women. The skin becomes less elastic and drier, with characteristic pigment patches, wrinkles, and jowls. Ecchymoses due to increased capillary fragility can be observed on the dorsum of the wrist. Age-related facial pallor, ptosis of the eyelids, and loss of the eyebrows must be differentiated from similar findings associated with pathological conditions in younger clients.

Upon completion of the general appraisal, the nurse begins a *systematic examination of the body.* The head, neck, chest, and back are examined with the client sitting. The client is then asked to lie down and the nurse proceeds to examine the anterior chest, the abdomen, the extremities, and the male genitalia. The examination for hernia may be performed with the client recumbent, but it will be more sensitive if the client is standing. At this time a more thorough examination of the back may be performed, the lower limbs may be examined for varicosities, and gait and balance may be checked. The entire neurological system may be tested at one time at the end of the examination, or each portion may be examined as the nurse appraises each region of the body. Finally, for men, a rectal examination is performed. For women, the genitalia and rectal examinations are performed last, with the client in the dorsolithotomy position.

The order of this examination is not fixed by necessity or tradition and can be modified; but the examiner must be systematic to perform a thorough health assessment.

EVALUATION OF PHYSICAL FINDINGS

Analysis and synthesis of assessment data culminate in the identification of functional disabilities that require nursing action or merit referral to a physician. In addition, particular attention should be given to the client's strengths as well as to the assets that should be maintained and fostered throughout the implementation of the prescribed health care regimen (Crane 1975).

94

Within the structure of nursing process, physical assessment findings provide the nurse with information essential for planning total health maintenance and management.

REFERENCES

AGATE, J. 1971. "The Natural History of Disease in Later Life." In I. Rossman, ed., *Clinical Geriatrics.* Philadelphia: J. B. Lippincott.

ANDERSON, E. A., B. J. LEONARD, and J. A. YATES. 1974. "Epigenesis of the Nurse Practitioner Role." *American Journal of Nursing* 74:1812–16.

BATES, B., and J. E. LYNAUGH. 1973. "Laying the Foundation for Medical Nursing Practice." *American Journal of Nursing* 73:1375.

———. 1975. "Teaching Physical Assessment." *Nursing Outlook* 23:297–302.

BENBASSAT, J., and A. SCHIFFMAN. 1976. "An Approach to Teaching the Introduction to Clinical Medicine." *Annals of Internal Medicine* 84:477–81.

BROWN, O. T., and F. W. WIGZELL. 1964. "The Significance of Span as a Clinical Measurement." In W. F. Anderson and B. Isaacs, eds., *Current Achievement in Geriatrics.* London: Cassell.

BUTTERWORTH, J. S., and E. H. REPPERT. 1960. "Auscultatory Acumen in the General Medical Population." *Journal of American Medical Association* 174:32–4.

CRANE, J. 1975. "Physical Appraisal: An Aspect of Nursing Assessment." In J. M. Sana and R. D. Judge, eds., *Physical Appraisal Methods in Nursing Practice.* Boston: Little, Brown.

ELSTEIN, A. S., N. KAGAN, and L. S. SCHULMAN. 1972. "Methods and Theory in the Study of Medical Inquiry." *Journal of Medical Education* 47:85–92.

ENGEL, G. L. 1966. "The Deficiencies of the Case Presentation as a Means of Teaching and Evaluating Clinical Skills." *Journal of Medical Education* 41:140–61.

FEINSTEIN, A. R. 1967. *Clinical Judgement.* Baltimore: Williams and Wilkins.

HARRIS, R. 1975. "Cardiac Changes with Age." In R. Goldman and M. Rockstein, eds., *The Physiology and Pathology of Human Aging.* New York: Academic Press.

HEJDA, S. 1963. "Skinfold in Old and Longlived Individuals." *Gerontologia* 8:201.

LEWIS, E. ed. 1974. "A Role by Any Name." *Nursing Outlook* 22:89.

LINN, B. S. 1975. "Chronologic vs Biologic Age in Geriatric Patients." In R. Goldman and M. Rockstein, eds., *The Physiology and Pathology of Human Aging.* New York: Academic Press.

LYNAUGH, J. E., and B. BATES. 1974. "Physical Diagnosis—A Skill for All Nurses?" *American Journal of Nursing* 74:58–59.

McCAIN, R. E. 1965. "Nursing by Assessment—Not Intuition." *American Journal of Nursing* 65:82.

ROSSMAN, I., ed. 1971. *Clinical Geriatrics.* Philadelphia: J. B. Lippincott.

TIMARIS, P. S. 1972. *Developmental Physiology and Aging.* New York: Macmillan.

WEINER, S., and M. NATHANSON. 1976. "Physical Examination: Frequently Observed Errors." *Journal of American Medical Association* 236:852–55.

WESEL, J. A., et al. 1963. "Age Trends of Various Components of Body Composition and Functional Characteristics in Women Aged 20–69 Years." *Annals of New York Academy of Science* 110:608.

UNIT 1: THE SKIN AND THE DERMAL APPENDAGES

The skin is composed of three primary layers: the *epidermis,* the *dermis,* and the underlying *subcutis* (see figure 6.2). These layers form a translucid envelope that has several important functions in maintaining the homeostasis of the body. The relatively impermeable epidermis, or outer layer, shields the organs from the outside world and minimizes water loss from the internal environment. Epidermal melanin protects the body against ultraviolet radiation. The extensions of the epidermis—the *hair follicles,* the *sebaceous glands,* and the *apocrine* and *eccrine sweat glands*—penetrate into the deeper layer of the dermis. The dermal layer contains a large number of sensory nerve endings and blood vessels. These vessels, in association with the eccrine sweat glands and the subcutaneous fat, play an important role in the regulation of body heat. The production of vitamin D and the formation of antibodies occur in the dermal layer. The subcutaneous fat cushions the body from injury and, along with stored subcutaneous water, forms a large part of the body's reserve stores of energy. This entire structure is supported by a dense underlying network of collagen fibers, which attach and maintain the skin to the underlying tissues, and associated elas-

FIGURE 6.2 Anatomy of the Skin.

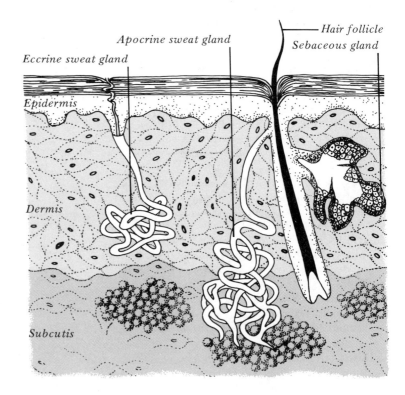

Eccrine sweat gland

Apocrine sweat gland

Hair follicle
Sebaceous gland

Epidermis

Dermis

Subcutis

tic fibers, which give the skin flexibility, elasticity, and strength. The dermal appendages—the hair and nails—are essentially vestigial in humans.

In spite of the accessibility of the skin to examination, clinicians have difficulty isolating and describing skin lesions. Skin lesions are often ignored or glossed over, and their clinical importance and relation to health are often unrecognized.

Changes in the skin due to aging cause a number of problems. These changes—atrophy of all skin layers, diminished vascularity, and decreased elasticity (Rossman 1976; Timaris 1972)—lead to loss of skin water. This desaturation causes the frequent pruritus and decubitus ulcers that complicate the lives of elderly clients. A thorough history and assessment of the skin permits the nurse to evaluate this organ and properly plan for preventive management and care. The use of proper terminology will insure greater precision and thus facilitate this care. This unit begins with the health history and subjective findings associated with skin problems in the elderly. The objective findings and specific techniques of assessment follow.

THE SKIN

HEALTH HISTORY AND SUBJECTIVE FINDINGS

The history of skin problems may be a primary complaint or may be obtained during the review of systems portion of the history (see chapter 5). As a dermatological problem is often polysymtomatic or is colloquially described, the nurse should obtain enough information to permit a pre-cise definition of the actual problem. Once the problem has been clearly defined, information is sought regarding the date of onset, the place on the body, and the presence of associated sensations, such as itch (pruritus), pain, burning, or dryness. Then the nurse inquires about the areas to which the lesions have extended, the length of time for this extension, and any treatment used, whether prescribed or not. Other important information includes a history of skin problems or other illness, skin color change, medication used prior to the onset, as well as the client's occupation, leisure activities, and place of residence. Finally the existence of any physical or mental factors that seem to aggravate the condition should be ascertained.

Date of Onset

Recording the date of onset not only serves to determine how fast the condition has evolved but also relates the lesion to the time of year. Lesions may be affected by seasonal conditions. The dry-skin syndrome is exacerbated by central heating in winter (Chernovosky 1976); tinea pedis infections tend to flare during summertime heat and humidity, as any sufferer of athlete's foot knows. Ascertaining the effect of sunlight and seasonal changes on the lesions will help both in assessment and in planning for care.

Place on the Body

Many lesions have a characteristic distribution. Senile seborrhea is manifested on the scalp, facial folds, eyebrows, postauricular area, sternum, axilla, and groin. Neurodermatitis is most commonly localized to the nuchal area, extensor aspect of the forearms, and anterior tibial region (Alexander 1971). Skin folds are a common site for intertrigo, and decubiti occur at well-known points of pressure.

Associated Sensation

Lesions may be without sensation, as are skin tumors, or they may be extremely painful, as are herpes zoster. Lesions may also be pruritic. Pruritus, however, may occur in the absence of any lesion. It may be a manifestation of the aging skin, due to a systemic disorder such as Hodgkin's disease, or associated with a definite dermatological disorder such as neurodermatosis (Cairns 1972; Alexander 1971).

Region of Extension

Identifying the region of extension further defines the distribution of the dermatitis and helps to indicate areas of risk. Observation of both of these areas will help in assessing the effects of management as well as in making the actual diagnostic assessment.

Client's Occupation, Leisure Activities, and Place of Residence

The implications of occupation, leisure activities, and place of residence in the occurrence and management of skin problems are apparent. Contact dermatitis requires that one be in contact with an offending agent. Poison ivy does not grow in England; yaws, pinta, and bejel are treponemal diseases seen only in tropical environments; and leprosy would be extremely rare in persons who have spent a lifetime in the northeastern United States.

EXAMINATION AND OBJECTIVE FINDINGS

The skin and its appendages must be systematically examined. Adequate lighting is essential, and indirect daylight is preferred. The entire skin surface may be examined or the skin may be attended to as each area of the body is examined. Skin folds, mucus membranes, hair, and nails must all be examined.

The examination begins with a general overview, which is followed by a more precise evaluation. The examination is systematic: it begins at the head and terminates at the toes. All findings are noted and each side of the body is compared with its symmetrical counterpart. The techniques of examination are inspection and palpation.

Inspection

Lesions are described according to their physical characteristics, distribution, and configuration. They have color, size, and shape and may be flat or raised, fluid-filled or solid. Lesions may be grouped, annular, or linear in placement.

Color is due to the pigment involved—hemoglobin, melanin, or carotenoids. Cyanosis and jaundice may be local or generalized; nevi and tattoos are generally localized lesions. In the elderly pallor is common because of the decreased vascularity of the skin.

Lesions may be divided into primary and secondary types (see figure 6.3). *Primary lesions* are induced by internal (intrinsic) disorders or by external (extrinsic) irritants. *Secondary lesions* evolve from, and generally overlie, primary lesions. Older lesions are usually characterized by scarring or scale.

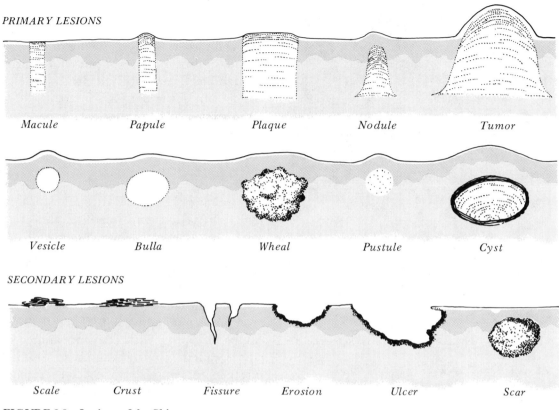

PRIMARY LESIONS

Macule Papule Plaque Nodule Tumor

Vesicle Bulla Wheal Pustule Cyst

SECONDARY LESIONS

Scale Crust Fissure Erosion Ulcer Scar

FIGURE 6.3 Lesions of the Skin.

Primary Lesions. *Macules* are flat, circumscribed areas of color change that are 1 cm or less in size. Larger areas are called *patches.* Flat moles, tattoos, freckles, and vitiligo are examples. Melanotic freckles and vitiligo are common in the older client.

Papules are circumscribed, solid elevations that vary from 0.1 to 1 cm in size. Larger elevations, called *plaques,* are exemplified by elevated nevi, warts, and localized neurodermatitis. Tiny, scarlet telangiectasia are vascular structures of the skin, which increase in number after middle age.

Nodules are circumscribed, solid masses no larger than 1 cm in diameter, which ex-

tend into the dermis. *Tumors* are larger and extend even farther. Lipomas, small epitheliomas, and erythema nodosum are examples of these lesions. Tumors may be malignant and require biopsy for diagnosis. Some clinicians may call any localized swelling a tumor. *Hyperkeratotic warts* are raised brown or black nodules (see figure 6.4). These greasy epithelial hyperplasias increase with age and have only a cosmetic significance. *Acrochordons* are soft, pedunculated, fleshy growths seen on the anterior and lateral aspect of the neck and axilla of the older client. These cutaneous tags vary from pinhead to pea size and have

99

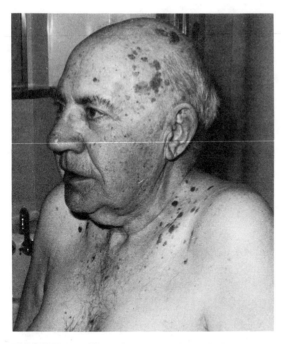

FIGURE 6.4 Hyperkeratotic Warts (Seborrheic Keratoses).
The color variation from brown to black and the raised, wart-like appearance are typical. Those on the neck are black, smooth, and dome shaped. These nodules are commonly distributed on the chest and at the hairline. They are also found on the back (see figure 6.1).

no significance except if injured (Malasanos et al. 1977).

Vesicles and the larger *bullae* are collections of free fluid in the outer epidermal layers. These lesions are often a reaction to toxins, as in poison ivy or in skin burns. They take the form of *wheals* or *hives* in urticaria and angioneurotic edema. If a vesicle or bullus becomes purulent, it is called a *pustule*. This superficial abscess of the skin is found in acne and infected second-degree burns.

Petechiae are small, pinhead-size blood deposits in the skin. They are commonly 1 to 3 mm in size. *Ecchymoses* are larger. Either type of lesion may be due to a hemorrhagic disorder. Ecchymoses are frequently due to trauma and may be present after the trauma has been forgotten. In the elderly the dorsum of the wrist is a frequent site of ecchymoses.

Cysts are encapsulated, fluid-filled masses in the dermis. Sebaceous cysts are examples of this lesion.

Secondary Lesions. Factors causing epithelial irritation may lead to abnormal shedding. This secondary lesion will appear as a fine *scale* or *squama* and is seen in dandruff and psoriasis. *Crusts* are dried exudate on the skin.

Dehydration of the epidermis, a common problem of aging skin (Tindall 1975), causes chapping with the appearance of cracks called *fissures*. Fissures are usually linear in appearance. Superficial scratches limited to the epidermis are called *erosions* and will heal without scarring. Deeper breaks, which extend into the dermis, are called *ulcers*. When these heal, they leave a scar.

Scar formation may take several forms. Extensive scars are sensitive to trauma and tend to break down and undergo malignant change. Scars may become hypertrophic. This enlargement causes a heaping up of the scar, which is a temporary phase of healing and will disappear. *Keloid* is a permanent scar hypertrophy caused by the hyperactivity of collagen formation. Blacks are particularly susceptible to keloid, although this condition may be found in people of other races. In clients with chronic dermatitis, the skin of the involved area takes on a thickened and coarse appearance called *lichenification*. This formation is frequently seen in neurodermatitis and in areas of recurrent-stasis ulcer of the ankle.

Scars must be differentiated from *striae*, which are scarlike stretch marks occurring in areas where the epidermis is intact. They are commonly seen subsequent to pregnancy, obesity, and Cushing's syndrome.

Special examinations of the skin may be performed under the light of a Wood's lamp (ultraviolet light). Scrapings may be taken for microscopical examination, and analysis of sweat may be performed. These procedures, as well as biopsies, are done in special situations requiring more definite information.

Palpation

After thoroughly inspecting a lesion, the nurse should palpate it. Palpation gives information about the temperature, moisture content, texture, and elasticity of the skin. The presence of increased fluid is revealed by *pitting*. Pitting is the persistence of a depression in the skin induced by the examining finger. Decreased fluid is demonstrated by the increased and persistent folding of the skin after it has been creased between the examining fingers. This condition is found in dehydrated clients but may be a normal finding in the elderly and is related to the diminished elasticity of aged skin (Rossman 1976). Gentle palpation with the back of the hand may reveal localized changes in skin temperature, including the warmth of inflammation and the coolness of ischemia. In the febrile client, diffusely warm, dry skin indicates a rising temperature; warm, moist skin usually indicates defervescence.

THE DERMAL APPENDAGES

The nails and hair are semivestigial remnants that apparently have only a cosmetic purpose in humans. The appearance and distribution of these structures are altered not only by artificial means but also by aging and disease. The nurse must be aware of all the possibilities that affect diagnostic judgment.

THE HAIR: EXAMINATION AND OBJECTIVE FINDINGS

Age, sex, race, and genetic background affect human hair growth. With age, total body hair diminishes with the single exception of facial hair, which increases in both sexes (Thomas and Ferriman 1957). Such increases are most apparent in Caucasians (Hamilton 1958).

Inspection

The nurse notes the quantity, quality, color, and distribution pattern of the client's hair. Although aging blunts the implications of body hair abnormalities, certain changes are useful indicators of health problems.

Loss of abdominal, pubic, and axillary hair seems directly related to hormonal changes, with a striking diminution occurring in women shortly after menopause and more gradually in men (Melick and Taft 1959). This loss of body hair must not be confused with the localized loss seen in peripheral vascular disease. Total hair loss in younger clients may be associated with alopecia totalis or with endocrinopathies such as panhypopituitarism. Melick and Taft (1959) also noted that one-sixth of a

101

group of elderly people had suffered loss of the outer third of the eyebrow. This change, usually associated with hypothyroidism, is commonly seen in elderly clients who do not have thyroid disease.

Generalized thinning of the hair of the scalp is common to both men and women. The male balding pattern with the anterior M-shaped hairline and vertex patch is genetically inherited and restricted to men (Rossman 1971). If found in women, it is probably abnormal and caused by a virilizing tumor of the ovary or adrenal gland. Patchy, irregular balding suggests *alopecia areata*. This usually self-limited balding may be due to a fungal infection or anxiety.

Graying of the hair results from the generalized loss of skin pigment that occurs with advancing years. The age of onset, as with balding, is genetically regulated. Isolated early graying has no clinical significance.

THE NAILS: EXAMINATION AND OBJECTIVE FINDINGS

Normal nail growth is approximately 0.1 mm per day and is related to the client's general state of health (see figure 6.5).

Inspection

Illness, which diminishes the body's albumin production or causes a severe stress, leads to a temporary arrest of nail growth. When growth resumes, this interruption is seen as a deep transversal line called *Beau's line*. The distance from the base to the line reflects the onset and duration of the illness.

Other changes relate to the texture and appearance of the nails. Iron deficiency causes a *spoonlike* deformity. The nails of clients with chronic pulmonary disease become clubbed. *Clubbing* is noted from the lateral appearance of the nail. Normally

FIGURE 6.5 Normal and Abnormal Nails.

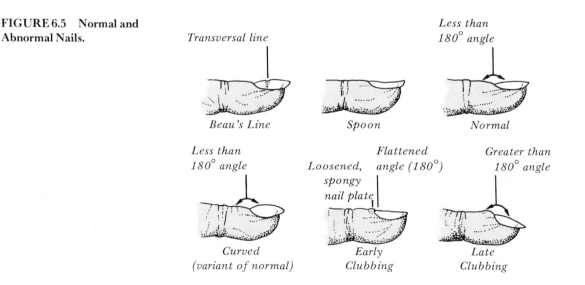

the angle of the nail with the finger is less than 180°. With clubbing, this angle becomes an obtuse angle of more than 180°. In this condition the nail plate is loosened and spongy and may be rocked, and the ends of the fingers and toes take on a rounded, bulbous appearance.

Nails may be deformed with thickening and lifting of the plate due to psoriasis or tinea pedis infection. Examination reveals a large amount of debris under the plate. When this debris is scraped and examined under the microscope, fungus will be seen if infection is present. Other causes of nail thickening are trauma and chronic ischemia of the extremity.

Normal nails contain longitudinal furrows. These furrows become more pronounced with age and may become so exaggerated that the nail develops a tendency to split along the affected furrow. If the splitting extends to the base, it may become painful and the nail may require taping to prevent further injury.

Color changes may be visible in the nail bed. Cyanosis appears as a dusky hue. Unfortunately, this condition is not reliable as an early sign of anoxia. It is masked by skin pigmentation and is absent in anemia. Cyanosis occurs when 5g of reduced hemoglobin per 100 ml of blood are present in the circulation.

REFERENCES

ALEXANDER, W. Y. 1971. "Skin Disease." In I. Rossman, ed., *Clinical Geriatrics.* Philadelphia, J. B. Lippincott.

CAIRNS, R. J. 1972. "The Causes of Pruritus." In A. Rook, D. S. Wilkinson, and F. J. G. Ebbing, eds., *Textbook of Dermatology,* 2d ed. Philadelphia: F. A. Davis.

CHERNOVOSKY, M. E. 1976. "Clinical Aspects of Dry Skin." *Journal of the Society of Cosmetic Chemistry* 27:365–426.

HAMILTON, J. B. 1958. "Age, Sex, and Genetic Factors in the Regulation of Hair Growth in Man: A Comparison of Caucasians and Japanese Populations." In W. Montagna and R. A. Ellis, eds. *Biology of Hair Growth.* New York: Academic Press.

MALASANOS, L., et al. 1977. *Health Assessment.* St. Louis: C. V. Mosby.

MELICK, R., and P. TAFT. 1959. "Observations on Body Hair in Old People." *Journal of Clinical Endocrinology* 19:1575–82.

ROSSMAN, I. 1976. "Human Aging Changes." In I. M. Burnside, ed., *Nursing the Aged.* New York: McGraw-Hill.

———. 1971. "The Anatomy of Aging." In I. Rossman, ed., *Clinical Geriatrics.* Philadelphia: J. B. Lippincott.

THOMAS, P. K., and D. G. FERRIMAN. 1957. "Variation in Facial and Pubic Hair Growth in White Women." *American Journal of Physical Anthropology* 15:171–93.

TIMARIS, P. S. 1972. *Developmental Physiology and Aging.* New York: Macmillan.

TINDALL, J. P. 1975. "Relieving Localized and Generalized Pruritus." *Geriatrics* 30 (3):85–92.

UNIT 2: THE HEAD

The head is an anatomical region containing structures of many systems (see figure 6.6). The eyes, ears, nose, mouth and pharynx, and central nervous system are particularly prominent and are discussed in separate units of this chapter.

This unit is devoted to the general assessment of the head, its appearance, size, and shape. Observation of the head is an important part of the general assessment. At all times the nurse observes facial mimic, the form of the head, and the freedom of movement of the head on the neck. In the course of the assessment, the nurse evaluates the two parts of the head—the cranium and the face.

THE CRANIUM

HEALTH HISTORY AND SUBJECTIVE FINDINGS

The nurse inquires whether the client is aware of any sores, lumps, itching, or tenderness in the cranium. Such areas must receive particular attention during the examination.

FIGURE 6.6   Structures of the Head.

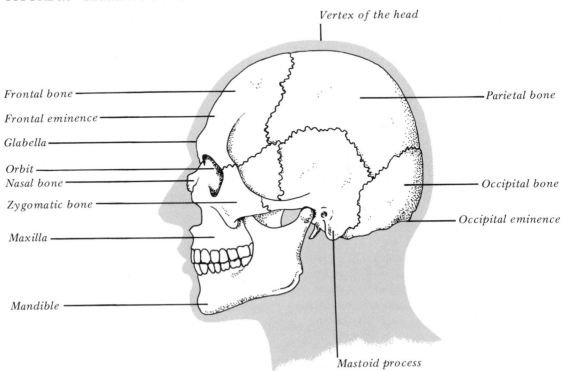

Vertex of the head

Frontal bone

Frontal eminence

Glabella

Orbit

Nasal bone

Zygomatic bone

Maxilla

Mandible

Parietal bone

Occipital bone

Occipital eminence

Mastoid process

EXAMINATION AND OBJECTIVE FINDINGS

The assessing techniques consist of inspection, palpation, and auscultation. The nurse observes the cranium for asymmetry and unusual size or masses and notes the color, distribution, and texture of the hair.

Inspection

The cranium may vary in size because of genetic variation, trauma, or systemic disorders. Its shape is most commonly ovoid, with the long diameter on the anteroposterior axis. The rounded, prominent, *occipital eminence* appears posteriorly; the *mastoid* process appears laterally, behind the ears; and the two *frontal eminences* appear anteriorly. The head is covered by the scalp, a loosely attached skin with variable amounts of hair.

Different patterns of baldness or *alopecia* may be observed. Aging is associated with a generalized thinning *(calvities)* and whitening of the hair in both men and women. *Alopecia areata* is a patchy, diffuse, and usually transient hair loss. *Alopecia totalis,* or total balding, is uncommon. More common, in men, is a sex-linked, genetically inherited pattern of hair loss. This male balding pattern is recognized by a symmetrical, M-shaped recession of the anterior hairline. It may be associated with a thinned patch on the *vertex.* The eventual result may be complete hair loss except for a line of hair extending from behind and above the ears and across the midline of the occipital region and nape of the neck (Rossman 1971). This pattern of hair loss is abnormal in women and may be due to a virilizing tumor.

Tumors and nonhealing sores are easiest to see on the bald scalp. If hair is present, the nurse must part it when inspecting the scalp.

Abnormal cranial enlargement is seen in *Paget's disease* (see figure 6.7). Facial size remains normal, resulting in a triangular-shaped head with a massive forehead. Further examination often reveals a thickened and bowed femur or tibia. A history of kidney stones is frequently obtained from these clients, and they may have noted an increase in hat size. Clients with acromegaly suffer enlargement of the bones of the head and face. Skull deformities due to an episode of rickets in childhood persist into adult life. This enlargement and flattening of the *frontal* and *parietal bones* gives a boxlike appearance to the head.

FIGURE 6.7   Paget's Disease of the Skull.
The forehead is disproportionately large for the face and thus causes a leonine appearance. The prominent facial wrinkles are a normal aging change (see figure 6.8 and section on inspection of the face), as are the enophthalmos (figure 6.10 and examination of the eye) and the prominent double skin-fold of the neck (unit 7, section on inspection of the neck).

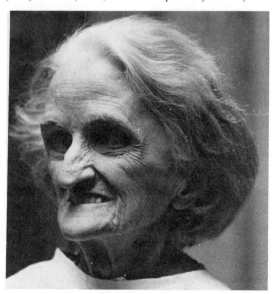

Palpation

Palpation is performed with the palmar surfaces of the fingertips gently touching the scalp with a slightly circular motion. When hair is present only the larger lesions will be felt. Tumors of the calvarium, such as wens and cysts, are firm and somewhat fluctuant. Osteomas and metastatic nodules are hard and fixed.

Sores are palpated to detect an underlying body or firmness, which usually indicates an invading tumor such as an epithelioma. Sores and tumors should be searched for in skin folds and in hidden areas behind the ears.

Auscultation

Auscultation of the cranium may reveal the bruit of an intracranial aneurysm or an abnormal arteriovenous communication.

THE FACE
EXAMINATION AND OBJECTIVE FINDINGS

The face is examined by inspection. All lesions are palpated.

Inspection

Anteriorly, below the cranium, are the frontal region and the face, which form an elongated oval. The frontal eminences sweep down to the superciliary ridges, which join at the *glabella,* above the nose (figure 6.6). Normally covered by the brows, these ridges cover the frontal sinuses in their medial third. Below the optic *orbits,* lateral to the nose, are the *maxilla,* or maxillary bones, which cover the maxillary sinuses. The chin is the inferior margin of the face and is composed of the *mandible,* or jaw bone, which sweeps back and up toward the ear.

The nurse notes the *condition of the brows and the distribution of facial hair.* With age facial hair increases in both men and women. In the very old the brows may not extend the full length of the superciliary ridge. In younger adults loss of the lateral third of the brow may be due to hypothyroidism or to cosmetic plucking (see the section on hair in unit 1).

The general appearance of the face is affected by intelligence as well as by degree of alertness, interest, and awareness. Age-related changes in appearance are due to changes of the facial skin.

The face of the older client is wrinkled, puffy, and pale. These changes are reminiscent of myxedema in younger clients. Characteristic wrinkles follow the frown lines and the pull of the muscles of motion (see figure 6.8). Older clients have crow's-feet at the corners of the eyes, prominent nasolabial folds extending toward the chin, and fine folds around the upper and lower lips. Jowls develop along with submental wrinkling and ptosis of the eyelids and ears. Ptosis of the upper lid may interfere with vision, requiring the client to tilt the head backward in order to see. Vascular changes and the usual depigmentation lead to intense paleness of the face.

Systemic and local conditions may affect facial appearance. *Acromegaly* causes generalized enlargement of the head and face as well as of the hands and feet. *Periorbital edema* may occur unilaterally due to trauma, infection of the cavernous sinus, or retro-orbital aneurysm, or it may occur bilaterally due to renal disease, myxedema, al-

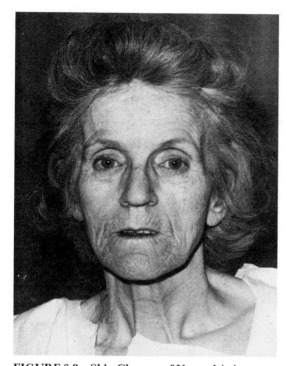

FIGURE 6.8   Skin Changes of Normal Aging.
The wrinkles follow the frown lines of the forehead. The pull of the orbicularis muscles causes folding around the mouth and eyes and between the nose and chin. Small jowls are seen on the jaw. In the neck the platysma forms a double vertical line and circular lines (see figure 6.7). The suborbital skin is puffy and enophthalmos is present (see also unit 3, section on examination of the eye, and figures 6.7 and 6.10).

lergy, or superior mediastinal tumor. This swelling affects the upper lids, which lose their normal folds.

Parkinson's disease (paralysis agitans) causes loss of facial expression, persistent drool, stiffness of the body, and a rhythmic tremor of the index against the thumb ("pill rolling").

Cushing's or *iatrogenic Cushing's syndrome* makes the face full and rounded ("moon face") with a rounded mouth ("fish mouth"). *Scleroderma* causes atrophy and tightening. Atrophied skin is taut and shiny, and facial expression is lost. The mouth may be tightly drawn, exposing the teeth.

Thyrotoxicosis is associated with an alert and startled expression caused by a bright-eyed *exophthalmos,* or protrusion of the eyes. This unblinking stare is due to a raised upper lid, which exposes the upper portion of the cornea and white sclera. Exophthalmos is usually associated with lid lag: the lid lags behind the globe when the eye rotates downward.

Although the intense pallor of age may be normal, other color changes may indicate disorders and should be noted.

Cyanosis, a blue discoloration seen in the lips, mucus membranes, nose, and ears, is due to an increased concentration of hemoglobin circulating in the blood. An increase in the total red cell mass (polycythemia) causes ruddiness and a plethoric appearance. The vasodilatation of acne rosacea and chronic alcoholism also cause a ruddy tinge.

Jaundice, or icterus, gives a yellow color that tints the sclera, unlike carotenemia, which causes the yellow skin of myxedema and the nephrotic syndrome. Jaundice is not visible under artificial light.

Erythematous rashes are produced by many conditions. A rash that extends across the bridge of the nose onto both cheeks and has a butterfly distribution may be due to lupus erythematosis. Seborrheic dermatitis is localized to the scalp and forehead.

Paleness, while associated with age, raises the possibility of anemia. Increased pigment is due to an increase in skin melanin,

107

which is most commonly caused by exposure to sunlight. In the elderly, melanotic freckles may appear as a localized papular patch of pigmentation. Increased pigmentation is also found in Addison's disease, hyperthyroidism, pituitary tumors, and sunlight and radiation injury.

Yellow deposits localized to the upper eyelids are called *xanthomata*. These lipid deposits are often associated with hyperlipidemia and diabetes mellitus.

Palpation

All lesions, whether sores or tumors, are palpated for consistency, firmness, and fluctuation. In addition, the nurse palpates with a fair amount of pressure the ridge overlying the frontal sinus and the bones overlying the maxillary sinus. Tenderness may indicate the presence of an acute sinusitis.

MOVEMENTS OF THE HEAD

Normally the head moves on the neck on an anteroposterior axis and rotates to the right and left. Combined, these impart a circular movement. Such motion may be active or passive: *active motion* is performed by the client; *passive motion,* by the nurse. Passive motion is always performed gently to prevent injury.

Full extension and flexion of the neck are limited by the chin touching the sternum anteriorly and the occiput touching the spine posteriorly. Full rotation is to 80° bilaterally. Further rotation requires movement of the shoulders and trunk. Inflammation of the cervical muscles, as in torticollis (wry neck), meningitis, and ar-

thritic conditions of the spine, limit the range of motion.

Congenital tremors and arteriosclerotic changes in the central nervous system can cause rhythmic tremors in the elderly. In clients with aortic aneurysms, a peculiar bobbing motion of the head may be noted.

REFERENCES

ROSSMAN, I. 1971. "The Anatomy of Aging." In I. Rossman, ed., *Clinical Geriatrics.* Philadelphia: J. B. Lippincott.

UNIT 3: THE EYE

The importance of the eye is underscored by the fact that 38 percent of the brain fibers relate to the eye and its tracts, while 50 percent of the cranial nerves subserve it.

Like the rest of the body, the eye changes with age. These changes affect not only appearance but ophthalmic function. Thorough assessment may isolate changes when the eye still functions well and may thus permit its maintenance. Roughly one-third of persons over age 80 have visual acuity of 20/50 or less (Anderson and Palmore 1974). Recent studies reveal that the incidence of primary-angle glaucoma rises from 0.5 percent of the population age 60 to 64 to 1.3 percent of the population age 70 to 74 (Kini et al. 1978). The relation of increased ocular pressure to visual loss is 1:6 or 1:7 (Schwartz 1978). Of greater significance is that simple assessment of the eye by examining with a flashlight, testing the visual fields, and using funduscopy provides well-trained examiners with a highly effective means of discovering early primary-angle glaucoma. One study showed that funduscopy was more effective than tonometry in the discovery of early glaucoma. The need for training in the funduscopic examination is thus apparent (Graham and Hallows 1966).

Changes induced by aging may affect the tissues surrounding the orbit or the eye itself. Externally the eye is seen between the two *eyelids* (see figure 6.9). These movable flaps are joined at both ends to form the *medial* and *lateral canthus,* or commissure. The lacrimal *punctum* or *nasolacrimal duct* opening is located on the edge of the lid near the medial canthus. Close contact of the punctum with the corneal surface is necessary to insure proper drainage of tears secreted by the *lacrimal gland.* At the medial canthus is a small elevation of tissue, the *caruncle.* The caruncle has a reddish hue and contains hairs and sebaceous glands, which increase with age. On the edges of the lids are the *eyelashes* or cils, just behind which are located a variety of small glands. Normally the cils sweep outward.

The eye is embedded in orbital fat, which resorbs with aging, leading to proptosis. At the anterior pole of the eye is the *cornea.* The posterior pole corresponds to the *fovea centralis* of the retina and not to the *optic disc.* A line joining these two poles is called the optic axis. The *retina,* or light-sensitive layer, is the innermost layer of the eye. Thinning or atrophy of the retina is common in older persons. The *sclera* is the outermost layer. Between these two layers lies the vascular *choroid.* The fusion of the retinal layers in the anterior portion of the eye forms the *iris* and the *ciliary body.* These overlap the *lens.* The canal of Schlemm and the circular vessels of the iris are derived from the choroid. The white sclera and transparent cornea are covered anteriorly by a membrane, the conjunctiva. This membrane extends from its bulbar portion to a *palpebral* portion, which passes into the inside of the eyelid. The *anterior chamber* of the eye lies between the cornea and the iris, the *posterior chamber* lies between the iris and the lens. These chambers are filled with a thin, circulating fluid called the aqueous humor. Behind the lens this fluid is thick and is called the *vitreous body.* With age the anterior chamber becomes shallow.

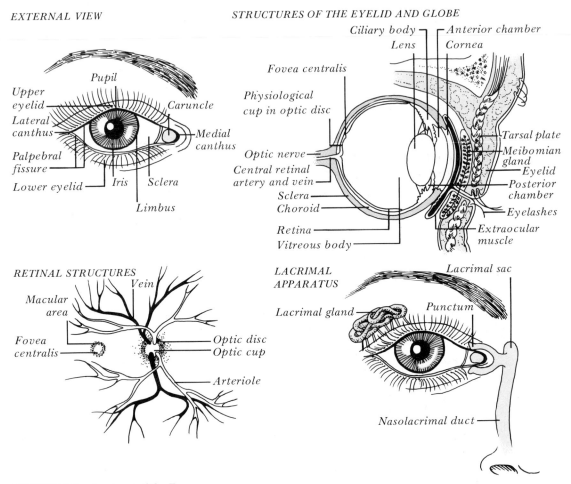

EXTERNAL VIEW

STRUCTURES OF THE EYELID AND GLOBE

Pupil

Upper eyelid
Caruncle
Lateral canthus
Medial canthus
Palpebral fissure
Lower eyelid
Iris
Sclera
Limbus

Ciliary body
Lens
Anterior chamber
Cornea

Fovea centralis

Physiological cup in optic disc

Tarsal plate
Meibomian gland
Eyelid
Posterior chamber

Optic nerve
Central retinal artery and vein
Sclera
Choroid
Retina
Vitreous body

Eyelashes
Extraocular muscle

RETINAL STRUCTURES

Vein
Macular area
Fovea centralis
Optic disc
Optic cup
Arteriole

LACRIMAL APPARATUS

Lacrimal sac
Lacrimal gland
Punctum

Nasolacrimal duct

FIGURE 6.9 Anatomy of the Eye.

HEALTH HISTORY AND SUBJECTIVE FINDINGS

Complaints relating to the eye usually consist of disturbances of vision or the presence of discomfort.

Visual Disturbances

If the client complains of visual disturbance, the nurse inquires about its nature, duration, and persistence or intermittency and notes the effect of time of day or conditions of lighting.

Transient blindness may vary from a few seconds in papilledema to five to fifteen minutes in a transient ischemic attack (amaurosis fugax).

Change of object size is found in temporal lobe epilepsy and tumors and in degeneration of the macular area.

Scintillating scotoma, often described as flashes, zig-zags, or rippling and associated with migraine in younger clients, is also indicative of occipital lobe tumors, lead intoxication, allergy, or overindulgence in tobacco.

Diplopia (double vision) may be binocular and disappears when the client closes one eye. This problem is due to palsy of a motor nerve of the eye and frequently is related to diabetes mellitus, strokes, or brain tumors. Monocular diplopia is the result of an ophthalmological disorder such as cataract.

Diurnal variation of vision may be found. In retinal detachment vision improves at night, whereas in glaucoma and cataract it worsens after sunset. Glaucoma may cause halos to appear around lights. In cataract cases, headlight glare at night may be blinding.

Discomfort

Headache is rarely associated with refractive error but may be associated with gross field defects or secondary and acute angle-closure glaucoma.

Asthenopia (eye fatigue) is more common with refractive problems and is often worsened by reading or watching T.V.

Sleepiness with reading indicates a problem of convergence.

Severe eye *pain* is usually caused by trauma, a foreign body, corneal erosion, or exposure to welding or arc light. It is also associated with acute glaucoma and iridocyclitis.

Recurrent and constant *tearing* is often due to blockage of the nasolacrimal duct or to ectropion. Clients complaining of unilateral *epiphora* (abnormal tearing) and ill-fitting dentures may have a cancer of the maxillary sinus.

VISUAL ACUITY: EXAMINATION AND OBJECTIVE FINDINGS

The nurse must approach the eye examination in a systematic manner. An effective method is to begin by testing visual acuity, then to proceed with the external examination of the lids and eyeball, followed by an evaluation of the pupillary reaction, the extraocular movements, and the visual fields. The examination is usually completed by the funduscopic examination, which is the most tiring one for the client.

Visual acuity decreases with age; only 5 percent of octogenarians have 20/20 vision (Slatapes 1950; Weale 1975). Near vision is checked by having the client read newsprint at twelve inches or less. The near point normally moves outward after age 40. All clients unable to read newsprint at twelve inches require refraction.

Distant vision is checked with standard charts, which are commonly placed twenty feet away from the client. Vision is recorded as a fraction whose numerator is the distance from the chart and whose denominator is determined by the smallest letters read at that distance. Thus if the client reads a line of letters that a normal eye sees at forty feet, the vision is recorded as 20/40. Clients who cannot read the largest letter are tested for perception of hand movements (HM), finger counting (FC), or perception of light (LP). Each eye is tested separately while the other is covered by a card.

Visual acuity tests disclose gross refractive errors and evidence of systemic health problems. If problems are found, the nurse should refer the client to an appropriate specialist for further testing.

EXTERNAL EXAMINATION AND OBJECTIVE FINDINGS

The techniques of external eye examination are inspection and palpation. Each eye is inspected separately, then both eyes are looked at together. The nurse checks to see that both are parallel. Next the brows are checked for lesions and scales as well as for quantity and quality of hair. The eyelids are examined when opened and closed. The nurse notes the position of the lid on the eyeball and the adequacy of separation, closure, and approximation. The lids must close completely to prevent drying. Failure of approximation may be due to exophthalmos, facial nerve paralysis, and acquired ectropion. Drooping, or ptosis, may develop because of aging tissue laxity or a third-nerve palsy. The nurse also notes color changes, lesions, edema, and the condition and direction of the lashes.

Color changes include xanthomas (localized yellow plaques) and redness, indicating inflammation. With aging, melanin deposits may increase, associated with the occurrence of melanotic freckles.

Lesions include *hordeolum* (sty), an infection of the lid margin; *chalazion,* an infection or cyst of the glands behind the eyelid; *crusting,* usually due to infection; and *keratoses,* related to aging skin.

Edema causes a puffiness that must be distinguished from the puffiness of aging (see figure 6.10). Edema may be due to local disease as well as to general health problems such as nephrosis, heart failure, allergy, and myxedema. Puffiness is also caused by the aging process: the resorption of orbital fat causes enophthalmos, and the lids sag, creating a puffy appearance.

Abnormal eyelid positions include *entropion,* in which the eyelids roll inward, and

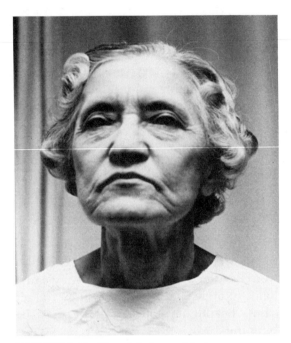

FIGURE 6.10   Enophthalmos of Aging.
Resorption of the orbital fat causes the eyes to sink into the orbits and is associated with ptosis and suborbital puffiness. Decrease of the lateral portion of the eyebrow and the presence of jowls give a myxedematous appearance. Ptosis of the upper lids may interfere with vision and thus force the client to tilt the head backward to see. This client has normal thyroid function. (See also figure 6.7.)

ectropion, in which the eyelids roll outward. Ectropion prevents normal closure; entropion causes corneal abrasion. These abnormal positions may result from tissue laxity due to age or they may be caused by scarring of the eyelids from infection.

Palpation

The nurse examines the lids by gently sweeping the palmar surface of the fingertip across them. After palpating any masses, the nurse then proceeds to inspect the eye.

Inspection

Lids and Eyeball. Inspection of the eyeball is performed by gently separating the lids (see figure 6.11). The index finger is placed on the upper lid and the thumb on the lower, at the points where each lid overlies orbital bone. To separate the lids, the nurse should gently press against the skin while parting the thumb and index finger. (In cases of trauma, the nurse should immediately halt the examination if eyeball penetration is evident and refer the client to a specialist.) Separation of the lids exposes the conjuctiva, cornea, and sclera. The client must look upward to expose the entire *inferior conjunctival sac* and from side to side for the lateral and medial portions.

The *superior conjunctival sac* is exposed by a special technique. The nurse asks the client to look downward, grasps the upper lashes between the thumb and index finger, and gently pulls them forward and down. A small stick or applicator, held in the other hand, is placed one centimeter above the lid margin and pushed down on the upper lid, causing it to invert. This inversion exposes the upper sac with its bulging lateral portion at the site of the lacrimal gland. The nurse's fingers can secure the lid against the brow. The inspection completed, the nurse gently grasps the lashes and pulls them forward while asking the client to look upward. The lid will return to its normal position.

Certain findings are common during the inspection. The points of penetration of the scleral vessels are often pigmented. These small black points should not be confused with foreign bodies. Just medial to the junction of the cornea and the sclera, a white or gray ring encircling the sclera may be seen. This *arcus senilis* is common in older clients and must be differentiated from the very white infiltrate of *hypercalcemic band keratopathy*. Arcus senilis has no

FIGURE 6.11 Separation of the Eyelids.
The thumb and index finger are placed where the lid overlies orbital bone. Separation of the fingers thus spreads the lids apart. No pressure is applied to the eyeball. Note the prominent insertions of the sternomastoid on the clavicle due to diminished subcutaneous fat (normal aging change, see page 94).

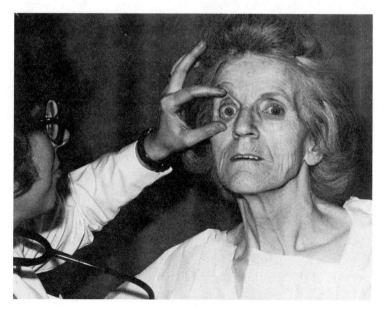

effect on vision and is probably not associated with an increased incidence of atherosclerosis (Macaraeg et al. 1968).

Conjunctival hyperemia, involving both the conjunctival and palpebral conjunctiva, may be due to fatigue, local irritation, or rhinitis. Redness associated with an exudate indicates conjunctivitis of bacterial or viral origin, an allergy, or a foreign body. *Hemorrhage* of the conjunctiva may be due to trauma or irritation. Subconjunctival hemorrhage is more common in older persons (Timaris 1972). Marked erythema of *keratoconjunctivitis,* an extremely painful condition, begins six to twelve hours after exposure to ultraviolet light, arc welding light, and excessive sunlight. Recurrent *unilateral conjunctivitis* may be due to an obstructed lacrimal duct.

Pterygium is a wing-shaped membrane extending from the nasal limbus toward the cornea. In the elderly it rarely invades the cornea or interferes with vision (Ehrlich and Keates 1978). *Pingueculum,* a small, yellow, fatty nodule at the nasal limbus, often precedes pterygium and is more frequently found in the older client (Timaris 1972).

The cornea, the clear portion of the eye, is often yellowed by age. Shining a light beam obliquely on the cornea will reveal superficial reflection irregularities. *Hypopyon*—pus in the anterior chamber of the eye—is seen as a yellow-white fluid; if present it is a medical emergency requiring treatment by a specialist. *Shallowness of the anterior chamber,* characteristic of an increased risk of angle-closure glaucoma, can be detected by shining a light beam on the side of the eye. Failure to illuminate the entire anterior chamber, with a substantial portion of the iris remaining in shadow, indicates the likelihood of a narrowed anterior chamber and an increased risk of glaucoma. Touching the cornea with a clean wisp of cotton should induce blinking and tests the integrity of the fifth and seventh cranial nerves (see unit 14).

Pulpillary Reaction. Next the nurse inspects the *pupil.* Its form, normally round and regular, is determined by the iris. With age the pupil tends to become smaller. The two pupils are usually of equal size and constrict in response to light and accommodation. In the elderly, pupil size may be somewhat unequal and the reaction to light is usually diminished. These reflexes are best tested in a partially dimmed room. A light beamed at the eye should cause it to constrict. This response is a *direct reflex.* If the nurse observes the other eye and again directs the light into the first eye, the other eye should constrict also. This response is the *consensual reflex.* Light perceived by an eye causes impulses in the nerve tissue on the appropriate side of the brain. The constriction reflex, however, is sent from the brain to both ciliary nerves. Injury to an eye may abolish the direct reflex, but the consensual reflex remains intact.

Accommodation is tested in a dimly lighted room by holding an unlighted object or a finger four inches from the client's eye. The nurse asks the client to look away and then to look at the finger. The normal response is constriction. Each eye is tested in turn.

Convergence is tested by moving an object from a distance toward the bridge of the nose while the client attempts to follow. Convergence is usually tested to a point three inches from the client's nose. Normally, as the object approaches the nose, both eyes rotate medially and focus on it. Failure to do so indicates a lesion of the brain stem.

Extraocular Movements. The extraocular movements are tested by asking the client to follow a finger or object through the six cardinal fields of gaze (see figure 6.12): straight nasal, upward and nasal, down and nasal, straight temporal, up and temporal, and down and temporal. Straight temporal movement is controlled by the *lateral rectus muscle* and the *sixth nerve,* while down and nasal is controlled by the *superior oblique muscle* and the *fourth nerve.* All other movements are controlled by the *third nerve* and the respective muscles. Lesions of the third, fourth, or sixth cranial nerves, the muscles, or the central nervous system cause a palsy (see unit 14). Nystagmus is a flicking motion of the eyeball that may be elicited by briefly pausing at the end of the lateral and the upward movements. Nystagmus occurs with lesions of the acoustic nerve, the inner ear, and the cerebellum (see unit 14).

Visual Fields. The visual fields are examined grossly by confrontation. The client covers the right eye with a card. The nurse takes a position two feet from and directly opposite the client so that their eyes are on the same level. The nurse closes the left eye so that the visual fields are approximately the same. Then, while observing the client's eye, the nurse brings a pencil or other brightly colored object from the periphery into the visual field. Eight equally spaced points should be tested around the visual field. The other eye is then tested in a like manner. The client must look at the nurse's eye at all times. Abnormalities should be confirmed by more precise perimetry.

Intraocular pressure is best tested by instruments that measure the displacement of the eye surface by pressure. Only gross impressions are obtained by palpation. With the client looking down, the nurse places an index finger on either side of the upper lid of one eye. The fingers then apply pressure alternately against the optic globe. The advancing finger fixes the globe, and the retreating finger feels the rebound of

FIGURE 6.12 Six Cardinal Fields of Gaze.

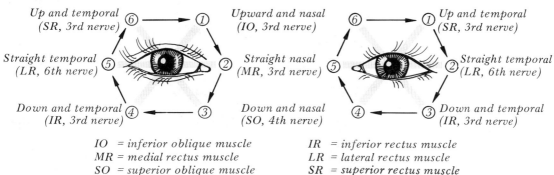

Circled numbers show sequence of examination.

115

the depressed sclera. The eye is harder in glaucoma. Tonometry is more accurate but requires first anesthetizing the eye with a drop of ophthalmic pontocaine. The tonometer is placed on the globe and the displacement pressure measured. Care must be taken not to scratch or infect the eye with the instrument.

FUNDUSCOPIC EXAMINATION AND OBJECTIVE FINDINGS

Through the use of the ophthalmoscope, the nurse can examine the posterior eye, or *fundus,* and evaluate the changes that occur in ophthalmological and systemic diseases. A more complete examination requires dilation of the pupil with one drop of 10 percent phenylephrine placed on the eye. This compound temporarily abolishes constriction and may precipitate an attack of glaucoma in susceptible clients. Without dilation the examination is limited but still useful.

The examination is performed in a dimly lighted room. Both the nurse and the client should remove corrective lenses and keep their eyes open. The client is asked to fix on a distant point. The instrument is set at 0 diopters, and the small white, round light aperture of the ophthalmoscopic head is used.

To examine the client's right eye, the ophthalmoscope is held in the right hand and the nurse uses the right eye (see figure 6.13). The nurse places the index finger of the right hand on the lens disc and holds the instrument firmly against the brow with the viewing aperture in front of the viewing eye. This relative position of examiner and instrument must not change during the entire examination. The nurse places the thumb of the left hand on the client's right brow. From a distance of 15 inches (45 cm) and on a line 15 degrees lateral to the client's line of sight, the nurse shines the light beam onto the client's pupil. An orange glow—the *red reflex*—is seen.

FIGURE 6.13 Ophthalmoscopic Examination of the Right Eye.
The nurse's right hand holds the instrument to her right eye. Her index finger is on the focusing wheel. Her left hand holds the client's head with the thumb elevating the upper lid. The client looks at a distant point with both eyes. The nurse is 15° lateral to the client's line of sight and observes the red reflex. Keeping the red reflex in view through the instrument, the nurse approaches the client's eye till the ophthalmoscope touches her left thumb.

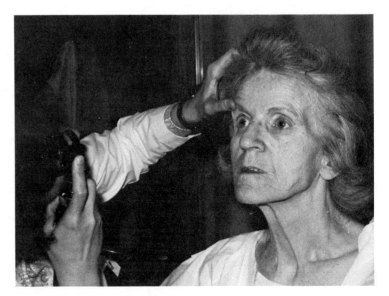

Black shadows interrupting this glow indicate opacities in the media between the cornea and the fundus. The nurse then approaches the client along the 15-degree line until the top of the instrument makes contact with the nurse's left thumb. At this point the fundus comes into view. The fundus is visible in the vicinity of the optic disc either as retinal pigment, a vessel, or the disc itself. If the disc is not seen, following a vessel centrally will locate it. The disc appears as a yellow-pink oval or round structure from which diverge the retinal arteries. If the image is blurred, rotating the lens wheel should focus it. The nurse must also look into the distance. In myopic (nearsighted) clients, the longer red-numbered lenses are used and are obtained by counterclockwise rotation of the lens wheel. In hypermetropic (farsighted) clients, the shorter black-numbered lenses are employed. Clients whose lenses have been removed are examined through black-numbered lenses. Using the left hand and the left eye, the nurse repeats this procedure to test the client's left eye.

The *optic disc* is examined for clarity, color, and the presence of rings and an *optic cup*. The normal disc margins are sharp except for the nasal border, which is blurred. The yellow-pink color fades into a gray central area. The margins may be accentuated by gray or dark crescents on the temporal margin. The optic cup is a depression seen on the temporal side of the center. It never extends to the disc margins.

The *fundus* is examined next. The *vessels* are identified: the arterioles are two-thirds smaller than the veins; they are also lighter and reflect light more. Venous pulsation near the disc is a normal finding. Each vessel is followed: first on the nasal side in the

upper and then in the lower quadrant, then on the temporal side in the upper and then in the lower quadrant. The *retina* is examined in each of these areas. The light is returned to the disc and then swung laterally to the *fovea centralis,* a small glistening point, two disc diopters (DD) temporally from the disc. The fovea lies within the *macula,* a finely pigmented avascular area, one DD in diameter. Glistening, moving reflections (light reflexes) are normal in the young but may indicate retinal detachment in the elderly. Fundal pigment, usually uniform, may be tessellated and show orange angiode streaks in some cases. A black ten or twelve lens will focus on the surface of the eye, and progressively smaller lenses will throw the focus farther and farther back through the anterior chamber and the lens, permitting examination of the *media.* In the elderly the media is subject to changes that decrease visual acuity. Lens opacifications (cataract) appear, as do hemorrhage and precipitations in the vitreous.

Abnormalities of the optic disc are shown by changes in appearance and demarcation (see figure 6.14). *Optic atrophy* causes a whitened appearance and may indicate disease of the central nervous system. *Papilledema* causes redness, blurred margins, and elevation. Glaucoma causes cupping and pallor of the disc. This depression changes the disc from an oval to a circular shape and *extends to the disc margins.* The earliest glaucomatous change is noted on the temporal side of the disc.

Fundal abnormalities include hemorrhages, exudates, drusen, and atrophy with loss of pigment (see figure 6.15). *Hemorrhages* are dark or red stains of varying size near vessels. They are found in hyperten-

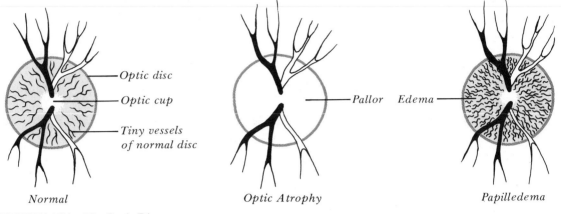

FIGURE 6.14 The Optic Disc.

Labels in figure: Optic disc, Optic cup, Tiny vessels of normal disc, Normal, Pallor, Optic Atrophy, Edema, Papilledema

sion, renal disease, diabetes, and atherosclerosis. *Exudates* are dense, gray, localized infiltrates. Soft exudates have fuzzy edges due to arteriolar microinfarction. They may totally disappear. Hard exudates, often associated with hemorrhage, are smooth and well demarcated. They indicate retinal disease. *Drusen* are characteristic of the aging retina. They appear as small, round, gray or yellow spots and are localized areas of hyaline degeneration. When they occur in the macula, they contribute to macular degeneration and interfere with vision. When exudates occur in the macula, they form a peculiar image called the *macular star figure.* Atrophic degeneration of the macula is more common to the elderly and is another cause of blindness.

Vascular abnormalities of the retinal structure are red and must be distinguished from hemorrhage (figure 6.15). *Microaneurysms,* common to diabetes and local *venous occlusion,* are tiny isolated red dots, smaller than vessels. Neovascularization appears as a compact mass of tiny, tortuous

vessels; it is often found in diabetic retinopathy, the most common form of blindness before age 60 (Kini 1978). In vascular obstruction, or occlusion, the vessel is narrowed distal to the obstruction. If this obstruction is in an arteriole *(arteriolar obstruction),* peripheral constriction will occur; in a venule, peripheral dilation will occur. The arterial wall thickens in hypertension and arteriosclerosis. This change causes a masking of the vein at the point of arteriovenous crossing and gives the appearance of a localized venous narrowing called *A-V nicking.* Other changes include gray deposits on the vessel wall called vascular sheathing or parallel streaking. These deposits are found in multiple sclerosis, leukemia, and retinal inflammation. A widening of the central arteriolar light reflex is found in atherosclerosis.

REFERENCES

ANDERSON, B., JR., and E. PALMORE. 1974. "Longitudinal Evaluation of Ocular Function." In E. Palmore, ed., *Normal Aging II. Reports from the*

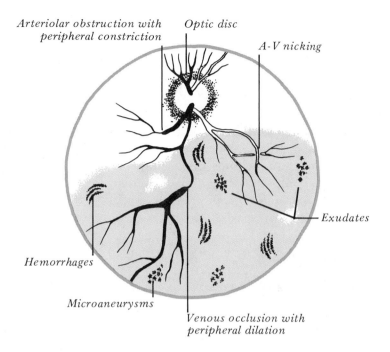

Arteriolar obstruction with peripheral constriction

Optic disc

A-V nicking

Exudates

Hemorrhages

Microaneurysms

Venous occlusion with peripheral dilation

FIGURE 6.15   Abnormalities of the Retinal Structure and Its Vessels.

Duke Longitudinal Studies. 1970–1973. Durham, N.C.: Duke University Press.

EHRLICH, D. R., and R. H. KEATES. 1978. "What to Do When the Elderly Patient Complains of External Eye Problems." *Geriatrics* 33(8):34–43.

GRAHAM, P. A., and F. C. HALLOWS. 1966. "A Critical Review of Detecting Glaucoma." In L. B. Hurt, ed., *Glaucoma: Epidemiology, Early Diagnosis, and Some Aspects of Treatment.* Edinburgh: Livingstone.

GUYTON, A. C. 1976. *Textbook of Medical Physiology,* 5th ed. Philadelphia: W. B. Saunders.

KINI, M. M., et al. 1978. "Prevalence of Senile Cataract, Diabetic Retinopathy, Senile Macular Degeneration, and Open Angle Glaucoma in the Framingham Eye Study." *American Journal of Ophthalmology* 85:28–34.

MACARAEG, P. V. J., JR., L. LASAGNA, and B. SNYDER. 1968. "Arcus Not So Senilis." *Annals of Internal Medicine* 68:345.

SCHWARTZ, B. 1978. "Current Concepts in Ophthalmology: The Glaucomas." *New England Journal of Medicine* 299:182–84.

SLATAPES, F. J. 1950. "Age Norms of Refraction and Vision." *Archives of Ophthalmology* 43:466–81.

TIMARIS, P. S. 1972. *Developmental Physiology and Aging.* New York: Macmillan.

WEALE, R. A. 1975. "Senile Changes in Visual Acuity." *The Transactions of the Ophthalmological Society of the United Kingdom* 95:36–38.

UNIT 4: THE EAR

Aging affects both the external appearance and the functional capacity of the ear. The 1964 National Health Survey (Public Health Service 1967) revealed that 30 percent of the population over age 65 suffered from a significant hearing impairment. Actual deterioration of the ability to understand speech under less than optimal conditions begins at age 50 (Bergman et al. 1976).

The external ear consists of an expanded oval, folded portion, called the *auricle,* and an ear canal, called the *external auditory canal* (see figure 6.16). The function of the external ear is to gather sound. The *helix* is the posterior outer fold of the auricle. In its inferior portion it merges with the *lobule.* In the elderly the lobule is elongated and often traversed by one or several oblique creases. Posterior to the auditory canal, or meatus, is a depression, the *concha;* anteriorly is a small, firm, triangular elevation, the *tragus,* which is often covered by tufts of hair in men over 40. The external auditory canal extends inward from the concha. The outermost portion of the canal is *cartilaginous* and flexible; its inner portion is *bony* and fixed. With age the wall of the canal falls inward, causing the passage to become narrowed. The S-shaped canal is closed at

FIGURE 6.16   Anatomy of the Ear.

EXTERNAL EAR   *EXTERNAL AUDITORY CANAL, MIDDLE EAR, AND INNER EAR*

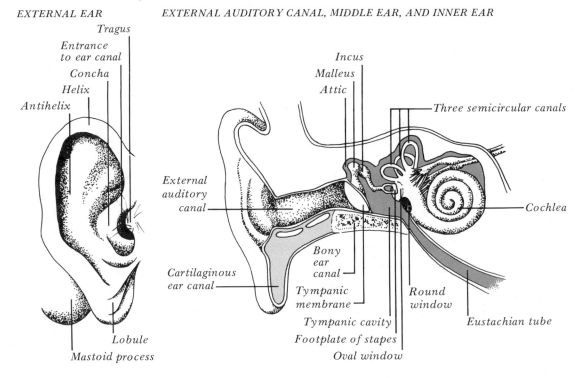

120

its inner end by an obliquely directed membrane, the *tympanic membrane,* or ear drum. In the elderly this membrane is often dull and white. This change has no apparent effect on hearing.

The *middle ear* consists of the *tympanic cavity* and the *attic* (figure 6.16). Its function is to increase the volume of captured sound. This cavity contains the three articulating ossicles, the *malleus,* which is attached to the tympanun, the *incus,* which articulates with the other two ossicles, and the *footplate of stapes,* which inserts into the *vestibular fenestra* (oval window) on the inner wall. Posteriorly the middle ear communicates with the air cells of the *mastoid process* and anteriorly it communicates with the nose through the *eustachian tube.* This communication serves to maintain equality of atmospheric pressure on both sides of the drum, which permits it to vibrate normally.

The *inner ear,* or *labyrinth,* is completely buried in the temporal bone (figure 6.16). Its auditory portion is called the *cochlea.* This part of the inner ear transforms soundwave energy into perceived nerve stimulation. The labyrinth is in contact with the middle ear through the vestibular fenestra (oval window), which is covered by a membrane and the base of the stapes, and through the *cochlear fenestra* (round window), which is covered by a membrane. The vestibular portion of the labyrinth is involved in spatial orientation. It is composed of the vestibule proper and the *semicircular canals.*

Direct examination of the ear is limited to the immediately accessible areas of the external ear. Changes seen in these areas or found by other simple, noninvasive techniques permit the assessment of the hidden middle and inner portions.

HEALTH HISTORY AND SUBJECTIVE FINDINGS

The usual complaints related to the ear are diminished hearing; buzzing, or tinnitus; drainage; dizziness, or vertigo; pain; and, rarely, facial paralysis.

Hearing Loss

Hearing loss is most troublesome for the elderly and frequently leads to social withdrawal. It should never be ascribed to aging without adequate evaluation. Deafness may be sudden or gradual, stable or progressive.

Sudden loss occurring after a shower or bath or on a rainy day is usually due to wax occluding the auditory canal. This problem is frequently intermittent and recurrent and can be resolved, after confirmation with speculum examination, by removal of the wax. In association with rhinitis, acute hearing loss is often due to a plugged eustachian tube. Complication by bacterial infection causes painful otitis media. In association with vertigo and tinnitus, sudden loss points toward labyrinthine disease. Acute vascular occlusion of the labyrinth, infection, and Ménière's syndrome are among the most prominent causes of labyrinthine disease in older clients.

Gradual loss may be due to presbycusis. This impairment does not progress to total deafness, and both ears are always equally affected (Keim 1977). Other causes of gradual hearing loss include genetically induced delayed-onset deafness, such as familial progressive deafness, and cochlear otosclerosis. Otosclerosis affects 1 percent of the population, is bilateral, and is the most common cause of progressive deafness in the middle-aged population with nor-

121

mal tympana (Meyerhoff and Paparella 1978). Typical bone changes are seen on x-ray tomograms. Accurate diagnosis requires audiograms and evaluation by an otorhinologist. Some other causes of gradual hearing loss include Paget's disease and chronic otitis media, as well as benign and malignant tumors. Infection is usually associated with recurrent drainage; examination should reveal a perforated eardrum and pus.

Tinnitus

Tinnitus may be described as a buzzing, chirping, or high-pitched sound. Any hearing problem may cause tinnitus. It is frequently associated with disorders involving the inner ear.

Vertigo

Vertigo is a sensation of rotation and must be clearly distinguished from a non-rotational sensation of imbalance, such as lightheadedness, giddiness, transient faintness, and what is often called dizziness. These sensations may relate to changes of posture, such as rotation of the head or changing from the recumbent to the upright position. When associated with deafness, nausea, and vomiting, rotational sensations are usually related to inner ear disorders. True vertigo may be due to wax or a foreign body in contact with the drum, to otitis media, or to disease of the labyrinth. Central nervous system disease and severe toxicity may also cause vertigo.

Pain

Pain, or otalgia, may be due to infection of the canal (otitis externa) or of the middle ear (otitis media). Many clients injure the skin of the canal and permit bacteria to grow by cleaning their ears with matches or fingernails. In otitis externa the auricle, lobe, and tragus are tender; in otitis media the tragus and the tip of the mastoid are sensitive. Chronic otitis externa may be associated with neuritis. Disorders of nearby structures, such as the base of the tongue, the posterior molars, and the larynx, may cause pain to be referred to the ear.

Drainage

The client may not complain directly of drainage from the ear, so the nurse should inquire about its presence. If drainage has occurred, the nurse should ask about its color and consistency and whether it is of recent onset, recurrent, or chronic. Pain, with or without fever, may be associated with drainage and caused by acute or chronic otitis media, cholesteatoma, or mastoiditis.

Paralysis

Facial paralysis may be related to injury of the facial nerve as it passes through the ear. It may also be due to tumor of the ear, mastoid, or temporal bone or to chronic otitis media.

EXAMINATION AND OBJECTIVE FINDINGS

Examination of the ear involves inspection and palpation, but rarely percussion. Each ear is examined separately.

Inspection

The nurse first inspects the outer ear. Abnormalities such as gouty tophi (small white deposits of uric acid) may be found on the margins of the auricle. Thickening due to trauma is called cauliflower ear. Crusting or ulcerated lesions should be suspected as malignant tumors and referred for biopsy (Keim 1977). To inspect the meatus, the nurse should pull the auricle up and back and push the tragus forward, then hold the auricle of the left ear up and back with the left hand. The right hand holds the otoscope fitted with the largest speculum that can comfortably enter the canal and guides the speculum into the canal. The client's head is tipped toward the right shoulder when the left canal is being examined, and vice versa. The speculum serves to straighten and dilate the canal and permits examination of the canal and drum head. The normal drum is pearly gray and shiny and somewhat transparent. It becomes dead white, dull, and opaque with age.

The normal orientation of the drum is oblique with a deeper, lower portion; it ap-pears as a cone with the point toward the examiner (see figure 6.17). The center cor-responds to the *umbo*, the *cone of light* is seen passing downward and forward, and the *manubrium* extends directly upward from the umbo. A flexible portion, the *pars flac-cida*, is seen above the *pars tensa*, the tense major portion of the drum. At the junction of the pars flaccida and tensa is the *short process of the malleus* and the *malleolar folds*. The drum is circumscribed by the white *annulus*.

Abnormalities cause changes of position, form, and color. Pus and increased middle ear pressure cause an outward bulging, which may obliterate all landmarks. Decreased middle ear pressure will cause tympanic retraction. If the drum is transparent, the malleus becomes more prominent and the short process becomes chalky white. In prolonged eustachian obstruction a transudate forms in the middle ear and gives the drum a yellow color. An

FIGURE 6.17 Right Ear Drum.

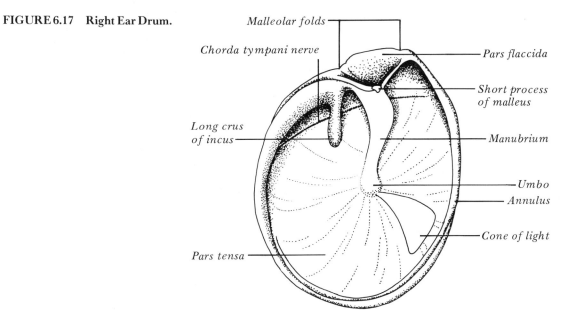

Malleolar folds

Chorda tympani nerve

Pars flaccida

Short process of malleus

Long crus of incus

Manubrium

Umbo

Annulus

Cone of light

Pars tensa

air fluid level or bubbles in the fluid may be seen. Drum perforations are commonly seen at the periphery and near the annulus. Healed perforations are translucid or transparent.

Color changes are significant. A yellow drum indicates serum, and a blue drum is due to blood (hematotympanum). A dull red or pink drum is associated with drum infections (myringitis). Old healed infections may leave dense white plaques (tympanosclerosis). If the plaques are associated with hearing loss, the nurse must consider the possibility of fusion of the ossicles.

Palpation

After completing a thorough inspection of the ear, the nurse should proceed with palpation. The auricle and lobule are palpated; the tragus and auricle are checked for tenderness. Tumors and nodules are noted, and all sores or visible lesions are palpated for soreness and evidence of infiltration. The antero- and posteroauricular areas are examined for nodules or glands, and the mastoids are checked for tenderness, irregularity, or masses.

Percussion

Mediate percussion is used primarily to evaluate the mastoid bone for tenderness as an adjunct to palpation. The normal mastoid is not tender to moderate percussion.

AUDITORY ACUITY: EXAMINATION AND
OBJECTIVE FINDINGS

A gross estimation of auditory acuity may be performed with minimal equipment. The two types of hearing loss are conductive and neurosensorial. *Conductive*

defects are due to external and middle ear disorders; *neurosensorial* or perceptive loss is related to the inner ear, the auditory nerve, or the brain. Combination deficits (mixed defects) occur. After age 50 perception of the higher pitched tones decreases progressively due to cell loss in the cochlea.

Each ear is examined in turn while the other is masked by means of a noise box, a moving finger in the external meatus, or the rubbing of a piece of paper near the masked ear. This distraction prevents the masked ear from perceiving the testing noise. The unoccluded ear may be tested by whispering numbers from a distance of one or two feet and asking the client to repeat them. The voice should begin softly and then increase in intensity if necessary. The lips are covered to prevent lip reading. A watch held at varying distances may be used, but since the tick is outside the pitch of human speech, this method is less helpful.

If hearing loss is present, gross differentiation is made through the use of a tuning fork. Forks of 512 or 1,024 cycles per second (cps) approximate human speech. The examiner sets the forks in motion by stroking them with the thumb and index finger or by tapping them with the knuckles. In normal hearing sound is conducted better through air (AC) than through bone (BC). This relationship is written as AC>BC. Normally the two ears hear bone-conducted sound equally well.

Gross Tests of Auditory Conduction

The Weber Test. The base of a vibrating fork is placed on the midline of the head (see figure 6.18), and the client is asked whether the sound is heard equally

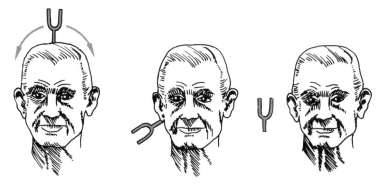

FIGURE 6.18   Gross Tests of Auditory Conduction.

Weber Test

Rinne Test

in both ears or in only one. In the presence of a unilateral conductive defect, the sound will be lateralized to the affected ear. If nothing is heard, the examiner should press the fork more firmly against the client's head.

The Rinne Test. The base of a vibrating fork is placed against the mastoid bone (figure 6.18), and the client is asked to indicate when the sound is no longer heard. Then the prongs are quickly placed near the external meatus. Both the person with normal hearing and one with perceptive loss will still hear the sound (AC>BC). Inability to do so (AC<BC) indicates a conductive defect. A pure conductive hearing loss indicates a disorder of the middle ear.

REFERENCES

BERGMAN, M., et al. 1976. "Age-Related Decrement in Hearing for Speech: Sampling and Longitudinal Studies." *Journal of Gerontology* 31:533–38.

KEIM, R. J. 1977. "How Aging Affects the Ear." *Geriatrics* 32(6):97–99.

MEYERHOFF, W. L., and M. M. PAPARELLA. 1978. "Diagnosing the Cause of Hearing Loss." *Geriatrics* 33(2):95–99.

PUBLIC HEALTH SERVICE. 1967. "Prevalence of Chronic Conditions and Impairments." *Data from the National Health Survey.* Washington, D. C.: Public Health Service Publication no. 1000, series 12, no. 8.

UNIT 5: THE NOSE

The anatomy of the nose allows it to function as a part of the respiratory system (see figure 6.19). In this role the nose moistens and warms inspired air and traps undesired particles. In its other role the nose is an olfactory sensory organ that samples the surrounding environment for noxious and pleasant odors and cooperates with taste in the perception of food. Diminution of these functions can be expected to have an impact on the entire organism. Anand (1964) demonstrated that smell sensitivity gradually decreases, a fact that becomes strikingly apparent by age 60. This decline in smell sensitivity, coupled with the age-related taste changes described by Hughes (1969), helps to explain the diminished and altered food preferences exhibited by the elderly.

An adequate examination of the nose may disclose organic factors that are either worsening the problem of decreased smell sensitivity or forcing it to occur prematurely. Certainly deterioration of respiratory or olfactory function should never be ascribed to aging without prior systematic evaluation.

HEALTH HISTORY AND SUBJECTIVE FINDINGS

The nurse inquires about the existence of nasal obstruction, drainage, and change in the sense of smell. Acute obstruction after trauma is often due to hematoma or to deviation of the septum. Allergic or spasmodic rhinitis causes intermittent or chronic obstruction that may be seasonal. Progressive obstruction is associated with polyps or tumors. Nasal drainage, or *rhinorrhea*, should be described in terms of color, consistency, and acuteness or chronicity. Serosanguineous drainage associated with an acute coryza usually indicates acute sinusitis. Unilateral purulent drainage is found in sinusitis and also with a retained foreign body. Rhinorrhea after a head injury may indicate a skull fracture and leakage of cerebrospinal fluid. This dangerous situation may cause bacterial

FIGURE 6.19   Anatomy of the Nose.

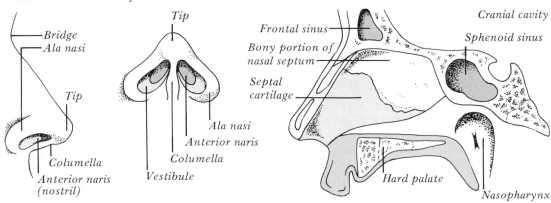

Bridge
Ala nasi
Tip
Tip
Columella
Anterior naris (nostril)

Tip
Ala nasi
Anterior naris
Columella
Vestibule

Frontal sinus
Bony portion of nasal septum
Septal cartilage
Cranial cavity
Sphenoid sinus
Hard palate
Nasopharynx

126

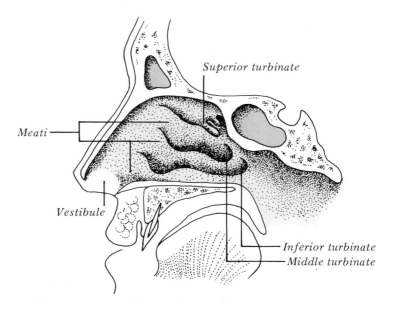

Superior turbinate

Meati

Vestibule

Inferior turbinate
Middle turbinate

FIGURE 6.20 **Lateral Wall of the Nose.**

encephalitis. Loss of the sense of smell may be due to simple coryza, allergic rhinitis, central nervous system disorders, or myxedema.

EXAMINATION AND OBJECTIVE FINDINGS

Inspection

The nurse first examines the *vestibule* of the nose by simply raising the tip of the nose with the thumb of the right hand and then directing a light into the exposed nares (figure 6.19). The *anterior naris* is bounded laterally by the flexible *ala nasi* and medially by the more rigid *septal cartilage*. The vestibule is frequently covered by inwardly projecting hairs, which function as a filter for large particles and become thicker with age. The client's head is tilted back for maximum exposure. The nurse looks for any deformity or obstruction that would interfere with the placement of the speculum. An otoscope, equipped with a short, wide nasal speculum, provides good light and magnification. The view is, however, somewhat more restricted than that provided by an independent mirror and speculum.

The nurse firmly grasps the client's head with the right hand while holding the otoscope with the left. The speculum is gently inserted about 1 cm into the nose while it rests against the ala nasi. The septum is both sensitive to pressure and highly vascular; thus it is a frequent source of anterior nasal hemorrhage (epistaxis). Pressing the left index finger against the outside of the ala stabilizes the instrument. The lower portion of the naris is inspected with the head upright; the head is then tilted back to expose the upper portions and from side to side to reveal the lateral regions. These maneuvers are guided by the right hand held firmly on the head.

Laterally, posterior to the *vestibule* are two rounded swellings, the *middle* and *inferior turbinates* (see figure 6.20). The *superior* 127 *turbinate* is invisible to anterior examination. The middle turbinate overlies the orifice of the maxillary antrum, and the inferior turbinate covers the nasal orifice of the nasolacrimal duct. The superior turbinate overlies the opening to the frontal sinus. Between the turbinates and the septum lie the respective *meati,* or passages.

The nurse notes the presence of deformities, masses, septal deviation, and drainage. If drainage is present, note is taken of its color, consistency, location, and uni- or bilateral occurrence. Drainage from the middle meatus is usually from the paranasal sinuses. Tilting the head helps expose the middle meatus; if nasal polyps are present, they are usually seen there. These polyps often originate in the sinus or near the antrum and are usually due to chronic infectious or allergic sinusitis. Other important observations include the presence of blood, the dilation of blood vessels, the condition of the septum, and the color and condition of the mucus membrane. Anterior perforations are due to trauma, infection, tuberculosis, or cocaine addiction. Posterior perforations are usually due to syphilis.

THE PARANASAL SINUSES: EXAMINATION AND OBJECTIVE FINDINGS

The paranasal sinuses are examined indirectly. Inspection of the face may reveal swelling overlying the frontal or maxillary sinuses. These areas may be tender when palpated. Simultaneous palpation of the frontal and maxillary sinuses may elicit differences in sensitivity, which may be helpful in diagnosing sinusitis. The palpating pressure should be directed upward toward the floor of the sinus, and the nurse should avoid pressing on the eye. The best technique for sinus evaluation is by means of sinus x-rays.

EVALUATING THE SENSE OF SMELL

Evaluation of the sense of smell is the assessment of the first cranial nerve (olfactory). The proper function of this nerve is affected by minor nasal conditions such as rhinitis; repeated evaluations may be necessary to form a true picture. Each nostril is tested separately. The other is held closed by firm digital pressure. A small bottle containing a volatile testing substance is held near the open nostril, and the client is asked to inhale deeply with the mouth shut. The same procedure is then repeated for the other nostril.

Pungent substances such as ether, ascetic acid, ammonia, and alcohol are avoided because they stimulate the trigeminal, or fifth cranial, nerve. Mild perfume, rose oil, orange or vanilla extract, coffee, and tobacco are acceptable as testing substances.

REFERENCES

ANAND, M. P. 1964. "Accidents in the Home." In W. F. Anderson and B. Isaacs, eds., *Current Achievements in Geriatrics.* London: Cassell.

HUGHES, G. 1969. "Changes in Taste Sensitivity with Advancing Age." *Gerontological Clinics* 2:224.

UNIT 6: MOUTH AND THROAT

The mouth and throat are the entrance to the digestive system (see figure 6.21). Significant changes in the oral cavity consist primarily of loss of teeth, diminished taste, and xerostomia. Effects of these changes—pain caused by loosened and infected teeth, the prolongation of chewing necessitated by dentures, decreased appetite caused by diminished taste, and difficult deglutition because of reduced salivary secretion—contribute to the nutritional problems of the older adult (Kart et al. 1978). Frequently these problems are compounded by a nurse's or physician's prescription of a bland low-residue diet for reasons that are sometimes obscure (Templeton 1978).

The examination of the mouth and throat should always be systematic and thorough. The detection of minimal disorders may permit a minor treatment that will prevent major disfigurement or further deterioration.

HEALTH HISTORY AND SUBJECTIVE FINDINGS

Clients' complaints include dry mouth, or xerostomia; sore gums, tongue, and throat; bleeding; change of voice; pain on swallowing; and loss or change of taste. Dysphagia, or difficulty swallowing, is more thoroughly discussed in unit 11, on the gastrointestinal system.

Dryness

Xerostomia is related to diminished salivary secretion. This change may be due to aging, Sjögren's syndrome, or sarcoidosis involving the salivary glands. Other causes

FIGURE 6.21   Structures in the Mouth and Throat.

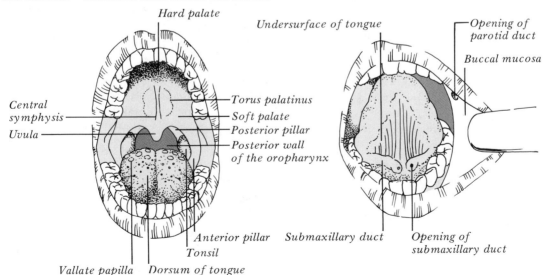

129

include many phenothiazine-related medications utilized by the older adult.

Soreness and Bleeding

Sore gums, tongue, and throat are usually related to local oral and pharyngeal conditions and are most commonly associated with local infection.

Bleeding, voice change, and painful swallowing must always be thoroughly investigated. If no cause is evident, the client must be referred to an otolaryngologist. The nurse should recall that pharyngeal pain may be referred to the ear.

Taste Loss or Change

Before taste loss or change is attributed to aging, neurological causes and alterations of smell should be considered. The sense of smell is mediated by the first cranial nerve and taste by the seventh.

EXAMINATION AND OBJECTIVE FINDINGS

Clients should be requested to remove their dentures prior to the examination. Dentures should be checked for gross fitting or breakage. All ulcerations or suspicious lesions of the mouth should be palpated with a gloved finger.

Inspection

Lips. The lips are inspected for changes in color as well as for moisture, ulcers, cracking, and masses. The edentulous state leads to absorption of maxilla and mandible, which produces shrinkage of the lower face. The client is asked to open the mouth so the nurse can inspect the *buccal mucosa* (figure 6.21). A tongue blade, held in the left hand, may be used to facilitate the

examination. The nurse directs a light into the cavity. Patchy hyperpigmentation is a normal finding; yellow sebaceous glands may be seen shining through the buccal mucosa. Opposite the site of the upper second molar, the nurse will see the *opening of the parotid duct.* Pressure over the parotid gland produces a clear secretion. In parotitis the duct may appear occluded or erythematous, and purulent material may be expressed. This discharge may occur as a complication of serious illness. A white line of keratin may be seen on the mucosa adjacent to the occlusive surfaces of the molars. This line results from sucking on the cheek or invaginating the cheek between the teeth.

Gingiva. The teeth and gums are inspected next. The nurse should note the presence of decayed or loose teeth and check the gingiva for evidence of swelling, bleeding, discoloration, retraction, or inflammation. Periodontitis is associated with softening, purulent discharge, and bleeding. Gum retraction due to bone resorption ordinarily occurs with aging. If gingival retraction is sufficient, the teeth may loosen and fall out.

Palate. The roof of the mouth is composed of a *hard* and a *soft palate* (figure 6.21). The posterior, soft palate is pink with visible blood vessels; the hard palate is paler with visible rugae running transversally. In heavy smokers tiny red dots scattered in the hard palate are seen. These dots are the orifices of inflamed mucus glands. Frequently a hard midline mass is present. This bony protuberance is called *torus palatinus,* an exostosis. Torus mandibularis occurs in the lower portion of the mouth.

Tongue. All visible surfaces of the tongue are inspected. The *dorsum of the tongue* normally is papillated and pink (figure 6.21). Abnormal smoothness and all color changes are noted. Coated tongue is due to keratinization of the filiform papillae. Elongation of the papillae gives a dark, hairy appearance to the tongue but has no other clinical significance. *Vallate papillae* are arranged in an inverted V at the posterior part of the tongue and usually are not visible without the use of a laryngeal mirror. The tongue should be raised and the *undersurface* and floor of the mouth examined. The ventral surface of the tongue is smooth. Rather prominent varicoselike veins may be noted. The frenum is at the *central symphysis,* in the midline. The U-shaped area under the tongue is a common site for malignancy; this area may be palpated with one gloved hand. Some tumors of the tongue can be detected only by palpation. Normally the tip of the tongue should be able to move easily in either direction; failure to do so usually indicates a disorder of the hypoglossal, or twelfth cranial, nerve.

Pharynx. The pharynx is inspected with the mouth open and the tongue in the mouth (see figure 6.22). The soft palate, *uvula,* glossopalatine folds, part of the tonsillar fossa and its *posterior pillar,* remnants of the *tonsil* (if present) and the *posterior wall of the oropharynx* are easily seen (figure 6.21). A more complete examination of the pharynx is performed by the use of a tongue blade, held in the left hand. The free end of the blade is firmly placed down on the midpoint of the arched tongue. The fingers holding the tongue blade are braced on the left cheek, out of the client's line of vision.

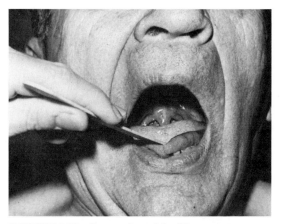

FIGURE 6.22   Inspection of the Pharynx.
The client's tongue is flat and behind the teeth or alveolar ridge. The blade, held in the left hand, is firmly placed on the midpoint of the tongue. Allowing the tongue to protrude or posterior placement of the blade will induce gagging. The normal soft palate is seen as a symmetrical arch with the uvula as its keystone.

The tip of the blade is firmly pressed against the tongue to scoop it downward and forward in the mouth and thus obtain maximum exposure. Care is taken not to place the blade too far posteriorly and excite a gag reflex. The client is then asked to say "ah!" This sound causes a symmetrical rise in the soft palate. No rise occurs if lesions of the ninth and tenth cranial nerves exist. White, cheesy material on an otherwise normal tonsil is due to epithelial debris. Vessels are visible on the tonsillar pillars and the posterior pharyngeal wall. Irregular areas of red or pink lymphoid tissue may also be seen in the pharynx. The nurse notes the presence of color changes, swelling, or masses in these areas. The tonsil may be palpated with a gloved finger if a tumor is suspected.

TESTING FOR TASTE

Taste sensations are mediated by the seventh cranial nerve in the anterior portion of the tongue and by the ninth cranial nerve in the posterior portion of the tongue. Only the anterior two-thirds of the tongue is accessible for testing. The client is asked to protrude the tongue and not to withdraw it until the substance being tasted is identified. Allowing the client to withdraw the tongue permits the material to pass to the other, untested side or to other taste buds in the palate. The nurse uses an applicator that has been dipped into a testing solution to rub the substance gently onto the tongue. The tongue itself must be moist. The four solutions are sodium chloride (salty), sugar (sweet), vinegar (sour), and quinine (bitter). Testing is performed first on one side, then on the other.

REFERENCES

KART, C. S., E. S. METRESS, and J. F. METRESS. 1978. *Aging and Health: Biologic and Social Perspectives.* Reading, Mass.: Addison-Wesley.

TEMPLETON, C. L. 1978. "Nutrition Counseling Needs in a Geriatric Population." *Geriatrics* 33(4):59–66.

UNIT 7: THE NECK

The neck is essentially an elongated cylinder that contains the passageways for major systems of the body and has intrinsic organs of its own (see figure 6.23). The neck is easily observed during the general inspection, and gross changes in position and external anatomy are readily apparent.

EXAMINATION AND OBJECTIVE FINDINGS

The techniques of examination are inspection, palpation, and auscultation. The examination is easily performed with the client sitting. However, because palpation of the carotids may elicit bradycardiac responses and auscultation requires relaxed silence, the vascular examination of the neck should be done with the client supine. The examination of the vessels of the neck is described in unit 10, on the cardiovascular system. The nurse must realize that age-related changes in the neck must be considered during the examination because they affect the nurse's interpretation of the anatomical findings.

Inspection

The nurse observes the neck for color changes, symmetry, masses, skin lesions, scars, and evidence of jugular enlargement. Gross enlargement of the *thyroid gland,* or goiter, may cause the gland to extend visibly upward from the base of the neck. The neck participates in the overall loss of height with aging. As a result, the thyroid gland shifts to a lower position in relation to the clavicles. Height loss occurs primarily in the vertebral column (Rossman 1971) and causes the neck to curve backward, thus shortening the space between

FIGURE 6.23 Structures in the Neck.

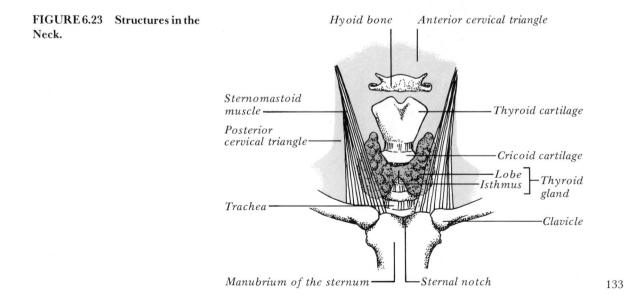

133

occiput and shoulder (see figure 6.24). Sagging tissues and fat deposition may lead to a double chin without other evidence of obesity. The pull of the subcutaneous platysma muscle causes the formation of a double line on either side of the midline and up the neck to the *mandible*. The pull of this muscle also leads to a reticulated skin pattern and the formation of accentuated circular skin lines. The frequency of acro-

chordons (small polyps of the skin) and other skin tumors in this area was discussed in unit 1, on the skin.

Normally the jugulars collapse when the client sits. Engorgement above the level of the clavicles indicates obstruction to venous blood flow toward the superior vena cava. This condition may be associated with tumors in the superior mediastinum, congestive heart failure, and other conditions. It is never a normal finding.

FIGURE 6.24   Cervical Lordosis of Aging.
A smooth, dorsal kyphosis and an associated backward tilt of the neck are evident. The occiput approaches the shoulders. The clavicles are higher and flatter than in youth, and the associated stooped shoulders and rounded back give the appearance of pulmonary emphysema (see pages 133, 143, and 205). The muscles appear prominent (see page 94).

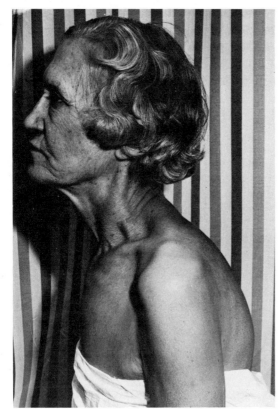

Palpation

All masses are palpated and described in terms of location, size and delimitation, depth, degree of fixation or mobility, consistency, tenderness, and inflammation, if any. The palpation of the *sternomastoid muscle* divides the neck into an *anterior* and *posterior cervical triangle* (figure 6.23). The posterior triangle lies between the anterior edge of the sternomastoid and the trapezius; the anterior triangle lies in front of the sternomastoid. As a general rule, lymphatics of the anterior triangle drain the face, pharynx, tonsil bed, and parotid gland; those of the posterior triangle drain the cranium.

Submental and Submaxillary Regions. Using the digital pads of the index and middle fingers, the nurse gently moves the skin over the submental and submaxillary regions, including first the pre- and post-auricular area, the mastoid, and the base of the occiput, then the area extending from the angle of the jaw along the medial aspect of the mandible and down from the point of the chin to the thyroid gland. The nodes of the angle of the jaw drain the tonsillar bed.

Anterior Triangle and Sternomastoid. The fingers are then directed to the anterior triangle and the sternomastoid. Nodes of the superficial cervical chain overlie the muscle. Nodes of the deep chain are palpated by hooking and palpating under both edges of the sternomastoid with the thumb and fingers. Palpation in the posterior triangle will locate enlarged nodes of the posterior chain. These nodes are found near the anterior edge of the trapezius.

Supraclavicular Region. Next the examination is directed to the supraclavicular space formed between the clavicle and the sternomastoid muscle. Palpation in this area must be deep. *Adenopathy* in a region requires searching for a lesion in the area drained by the chain. Nodes may be discrete, prominent, or matted together. Hard or fixed nodes suggest malignancy; discrete or tender nodes are signs of inflammation. Adenopathy due to chronic infection may cause matting, fixation, and local inflammation or even sinus tracts. Malignant adenopathy, often hard and fixed, may be due to extension of a local carcinoma or to a systemic disease such as lymphoma or leukemia.

Glands. The submandibular salivary gland is palpated as a flat, firm mass one or two centimeters in front of the angle of the jaw and is checked for bilateral equality. This gland may be felt by the client and give rise to unfounded fear of a tumor. The other salivary glands normally are not palpable. Enlargement of the salivary glands may be due to a stone or calculus in the duct. The involved gland swells during a meal. *Parotid enlargement* is palpated on the ascending ramus of the mandible. It is seen as an upward and outward displacement of the ear lobe. Acute suppurative parotitis is usually associated with wasting diseases but may be found in the debilitated older adult. The gland is hot, reddened, tender, and enlarged. Pressure on the gland will often express pus from the duct. This abscess causes severe generalized toxicity. Among other causes of parotid enlargement is the mixed tumor, which has a malignant potential. In parotid enlargement the examiner cannot grasp the ascending ramus of the mandible.

Trachea. The *trachea* is examined for deviation in the jugular or *sternal notch* (figure 6.23). A finger is placed on the trachea in this area and then is slipped off the trachea to either side. Any deviation from the midline is noted. A pulsating swelling behind the sternomastoid may be due to a buckling of the innominate and right carotid arteries. This swelling is more common in older women than in younger ones (Honig et al. 1953). The head is then extended and the nurse places thumb and index finger on the cricoid with gentle, upward pressure. The finding of a *tracheal tug* raises the possibility of an aortic aneurysm. *Tracheal deviation* may be due to an aortic aneurysm or substernal mass or goiter as well as pneumothorax or pulmonary fibrosis.

Thyroid. The nurse inspects the thyroid gland by asking the client to extend the neck slightly and swallow. (The thyroid gland moves with swallowing; lymph nodes and vessels remain fixed.) Giving the client some water to swallow, on command, may be helpful. Palpation is performed either from in front or from behind. The thyroid gland is composed of two lateral *lobes*

135

joined by a central *isthmus* (figure 6.23). The aspect is grossly that of a fat letter H. The isthmus is anterior to the trachea and just below the *cricoid cartilage.*

To palpate the thyroid *from in front* (see figure 6.25), the nurse places the pads of the right index and middle fingers just below the cricoid cartilage and asks the client to swallow. The isthmus is felt rising upward under the fingers. The fingers are then moved laterally and deeply to the edge of the sternomastoid in an attempt to feel each lobe both during and after a swallow. To examine the right lobe, the client's head is inclined slightly forward and to the right. The nurse's right thumb gently pushes the lower portion of the client's *thyroid cartilage* to the client's right. The tips of the index and middle fingers of the left hand grasp the posterior edge of the sternomastoid and press it forward while the left thumb examines the front of the muscle. The fingers are placed below the level of the thyroid cartilage; while the nurse holds this position, the client is asked to swallow. The left lobe is palpated by the same technique but with the positions of the hands reversed.

To palpate the thyroid *from behind* (see figure 6.26), the nurse first asks the client to extend the head slightly. Then, using the digital pads of the right index and middle fingers, the nurse palpates the front of the neck for masses or nodules. These fingers are then placed below the cricoid cartilage, and the nurse attempts to palpate the isthmus and the anterior surfaces of the lateral

FIGURE 6.25   Thyroid Palpation from in Front.

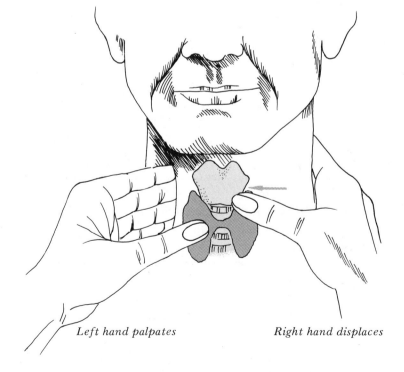

Left hand palpates   *Right hand displaces*

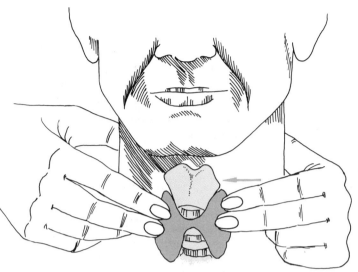

FIGURE 6.26 Thyroid Palpation from Behind.

Right hand palpates

Left hand displaces

lobes. The client's head is then inclined forward toward the side to be examined. On the right side, a push with the fingers of the left hand displaces the thyroid cartilage toward the right. The right thumb is placed behind the sternomastoid and the palpating fingers are placed in front. The client is asked to swallow, and the right lobe is palpated while sliding between fingers and thumb. The other lobe is examined by the same procedure but with the positions of the hands reversed.

The normal thyroid gland weighs approximately twenty-five grams—the isthmus weighs five grams; and each lobe, ten grams (Prior and Silberstein 1973). Enlargement of a lobe or of the isthmus is usually described in terms of estimated total weight of the gland as well as in terms of type of enlargement. Thus a gland whose isthmus and right lobe are twice the normal size would weigh about forty grams, with the isthmus weighing ten grams; the

right lobe, twenty grams; and the left lobe, ten grams. The nurse also observes whether the enlargement is diffuse or circumscribed; smooth or nodular; soft, hard, stony, or rock hard; firm or fluctuant. Clients with short, stocky necks are difficult to examine, particularly if the gland is normal in size or only minimally enlarged. In the older adult the lobes may slip near or behind the clavicle, and palpation may be difficult.

A variety of conditions can cause thyroid enlargement. Inflammation of the gland is known as *thyroiditis.* In the acute and subacute forms of thyroiditis, the gland is usually tender. In the chronic form the gland may attain great size and is usually quite firm. *Graves's disease,* or thyrotoxic goiter, is another cause of increased size. This condition is associated with hyperthyroidism. The soft, irregular mass occasionally palpated near the midline, between the isthmus and the hyoid bone, is a remnant of a

137

thyroglossal duct that has undergone cystic degeneration. The vestigial fibrous thyroidal pyramidal lobe is rarely palpated in the midline between the isthmus and the thyroid cartilage.

Any abnormally forceful vascular pulsations will have been observed during the inspection. Gentle palpation of the vessels is performed with the client supine to avoid precipitating reflex bradycardia. A carotid artery aneurysm may be visibly pulsatile. Careful palpation will reveal that the enlargement expands equally in all directions, in rhythm with the pulse. A mass overlying an artery and transmitting the pulsation will expand only in a single direction.

Auscultation

If the nurse suspects thyroid enlargement, the base of the neck should be carefully auscultated. A venous hum may be associated with hyperthyroidism.

Auscultation of the vessels is performed with the client's head extended. The client is asked to inhale, then to exhale, and then not to breathe. The bell of the stethoscope is placed over the artery. High-pitched bruits over the carotid bifurcation may indicate internal carotid stenosis; low-pitched murmurs at the base of the neck often reveal atherosclerosis of the subclavian artery.

MOTION OF THE NECK

The range of motion of the neck was discussed in unit 2 in the section on movements of the head. Head rotation and shoulder shrug are controlled by the eleventh cranial nerve (spinal accessory). This nerve may be tested by asking the client to make the appropriate movement while the examiner resists it with the hand.

Limitation of neck motion is occasionally' found in older adults. This rigidity may render all motion of the neck impossible and thus prevent all maneuvers permitting evaluation of meningeal inflammation (see the section on neurological evaluation in unit 14).

REFERENCES

HONIG, E. I., W. DUBILIER, and I. STEINBERG. 1953. "Significance of the Buckled Innominate Artery." *Annals of Internal Medicine* 39:74–85.

PRIOR, J. H., and J. S. SILBERSTEIN. 1973. *Physical Diagnosis: The History and Examination of the Patient.* St. Louis: C. V. Mosby.

ROSSMAN, I. 1971. "The Anatomy of Aging." In I. Rossman, ed., *Clinical Geriatrics.* Philadelphia: J. B. Lippincott.

UNIT 8: THE RESPIRATORY SYSTEM

Age-related changes in the respiratory system diminish the accuracy of the chest x-ray and respiratory testing. Because of this problem, considerable expertise and sensitivity in physical assessment must be attained (see figure 6.27). X-ray and respiratory test results have to be interpreted in light of the findings of a health assessment. Sometimes a modest change from a baseline evaluation may be the only indication of a deteriorating respiratory status; but if the nurse has assessed the client's respiratory system in a health evaluation and is aware of the client's limitations, a program of amelioration may be formulated.

HEALTH HISTORY AND SUBJECTIVE FINDINGS

The following complaints volunteered by the client or elicited by the nurse during the interview suggest the possibility of a respiratory problem: aphonia and hoarseness, sneezing and nasal drip, weight loss and night sweats.

Other, more definite complaints include *cough,* with or without expectoration; *breathlessness;* and, rarely, *pain.* None of these complaints is necessarily of respiratory origin; they may be caused by cardiovascular, musculoskeletal, neurological, or hematological disorders.

Cough

Cough is the primary respiratory complaint and indicates an abnormality somewhere in the system. The nurse inquires whether it is dry or productive of sputum and notes its frequency and character. A *dry cough* indicates a congested mucus membrane with little or no secretion. *Expectoration* indicates secretion, and a loose cough indicates that the secretions lie free in the bronchial tubes. In acute bronchitis an initially dry cough becomes productive; in acute coryza or laryngitis the cough usually remains dry.

Coughs may occur in fits, or paroxysms, or they may occur as a constant tickle. Paroxysms provoked by position change are typical of chronic bronchitis and bronchiectasis.

Acute illness is usually marked by an acute onset of coughing. If the client has a prolonged history of coughing, the nurse must suspect chronic illness, such as chronic bronchitis, bronchogenic carcinoma, and tuberculosis. Finally the nurse should inquire about problems such as pain, vomiting, or fainting, which are more commonly associated with protracted, paroxysmal coughing.

Expectoration. Information about the quantity, color, and consistency of expectoration and the effect of postural change is necessary.

Scanty sputum indicates a primarily inflammatory phase, whereas the production of large quantities of foul-smelling sputum is indicative of pulmonary abscess or infected bronchiectasis. Thick mucoid sputum is common in the chronic bronchitis of smokers. Thick bronchial casts are occasionally found at the end of an attack of bronchial asthma.

Sputa are classified by appearance. *Mucoid* sputum is clear, jellylike, and of

139

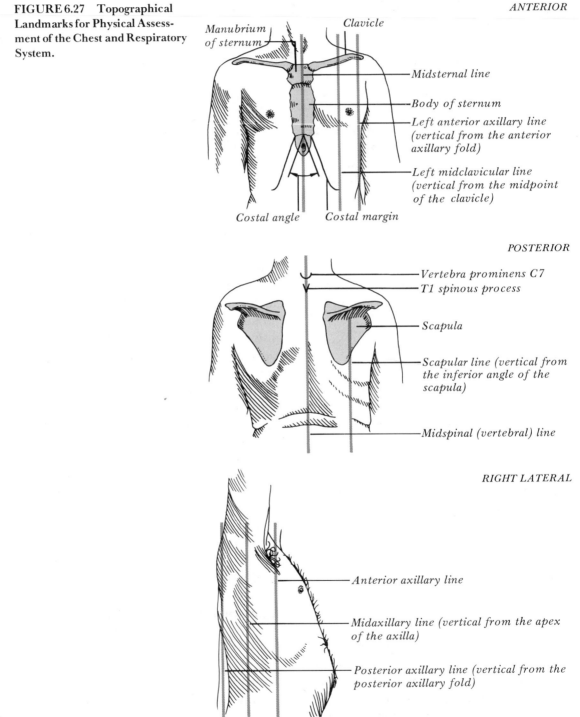

FIGURE 6.27   Topographical Landmarks for Physical Assessment of the Chest and Respiratory System.

ANTERIOR

Manubrium of sternum

Clavicle

Midsternal line

Body of sternum

Left anterior axillary line (vertical from the anterior axillary fold)

Left midclavicular line (vertical from the midpoint of the clavicle)

Costal angle

Costal margin

POSTERIOR

Vertebra prominens C7

T1 spinous process

Scapula

Scapular line (vertical from the inferior angle of the scapula)

Midspinal (vertebral) line

RIGHT LATERAL

Anterior axillary line

Midaxillary line (vertical from the apex of the axilla)

Posterior axillary line (vertical from the posterior axillary fold)

varying color and consistency. *Mucopurulent* sputum is creamy yellow or green. *Purulent* sputum or *frank pus* indicates pulmonary suppuration. *Hemorrhagic* sputum is either totally bloody or blood streaked. The most common cause of hemorrhagic sputum is bronchitis, but lung tumor and tuberculosis must also be considered. In lobar pneumonia the sputum may have a rusty appearance.

The production of hemorrhagic sputum, called *hemoptysis,* must be differentiated from *hematemesis,* which is the vomiting of blood. Hemoptysis is usually preceded by cough, the material is usually frothy, blood is often present for a few days, and the client frequently has a history of respiratory illness. Hemoptysis requires an evaluation of the entire respiratory tract, from nose to lungs. Some causes of hemoptysis include pulmonary embolism and, more rarely, congestive heart failure and mitral stenosis.

A special type of copious, frothy, watery blood-tinged sputum is associated with *acute pulmonary edema.* This kind of sputum may be due to heart disease, pulmonary infection or embolism, or other severe pulmonary or systemic conditions. It is discussed more thoroughly in unit 10, on the cardiovascular system.

Dyspnea

Breathlessness, or *dyspnea,* implies that the respiratory effort is conscious and excessive; it may also be extremely uncomfortable. Rapid breathing is called *tachypnea;* slow breathing is known as *bradypnea.* Dyspnea aggravated by recumbency is called *orthopnea.* Dyspneic clients complain of a decreased ability to perform a previously simple effort. Dyspnea is more common in cardiac disorders. When associated with respiratory disease, it indicates severe respiratory impairment. The nurse ascertains whether the dyspnea is continuous, paroxysmal, or precipitated by changes of posture or activity.

Dyspnea is also caused by systemic acidosis, as in renal failure and diabetic ketosis; airway obstruction from an inhaled foreign body; a tumor of the larynx or trachea; asthma; bronchial infection; and anemia. In the elderly it may be related to obesity or simply to poor physical conditioning. Poor mechanical functioning of the lung due to emphysema or splinting of the chest will diminish air flow and cause dyspnea. Additional causes include those associated with a loss of alveoli, as in pneumonia, pulmonary embolism, collapsed lung, atelectasis, and pleural effusion. The amount of dyspnea is directly related to the speed of onset of the collapse or consolidation and is due to the induced degree of hypoxia.

Pain

Pain is not common in respiratory disorders. Lung tissue is insensitive; pain is felt only in the pleura and the upper air passages. Pain is also less common in the elderly. Acute tracheitis and bronchitis may cause a rawness felt behind the sternum. Pleural irritation is painful regardless of the cause. The distribution is that of the appropriate intercostal nerve and may be referred to the abdomen and the back. In the older client these pains are atypical and blunted. Apical lung tumors extending into the cervical plexus may cause pain in the arm, and diaphragmatic pleurisy is felt at the origin of the phrenic nerve in the neck.

Chest pain may be due to a variety of conditions, including diseases of the heart, chest wall, and breasts. In all cases the nurse should ask the client about precipitating causes such as employment, interpersonal contacts, and cigarette use.

EXAMINATION AND OBJECTIVE FINDINGS

The portions of the respiratory tract located in the head and neck were discussed in units 2 and 7. Certain objective findings—namely, *cyanosis* and *clubbing* of the fingers—should alert the nurse to the possibility of respiratory disease. If the client has a productive cough, the sputa should be examined.

Cyanosis is a blue discoloration of the skin and mucus membranes caused by the presence of at least 5 grams of reduced hemoglobin circulating per 100 milliliters of blood. Cyanosis is more severe in heart disease but is also found in a variety of respiratory conditions. It is most easily seen in the lips, ears, cheeks, and nose and imparts a dusky red to deep purple coloration. Frequently associated with dyspnea, it is aggravated by cold and physical effort.

Clubbing of the fingers is frequently seen in clients with chronic lung disorders or with heart disease. It is most striking in association with bronchiectasis or pulmonary carcinoma, and in the elderly it is almost always due to bronchogenic carcinoma. Occasionally clients with chronic pulmonary disease complain of an associated, painful swelling of the wrists and ankles called *hypertrophic pulmonary osteodystrophy.* Clubbing was described in unit 1, in the section on dermal appendages.

Examination of the chest is best performed when the client is sitting, but it may be done when the client is lying down. The examination must be complete. Good lighting is essential to prevent shadows across the chest, and the room temperature must be comfortable to prevent shivering. The client undresses to the waist. For women a paper garment, open in the back, preserves dignity. The nurse's hands are washed before and after the examination. The order of examination is inspection, palpation, percussion, and auscultation. The nurse compares one side of the chest with the other and proceeds from the top downward.

Inspection

Initially the client's respiratory rate is measured. The normal rate is sixteen to eighteen breaths per minute; fever increases the rate by four breaths per minute per degree Celsius.

Respiration. Respiration is classified by pattern and rate. Normal respiration is free and easy. For the client with *dyspnea,* respiration is a conscious effort. If the dyspnea occurs on inspiration, large-airway obstruction may be the problem; if it occurs on expiration, a small-airway disorder is likely. *Stridor,* a low-pitched sound, is often heard with tracheobronchial disorders. *Hyperpnea* is an increase in the respiratory depth. *Hyperventilation* is an increase in both rate and depth. *Apnea* is a temporary cessation of respiration. *Periodic respiration* is characterized by alternating apnea and hyperpnea: the period of apnea is followed first by a period of increasingly rapid respirations of increasing depth and then by a period of slower respirations of decreasing depth, followed by another period of apnea (Cheyne-Stokes respirations). In an elderly client this condition probably indicates a central nervous system disorder. Although in younger clients periodic respiration is associated with a poor prognosis, older persons may tolerate the condition for years (Agate 1971).

Stertorous respirations are noisy breathing due to an accumulation of secretions in the upper air passages. Such breathing is frequently heard in the dying and has been called the *death rattle.* Sighing respirations are usually prolonged and terminate in an audible sigh; they often are manifestations of an emotional state.

Air trapping is usually associated with obstructive lung disorders. Trapping of air in the lungs occurs during rapid respiration and results in an increase in the residual air remaining at the end of each expiration.

Ataxic respiration is characterized by total irregularity of rate, depth, and frequency; it is due to severe central nervous system problems involving the respiratory centers.

Chest. After noting the pattern and rate of respiration, the nurse begins the inspection of the chest. The general appearance of the skin is observed, including the distribution of hair; the state of nutrition, hydration, and general development; and any sores, nodules, and abnormal vascular patterns or engorgement.

The nurse can best perceive thoracic asymmetry and deformities by looking from above downward and by observing from the sides. Normal thoracic excursions consist of an upward and outward movement on inspiration. The anteroposterior diameter is normally one-half of the side-to-side diameter. In older clients the anteroposterior diameter is larger and the thoracic excursions are diminished, mimicking pulmonary emphysema with a fixed outward thoracic expansion. This expansion is associated with a change in the angle of the ribs from forty-five degrees toward the horizontal.

The nurse observes the intercostal spaces for retraction during inspiration and for bulging during expiration. Retraction indicates obstruction to air flow. Bulging is found with massive pleural effusion or during forced expiration in a client with an obstructive lung disorder such as asthma or emphysema. Normal aging is not associated with evidence of airway obstruction.

Gross differences in chest expansion from side to side are found in unilateral fibrosis, chest trauma, and pleurisy with splinting. Bilateral disorders cause bilateral restriction. Seen from the side, the normal thoracic spine imparts an anterior concavity to the back of the chest. Lateral deviation is minimal. Exaggeration of this curvature is called *kyphosis.* A sharp angulation is called a *gibbous.* If kyphosis is associated with a marked deviation, the combination is called *kyphoscoliosis.* Excessive straightening occurs in arthritic conditions and causes a *poker spine.*

Normal aging is associated with kyphosis. The association of a gibbous or a scoliosis is definitely abnormal. Other deformities include excessive sternal depression, called *funnel chest,* and excessive sternal prominence, called *pigeon breast.*

Finally the nurse visualizes the probable projections of the lobes of the lungs on the chest wall (see figure 6.28). Initially it may be helpful to mark these lobes on the client's skin as reference points for pulmonary evaluation.

143

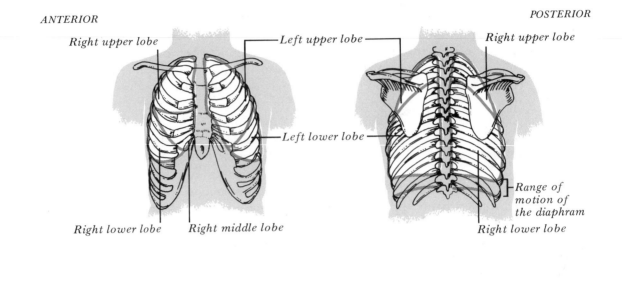

ANTERIOR

Right upper lobe

Left upper lobe

Left lower lobe

Right lower lobe

Right middle lobe

POSTERIOR

Right upper lobe

Range of
motion of
the diaphram

Right lower lobe

RIGHT LATERAL

Right upper lobe

Right middle lobe

Right lower lobe

LEFT LATERAL

Left upper lobe

Left lower lobe

FIGURE 6.28   Position of the Lungs.

Palpation

Palpation permits the nurse to evaluate skin texture while feeling for areas of tenderness, crepitation, pulsation, and masses.

The excursions of the two hemithoraces are best evaluated by palpation.

From behind, the nurse places both hands over the apices. The client is seated with the head tilted forward and down while the nurse stands behind and looks down over the client's shoulders. The bases of the chest or thorax are examined by placing the hands along the lowest palpable ribs with the fingers on the rib and the thumbs pointing toward the vertebral column.

From in front, the client is recumbent and the nurse's hands are placed so that the thumbs are on the costal margins at the costal angle and point toward the xyphoid. The fingers extend along the ribs and point toward the axilla. Once the hands are placed, the client is asked to breathe in and out slowly and deeply. Inequality or limitation of expansion is usually more obvious from the anterior position.

Next the nurse evaluates *fremitus* (see figure 6.29). Fremitus, or vibration within the thoracic cavity, must be felt by the examining hand. Laryngeal phonation will cause *vocal fremitus;* a deep cough, *tussive fremitus;* a pleural rub, *pleural fremitus;* and sonorous rhonchi, *rhonchial fremitus.*

Vocal fremitus is a palpable vibration of the thoracic wall induced by phonation and transmitted to the palpating hand from the larynx through the bronchi and lungs and the chest wall. The client is asked to say "Ninety-nine" or "One, one, one," and the same hand is placed on the chest in identical places on each of the two sides in turn. The flat of the hand or, for more accurate localization, the ulnar border of the hand is used. The intensity of the vibration varies with the character of the media and the portion of the chest through which it is transmitted. The lower the pitch of the voice, the better the transmission. Normally fremitus is increased posteriorly in the intrascapular region and anteriorly at the second right costal cartilage, where the bronchi are close to the surface. A high-pitched voice or a chest wall unusually

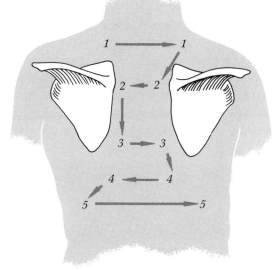

POSTERIOR

FIGURE 6.29   Sequence of Examination for Fremitus.

thickened by fat or muscle will diminish fremitus.

Fremitus is abnormally decreased by bronchial obstruction from foreign bodies or tumors; by asthmatic bronchial spasm; or by damping due to a pleural effusion or pneumothorax, particularly if the lung is collapsed below the effusion or intrapleural air.

Fremitus is increased when a solid or collapsed lung is in contact with air passages and chest wall. This consolidation may occur with pneumonia or a tumor.

Percussion

Percussion is performed from the apices of the thorax downward; one side is compared with the other, intercostal space by intercostal space. The pleximeter finger is always held parallel to the ribs (see figure 6.30). In the posterior examination the client is erect with head tilted forward and

145

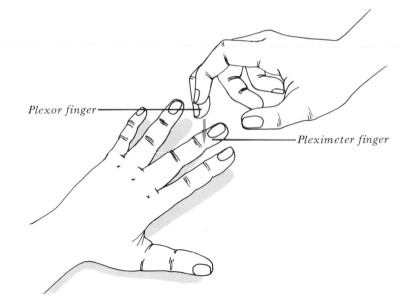

Plexor finger

Pleximeter finger

FIGURE 6.30 Mediate Percussion.

arms crossed at the waist. This position moves the scapulae as laterally as possible. The width of resonance at each apex is noted and compared with the others. Normally width is five centimeters.

Percussion of the anterior chest begins in the supraclavicular spaces and proceeds downward. The axillae are examined with the arms raised and resting on the head. Percussion proceeds from the armpit to the costal margin. A thick chest wall decreases normal resonance.

Normally dullness in the anterior left chest is due to the heart and the liver. A transition from resonance to tympany at the anterior left base is caused by the air-filled stomach.

Diaphragmatic motion may be percussed by instructing the client to take a deep breath and to hold it. The nurse determines the lowest level of resonance by percussion from above downward. Next the client is told to exhale as far as possible

and the nurse repeats the examination. If the skin is marked after each phase, the two sides may be compared and the degree of motion noted. Normally motion is from three to five centimeters. Pleurisy and emphysema tend to diminish motion, and intraabdominal masses or ascites tend to raise the diaphragms.

The percussion note of the lungs is modified by various conditions. *Tympany* occurs when air fills the pleural space or is found above a pleural effusion over a collapsed lung. *Dullness* is caused by a solidified lung, as in pneumonia; by a tumor; or by pulmonary fibrosis. *Flatness* is found with pleural effusion or tension pneumothorax or over a solidified lung with an obstructed bronchus.

Auscultation

For successful auscultation the nurse must learn to disregard the heart when listening to the lungs. Identical points on each side are examined, and the examination proceeds from the top down. The client is asked to breathe somewhat more deeply than usual through an open mouth. Too deep a breath may produce confusing muscle sounds. The open mouth decreases extraneous sounds due to air flow. The nurse determines the character of the breath sounds and their bilateral equality, and the presence of other sounds and their location.

Character of Breath Sounds. Breath sounds are evaluated for pitch, intensity, quality, and duration. These sounds are composed of three elements: a *vesicular* element—a soft, rustling sound caused by the passage of air into millions of alveoli; a *tracheal* element—a harsh sound caused by the vibration of air passing through the vocal cords and trachea; and a *bronchial* element— a softer sound formed when the tracheal element passes into the bronchi. In areas where the bronchi approach the lung surface, at the apices and between the scapulae, the elements combine to form a *bronchovesicular* sound.

Bronchovesicular breathing is harsh with a short pause between inspiration and expiration and a prolonged expiration. Because this kind of sound is often heard over areas of abnormal lung, the nurse must remember that it normally occurs at the apices and between the scapulae.

Other Sounds. The nurse listens for (1) abnormal breath sounds, (2) changes in vocal resonance, and (3) the presence of adventitious sounds.

1. *Abnormal breath sounds* are varieties of bronchial breathing in which the bronchial

element becomes more or less prominent. *Bronchial* breathing is simulated by placing the stethoscope on the occiput and breathing through the nose. It is caused by suppression of the alveolar component and occurs in consolidation due to pneumonia or a tumor. The sounds of bronchial breathing seem to be louder than normal.

Tubular breathing is a higher pitched form of bronchial breathing. It has a metallic quality similar to the sound made by blowing across the mouth of a narrownecked bottle. Tubular breathing is often heard over thin-walled lung cavities and occasionally over a pneumothorax with a pulmonary-pleural fistula and a free flow of air. If the tone is similar but of lower pitch, it is called *cavernous* or *amphoric*. The causes are the same. The sound of cavernous breathing is similar to that made by breathing into a glass. Findings localized to one lung, or a portion of one lung, have greater significance and are more likely to indicate pathology. Bilateral, diffuse changes may be only qualitative differences or transient conditions.

Auscultation requires that the breath sounds be well produced and well transmitted. A variety of conditions may decrease or eliminate the breath sounds. The presence of fluid or air in the pleural space or a thickened pleura will decrease the breath sounds over that lung. The breath sounds will also be decreased in clients with pulmonary emphysema or bronchial obstruction, in aged clients with feeble respirations, and in clients who are splinting the chest wall. Diminished or absent sounds, especially if localized to one lung or to a portion of a lung, are a most important finding and usually indicate a pathological condition.

147

2. *Voice transmission* through the chest wall may also be evaluated through the stethoscope. This sound is called *vocal resonance* and is the audible equivalent of vocal fremitus. Higher pitched sounds are heard best, particularly when transmitted through the interscapular region and the right apex. These tones are more clearly perceived in men because of their generally more resonating thorax.

Vocal resonance that is increased over solid lung or resonating cavities is called *bronchophony*. If the increased resonance is such that actual syllables are discernible, it is called *pectoriloquy;* and if the whispered voice produces this result, it is called *whispering pectoriloquy,* which always indicates a consolidation as in pneumonia. In the feeble aged, the whisper may be the only voice transmission attainable.

Egophony is a special kind of bronchophony causing the voice to take on a bleating quality. It is particularly audible if the client is asked to say "e-e-e." If egophony is present, this pure tone is transformed into "ā-ā-ā." The change from "e" to "ā" is usually heard over a consolidated lung at the upper limit of a pleural effusion. Vocal resonance is decreased under the same conditions that cause decreased tactile fremitus.

3. *Adventitious sounds* are superimposed on the breath sounds. They are usually abnormal and may accompany normal or abnormal breath sounds. Those most commonly heard are rhonchi, rales, and the pleural friction rub. Less frequently encountered is the hippocratic succussion splash.

Rhonchi and rales are generally produced by the passage of air through a narrowed or partially blocked respiratory tract (see figure 6.31).

Rhonchi are musical sounds produced by the passage of air through the narrowed *trachea, bronchi,* or *bronchioles.* These sounds are continuous and are usually more pronounced during expiration. *Sonorous rhonchi* are produced in large air passages and have a deep-toned note. *Sibilant rhonchi* are produced in the smaller bronchioles and have a high-pitched squeak. Rhonchi vary from breath to breath and are usually partially clearable by coughing. They are found in bronchitis and other secretory or purulent conditions of the bronchial tubes as well as in the presence of tumors or foreign bodies. They may also be found in obstructive lung disorders and are associated with bronchospasm. The turbulence of the air flow through the passageway causes the sound.

Rales are coarse, abnormal sounds of varying quality. Produced by the bubbling of air through a fluid, they are added onto the breath sounds and are most distinct at the terminal phase of inspiration. The client must inhale deeply if these sounds are to be heard. The quality of rales is similar to that of sounds heard from a freshly poured glass of carbonated water. Rales are of three types: coarse, medium, and fine. *Coarse or bubbling rales* are low toned and moist. Originating in the trachea, bronchi, or even the bronchioles, they can often be cleared with a strong cough. In moribund clients who cannot clear secretions, these sounds become audible and form the *death rattle.* These loud, coarse, gurgling sounds are produced by the passage of air through viscid secretions in the larger air passages.

Medium or crackling rales (subcrepitant rales) are somewhat less bubbling. The sound is not unlike that produced by rolling a dry cigar between the fingers. Medium rales are produced by air bubbling

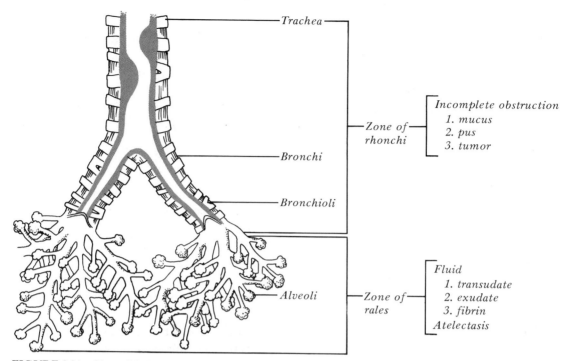

Trachea

Bronchi

Bronchioli

Alveoli

Zone of rhonchi
Incomplete obstruction
1. *mucus*
2. *pus*
3. *tumor*

Zone of rales
Fluid
1. *transudate*
2. *exudate*
3. *fibrin*
Atelectasis

FIGURE 6.31   Sites of Origin and Causes of Adventitious Sounds.

through exudate in the alveoli and the smaller bronchioles.

Crepitations or fine rales (crepitant rales) are the finest rales; their sound may be imitated by rolling hairs between fingers held close to the ear. They have a finer, more metallic quality than the coarser rales and occur in late inspiration. Fine rales are due exudate in the alveoli and thus indicate pulmonary involvement. They also may be caused by the opening of the adherent alveolar walls; in such cases they indicate alveolar collapse. They are present with simple atelectasis and are produced at the base of the lung in the bedridden or feeble client and often in the elderly client with a shallow tidal volume.

The nurse must make every effort to have the client clear these rales by vigorous coughing and deep inspirations prior to auscultation. On occasion the nurse will hear medium rales that appear after coughing. These posttussive or latent rales always indicate lung involvement, most commonly tuberculosis.

The clinical implication of persisting rales is that they often provide objective data for the presence of lung disease. Fine rales are found in pneumonia, pulmonary inflammation, and congestion. Medium rales are audible in congestive heart failure and in bronchitis involving the smaller bronchioli. Finally, coarse rales are more common in bronchitis and over cavities.

Pleural friction rub is produced by the rubbing of roughened, inflamed pleural surfaces as they ride over each other during respiration. This characteristic creaking or grating quality is similar to that produced by creaking leather and is usually heard during both phases of respiration. It has a very superficial quality and seems to be just under the stethoscope. It is most frequently found in the anterolateral chest in the areas of greatest excursion. The nurse must not confuse pleural friction rub with coarse rales. Occasionally a friction rub may be heard only at the end of inspiration and may not be audible with shallow breathing.

Hippocratic succussion is a splashing sound produced by shaking the client. It is due to the presence of air and fluid in the pleural space.

EVALUATING RESPIRATORY PROBLEMS

A combination of subjective and objective data permits the nurse to form a mental image of the condition of the respiratory system and the possible disorders that may be affecting it. This image is clarified through certain tests that may be requested from the laboratory. Pulmonary function studies, the use of blood gases, and some of the uses of chest x-ray are described in chapter 9.

Snider's test permits a quick evaluation of a client's peak flow and forced expiratory volume. In this test the client is instructed to hold the mouth open, after removing any false teeth. The nurse holds a lighted match six inches from the client's mouth, and the client is asked to take a deep breath and blow out the match without pursing the lips. Ability to do this indicates a forced expiratory volume of at least 1 liter and a peak flow of at least 130 liters per minute; failure to do it indicates diminished pulmonary function.

Table 6.1 summarizes the subjective and objective findings and assessment considerations that alert the nurse to the existence of a respiratory health problem. For convenience these data are grouped under conditions affecting the bronchi, the lungs, and the pleura.

TABLE 6.1
Summary of Subjective and Objective Respiratory System Findings

| Site of Health Problem | Findings | | Assessment Considerations |
	Subjective	Objective	
Bronchial	Cough Sputum	Auscultation rhonchi stridor	Acute Conditions sharp onset short course Chronic Conditions course prolonged over three months
Lung Parenchyma Congestion and Edema	Dyspnea Cough Sputum	Percussion dull Auscultation diminished breath sounds fine to medium rales	Cardiac Conditions Pulmonary Conditions

| Site of Health Problem | Findings | | Assessment Considerations |
	Subjective	Objective	

Consolidation	Dyspnea
	Cough
	Sputum
		Palpation
		    increased vocal fremitus
		Percussion
		    dull
		Auscultation
		    bronchial breath sounds
		    increased vocal resonance
		    medium rales
			Pulmonary Infection
			    or Tumor
			Vascular Conditions:
			    Embolism

Atelectasis	Dyspnea
	Cough
		Percussion
		    dull to flat
		Auscultation
		    breath sounds absent
		    diminished vocal resonance
			Prolonged Bed Rest
			Infection
			Tumor

Emphysema	Dyspnea
	Cough
		Inspection
		    increased
		    anteroposterior diameter
		    diminished excursion
		Percussion
		    hyperresonant
		    low diaphragms
		Auscultation
		    diminished and bronchial
		    breath sounds
		    sibilant rhonchi
			Compensatory—
			    Reversible
			Chronic Obstructive
			    Lung Disorders

Pleura
    Pleurisy
	Pain
	Dyspnea
		Fever, Tachycardia
		Inspection
		    splinting same side
		    respiratory grunt
		Auscultation
		    friction rub
			Acute Conditions:
			    Dramatic Complaints
			    infection
			    embolism

Pleural Effusion	Dyspnea	Inspection
		    diminished excursion,
		    same side
		    heart & trachea deviated
		    toward opposite side
		Palpation
		    decreased vocal fremitus
		Percussion
		    flat
		Auscultation
		    diminished and bronchial
		    breath sounds
		    diminished pectoriloquy
		    and vocal resonance
			Acute Conditions
			    infection
			    embolism
			    malignant neoplasm

151

| Site of Health Problem | Findings | | Assessment Considerations |
	Subjective	Objective	

Pneumothorax	Pain
	Dyspnea
		Inspection
		  diminished excursion,
		  same side
		  heart and trachea
		  deviated toward
		  opposite side
		Palpation
		  decreased vocal fremitus
		Auscultation
		  diminished and
		  amphoric breath sounds
		  diminished vocal
		  resonance
		  succussion splash
			Trauma
			Ruptured Cyst
			Chronic Infection
			  with Cavities
			Malignant Neoplasm

REFERENCES

AGATE, J. 1971. "Common Symptoms and Complaints." In I. Rossman, ed., *Clinical Geriatrics.* Philadelphia: J. B. Lippincott.

UNIT 9: THE BREASTS

As mentioned in the description of the general examination in the first part of this chapter, the breasts participate in the generalized process of aging (see figure 6.32). The outward contour changes associated with the loss of subcutaneous fat and the pull of gravity are well known to aging people of either sex and to their health workers. Involutional internal changes also occur. These changes are related to the postmenopausal decrease of gonadal hormones and to intracellular aging itself (Herman 1971). The thinner skin, diminished muscle mass, and tissue fibrosis cause changes in the findings of the health assessment. The nurse's responsibility lies in correctly evaluating these findings so that appropriate decisions can be made.

HEALTH HISTORY AND SUBJECTIVE FINDINGS

Complaints related to breast problems include changed appearance or the presence of a mass, tenderness, or discharge.

FIGURE 6.32 Structures of the Female Breast.

INTERNAL STRUCTURES   *SUPPORTIVE TISSUES*

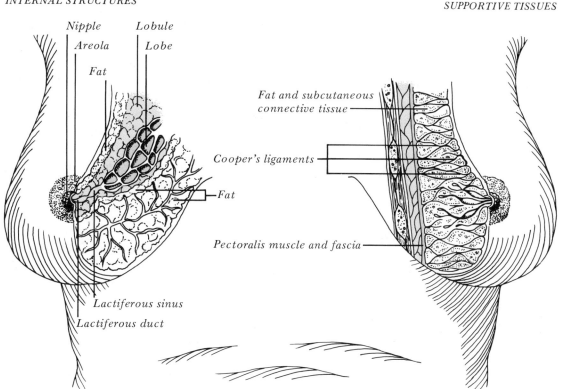

Changed Appearance or Mass

The nurse determines when change in the appearance of the breast was first noted; the exact nature of the change; whether it is stable, variable, or progressive; and whether it is uni- or bilateral. Unilateral change is of particular concern, but in the elderly any increase in breast size must not be ignored. Possible causes include benign or malignant tumors and medications such as spironolactone, which can cause breast tenderness and gynecomastia in men.

Trauma may initially cause swelling and, later, breast retraction induced by fat necrosis and scarring. Involutional changes of aging cause nipple retraction and fibrotic linear stranding. These changes must be carefully differentiated from those due to malignancy.

Tenderness

Because cyclic hormonal stimulation is diminishing, tenderness not associated with trauma must be carefully evaluated. Medications or a tumor, with associated hemorrhage or necrosis causing internal swelling and pain, may be responsible.

Discharge

Discharge must be carefully evaluated in all clients. The nurse ascertains its appearance as well as character and date of onset.

Certain medications, such as the tricyclic antidepressants, may cause galactorrhea. Bloody discharge is commonly due to a benign intraductal papilloma. Pus mixed with blood or a sanguineous discharge must raise the nurse's suspicion of a possible ductal carcinoma. Breast secretion requires evaluation at any age.

EXAMINATION AND OBJECTIVE FINDINGS

A systematic examination of the breasts must be performed in all clients regardless of age or sex. The usual order of procedure is inspection followed by palpation. Both breasts are examined with the client sitting and in a recumbent position. Upon completion of the breast examination, the nurse examines the axillae and the supraclavicular areas.

The client disrobes to the waist. Embarrassment is diminished by the use of a towel or sheet to cover the breasts until the moment of examination. Adequate light is essential.

For purposes of orientation, the breast is divided into four quadrants by horizontal and vertical lines crossing at the nipple. These areas are identified as the *upper inner* and *outer* and the *lower inner* and *outer quadrants* (see figure 6.33). Alternatively the breast is visualized as a clock face with twelve o'clock situated at the upper pole. Lesions are described in terms of their position on the clock and number of centimeters from the nipple.

Inspection

With the client seated and the arms at the sides, the nurse inspects the breasts for symmetry, size, contour, and appearance of the skin and nipples.

Symmetry and Size. The breasts may not be symmetrical or identical in size. Although consistent with normality, inequality may serve to alert the nurse to the possi-

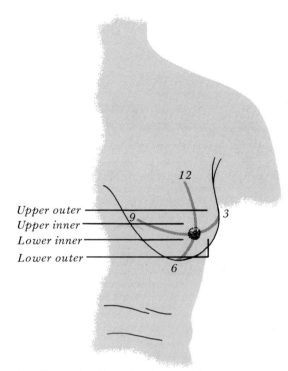

Upper outer
Upper inner
Lower inner
Lower outer

12
9
3
6

FIGURE 6.33   Four Quadrants of the Breast.

The nipples are also examined for size and shape, for the direction in which they point, and for the presence of rashes and ulcerations. Nipples normally point in the same direction. Inversion may occur normally in the elderly but is definitely significant when fixed. Like unilateral rashes and ulcerations, inversion may indicate a malignancy.

Contour. Shape and form are carefully examined. Dimpling indicates retraction related either to subcutaneous scars or to infiltrating tumors. In the absence of inflammation, skin retraction is evidence of carcinoma (Prior and Silberstein 1973). To exaggerate early dimpling or skin retrac-

FIGURE 6.34   "Pig Skin" or "Orange Peel" Appearance.

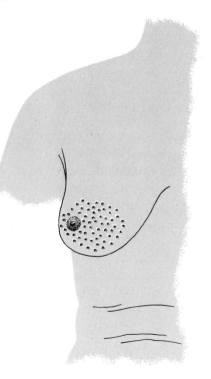

bility of tumors, inflammation, or congenital anomalies.

Appearance. The nurse observes the breasts for color, presence of skin thickening or edema, and existence of an abnormal venous pattern. Erythema may be due to inflammation or neoplastic involvement of the lymphatic drainage. The lymphatics of the breasts drain toward the axilla, the subclavicular nodes, the internal mammary chain, the other breast, and the deep lymphatics of the abdomen.

Prominent hair follicles and pores, which give the skin a "pig skin" or "orange peel" appearance, are due to edema and are commonly associated with carcinoma (see figure 6.34).

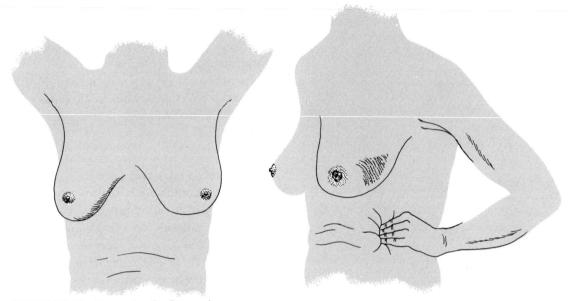

FIGURE 6.35   Inspection for Retraction.

tion, the nurse should ask the client to raise arms overhead, then to place hands on hips and firmly press down (see figure 6.35). These maneuvers activate the underlying muscles and suspensory ligaments, thereby augmenting retraction.

Palpation

Breasts vary greatly in their "feel." In elderly women breast tissue feels stringy and nodular. Similar changes occur in men with any degree of gynecomastia. Abundant subcutaneous fat alters this consistency. A large, pendulous breast is more difficult to evaluate than a smaller one. Because of the diminished fat, breast masses are more easily palpated (Rossman 1971).

Palpation must be systematic so that no area is overlooked. It is best performed with the client recumbent and the breast tissue evenly distributed over the chest. The technique consists of compressing the breast between the flat of the fingers and the chest wall. The fingers are lightly applied in a slight rotational motion.

Small shoddy granules are normal lobulations and may be quite pronounced in the elderly. In elderly men little or no breast tissue is palpated in the absence of gynecomastia. The axillary tail is carefully examined. It may be quite atrophic in the elderly. The nurse searches for induration, tenderness, and nodules. All findings are described in terms of location, size in centimeters, contour, consistency, mobility, discreteness, and tenderness.

Location of Lesions. Recording the location of a tumor or other lesion in the breast not only identifies lymphatic drainage but also makes relocation easier. The majority of breast tumors occur in the upper outer quadrant and in the axillary tail (Malasanos et al. 1977).

Size. Recording the size of a lesion permits future comparisons and is most helpful in determining the evolution of the lesion.

Contour and Consistency. The outline and consistency of a lesion may be quite helpful in identifying malignancy. Benign lesions often have smooth, regular contours; malignant lesions, firm and irregular ones. Cystic lesions are usually soft; malignant lesions, stony hard.

Mobility. Inflammatory or malignant lesions are fixed; benign ones are usually mobile.

Tenderness. Tender lesions are unusual in elderly men and in postmenopausal women. In the absence of cyclical hormone stimulation, cystic mastitis does not occur. Areas of tenderness not related to trauma must be carefully evaluated.

EXAMINATION OF THE AXILLAE AND SUPRACLAVICULAR AREAS

The axillae and supraclavicular areas are examined after the nurse completes the examination of the breasts. The axilla is palpated with the slightly cupped fingers of one hand while the other hand holds the client's arm at the side. The nurse reaches as high as possible into the axilla, exploring both anterior and posterior portions of the region. The examination is continued as the hand passes downward. The client's arm is then abducted and the examination is repeated on the other side.

Axillary lymphatics drain the arm, back, and shoulder in addition to the intercostal spaces and the breasts.

After the examination of the axillae, the nurse palpates both supraclavicular spaces. As in the axilla, adenopathy may be of inflammatory or neoplastic origin. The left supraclavicular space receives lymphatics from the abdomen and the upper lobe of the left lung in addition to those of the left side of the neck, the left axilla, and the left breast. The right supraclavicular space receives drainage from its side of the neck, axilla, and breast along with deeper lymphatics from the left and right lungs.

REFERENCES

HERMAN, J. B. 1971. "Personal Communication." Cited in I. Rossman, "The Anatomy of Aging," in I. Rossman, ed., *Clinical Geriatrics.* Philadelphia: J. B. Lippincott.

MALASANOS, L., et al. 1977. *Health Assessment.* St. Louis: C. V. Mosby.

PRIOR, J. A., and J. A. SILBERSTEIN. 1973. *Physical Diagnosis: The History and Examination of the Patient.* St. Louis: C. V. Mosby.

ROSSMAN, I., ed. 1971. *Clinical Geriatrics.* Philadelphia: J. B. Lippincott.

UNIT 10: THE CARDIOVASCULAR SYSTEM

The various portions of the cardiovascular system are examined at different moments during the health assessment: funduscopy permits visualization of the vessels of the eye; peripheral pulses and veins are checked when the nurse examines the limbs; the abdominal exam permits evaluation of that portion of the aorta; and although described in this unit, the jugulars and carotids are examined with the neck. The heart and great vessels (see figure 6.36) are usually evaluated after the examination of the lungs.

HEALTH HISTORY AND SUBJECTIVE FINDINGS

Clients with cardiovascular disease may have either no complaints or some that appear totally unrelated to any illness of the heart and vessels. Certain subjective findings are extremely common and point toward this system. Clients with complaints of dyspnea, palpitations, and pain should be encouraged to describe them completely in their own words before the nurse begins any extensive questioning. Other complaints referable to the central nervous, digestive, and urinary systems help complete the picture.

Dyspnea

Dyspnea was well described in unit 8, on the respiratory system. It is initially effort related and out of proportion to the effort. It must be distinguished from the effort dyspnea of obesity and lack of muscular conditioning that often occurs in the elderly. Effort dyspnea frequently indicates

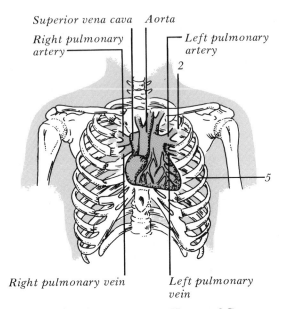

Superior vena cava   Aorta

Right pulmonary artery

Left pulmonary artery

2

5

Right pulmonary vein   Left pulmonary vein

FIGURE 6.36   Location of the Heart and Great Vessels.

congestive failure when other causes and anemia have been excluded. The amount of effort needed to produce the dyspnea is a valuable clue to the degree of decompensation. *Orthopnea* is evidence of a more advanced degree of failure: the client can no longer lie flat without becoming dyspneic. *Paroxysmal noctural dyspnea* awakens the client in the middle of the night with a smothering sensation. Frequently the client sits up at an open window in an attempt to obtain relief. Breathing is labored; a wheeze may be audible. These episodes may progress to acute pulmonary edema with a cough productive of foamy, blood-tinged sputum. These complaints usually indicate progressive left ventricular failure.

Cheyne-Stokes, or periodic, respirations may be associated with heart disease in the elderly. This syndrome was discussed in unit 8 in the section on respiratory assessment.

Palpitations

Palpitations, or conscious sensations of the heartbeat, are usually described as a bumping, throbbing, or fluttering in the chest or at the base of the neck. They may originate in an increased force or rate of contraction or in an irregular rhythm. They are more common to hyperthyroidism and anxiety than to organic heart disease. Clients with grossly abnormal rhythms are often totally unaware that they have this condition.

Pain

The pain of heart disease is due to myocardial ischemia. In the elderly this pain is usually blunted, less severe, and less well described, making evaluation all the more difficult (Rodstein 1956). Cardiac problems in the absence of ischemia are painless. All chest pain must be carefully evaluated to avoid improper decisions that not only might threaten the client's life but also might impose unnecessary restrictions and cause anxiety.

When present, ischemic pain is usually well described and may be associated with considerable apprehension. The pain is situated behind the sternum in the mid, upper, or lower chest. At times it is felt in the epigastrium; it may radiate to the jaw, the neck, or across the chest to the left shoulder and down the arm to the fingers.

This pain is provoked by effort or excitation. If related to effort, the same effort provokes the pain at the same point and usually forces the sufferer to cease the activity. This imposed rest relieves the pain. The pain is short lived, rarely lasting more than five or ten minutes. It is steady and described as crushing, burning, or pressing. If the pain is brought on by effort and relieved by rest, a cardiac origin must be considered. In the elderly, anginal pain often induces such fear that sufferers intentionally diminish their activity.

Similar pain may be provoked by lying down and eased by sitting. This angina of recumbency (decubitus) is found in clients with congestive failure and coronary atherosclerosis. The pain of myocardial infarction, another manifestation of myocardial ischemia, is also blunted in the older client; the episode of pain is similar but more prolonged.

Chest pain related to movements of the chest wall is due to other conditions, such as costochondral arthropathy or pectoralis muscle strain. Pleurisy and diseases of the chest wall cause a pleuritic type of pain. Disorders of other intrathoracic organs must also be considered in the assessment of chest pain.

Pain is often associated with vascular disorders. A dissecting aneurysm is associated with severe pain along the path of the vessel. Acute vascular obstruction is painful, and the pain usually localizes the area of the obstruction. Numbness, coldness, and heaviness are commonly associated with the pain of arterial occlusion. Painful swelling points to thrombophlebitis.

Chronic or progressive arterial occlusion in a lower limb causes complaints reminiscent of angina. This syndrome of *intermittent claudication* causes pain provoked by effort and relieved by rest. Usually described as a cramp, this pain is aggravated by cold; its severity is related to the amount of the effort.

Night pain and rest pain are also related to arterial ischemic disorders.

Complaints Relating to Other Organ Systems

Complaints relating to organ systems other than the heart may occur in clients with congestive heart failure. Such complaints include dyspepsia, anorexia, and bloating due to congestion in the gastrointestinal tract; scanty, dark urine due to decreased glomerular filtration; and dizziness, headache, confusion, and insomnia due to cerebral anoxia.

Syncope may occur because of Stokes-Adams attacks and may be due to heart block and a bradycardia or to tachyarrhythmia with decreased cardiac output. In these cases the client is usually standing and feels giddy and light headed. Occasionally the client feels a kind of stumbling sensation. Often the client faints and may have a seizure if cerebral ischemia is sufficient.

PERIPHERAL AND CENTRAL VASCULAR SYSTEM: EXAMINATION AND OBJECTIVE FINDINGS

Blood Pressure Assessment

The determination of *blood pressure* is an important part of every health assessment. This test provides more information about the cardiovascular system than its simplicity would suggest. The taking of blood pressure involves more than simply raising the cuff pressure and then listening for the two points of systole and diastole. Performed with care, this procedure provides valuable information regarding cardiac output and vascular competence.

The completely deflated cuff is applied firmly and evenly to the arm. The client is seated or recumbent and, above all, comfortably relaxed. The cuff must be adequate for the size of the arm.

If the sounds are too low to be audible, they may be augmented by (a) keeping the arm directly overhead during the raising of the cuff pressure, (b) insuring that the pressure registers 0 before the cuff is inflated, and (c) having the client open and close the fist, with the cuff inflated and the arm overhead. This procedure pumps blood out of the artery, accentuates the difference in vascular pressure above and below the cuff, and augments the sounds.

Occasionally the sounds are heard at a high level only to disappear and then reappear at a lower level. This phenomenon is called the auscultatory gap. If the cuff pressure is raised into the gap and then lowered, the first audible sound is interpreted as systolic pressure and gives a falsely low reading. This distortion can be avoided if the nurse palpates the radial pulse while raising the cuff pressure high enough to abolish the pulse. This gap corresponds to the second phase and may be abolished by the techniques of augmentation described above.

At the time of the initial data base assessment, the nurse obtains the blood pressure in both arms. Certain conditions, such as obstruction of the innominate artery or an aortic aneurysm, may cause a difference in pressure levels in the two arms.

Pressure readings may be obtained in the lower extremities by placing an appropriate-sized cuff on the lower third of the thigh and auscultating in the popliteal space, over the popliteal artery. This examination is particularly useful in clients with hypertension. By this simple step the nurse evaluates for *coarctation of the aorta*. This rare cause of elevated blood pressure causes the pressure in the lower extremities to be lower than that in the upper ones. Normally systolic pressure readings are higher in the lower extremities. Other causes of reduced blood pressure are associated with thrombotic vascular occlusions of the aorta and its branches.

Assessing the Pulse

The assessment of the *pulse* is equally important. The radial artery is most commonly used to evaluate the pulse rate. However, other pulses—the brachial, axillary, femoral, popliteal, pedal, carotid, and temporal arteries—should be evaluated as part of the vascular examination. The beating of the radial artery, palpated in the wrists, is called "the pulse."

The nurse palpates the pulse in both wrists simultaneously and notes any differences in the force of the beat. An inequality is palpatory evidence of the pressure differences described above. In palpating the pulse, the nurse notes the rate, rhythm, and form of the pulse and the condition of the arterial wall.

The pulse is counted for thirty seconds. If the pulse is irregular, it should be counted for one minute. Frequently the heart rate decreases with age (Harris 1970). Rates between 60 and 100 beats per minute are normal. If the rate is above 100, it is called a *tachycardia;* a rate below 60 is called a *bradycardia*. The pulse rate is compared to the auscultated apical heart rate. These

rates normally occur synchronously. A *pulse deficit* exists if the apical heart rate is greater than the peripheral pulse rate.

The pulse rate is increased by effort, emotional stress, thyrotoxicosis, and certain heart conditions such as congestive failure. Slow rates are found in heart block and myxedema. These problems will be discussed in the section on the examination of the heart.

The normal rhythm is perfectly regular. Occasionally the pulse quickens with inspiration and slows with expiration. This sinus arrhythmia is rare in the elderly.

A variety of irregularities may be noted; however, usually the heart must be auscultated before a correct assessment can be made. Occasionally the pulse appears to skip, or a weaker than normal beat is felt sooner than expected, followed by a longer than normal pause. These irregularities are found in the presence of *ventricular extrasystoles,* which are common in the elderly (Kennedy and Caird 1972). The occurrence of a slightly longer than normal pause followed by a regular rhythm or of an early weak beat followed by a normal interval is indicative of atrial extrasystoles. These irregularities often disappear with exercise. In *atrial fibrillation* the pulse is irregular with a varying rate, rhythm, and strength from beat to beat. This type of irregularity is often increased by exercise and is the most common arrhythmia in old age (Kennedy and Caird 1972). Cardiac auscultation and electrocardiography, which will be more fully discussed later, assist in the assessment of rhythm abnormalities.

The nurse assesses the form of the palpated pulse wave. This wave is not due to the flow of blood from the heart but is actually the transmission of the kick of the

161

ventricular beat, or pressure wave, through the arterial wall. The wave relates to the state of the wall and the force of the ventricular thrust. A pulse may be thready or bounding or of some intermediate grade.

A number of wave forms have been described and confirmed by direct graphing (see figure 6.37). Wave forms may often be palpated in the peripheral artery but are more prominent in the carotids, particularly if the examiner simultaneously palpates the carotid and auscultates the heart. The wave form is composed of a quick, smooth upstroke; a rounded, smooth peak; and a gradual, smooth downstroke. The small notch on the peak of the upstroke (anacrotic) and the similar notch on the downstroke (dicrotic) are not normally palpable.

Assessing the Arteries

During the examination of the pulse, the nurse also assesses the condition of the arterial wall. This assessment is best accomplished by occluding the vessel with digital pressure and emptying it of blood distal to the occlusion. The wall may then be palpated. In older clients the wall is distinctly palpable, and in the presence of arteriosclerosis the artery is tortuous or irregular with beaded ringlike structures. Pulsations diminish or disappear, and the artery has a "pipestem" appearance. The brachial arteries may exhibit snakelike pulsations, which are easily seen under the skin of the arms. This phenomenon is particularly apparent if the nurse flexes the elbow slightly while looking at the medial aspect of the limb (see figure 6.38).

FIGURE 6.37 Jugular and Carotid Pulses.

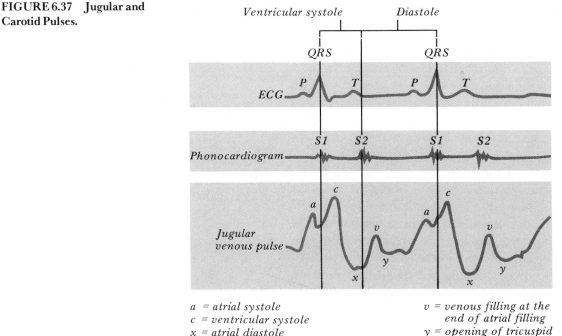

a = atrial systole
c = ventricular systole
x = atrial diastole

v = venous filling at the end of atrial filling
y = opening of tricuspid valve

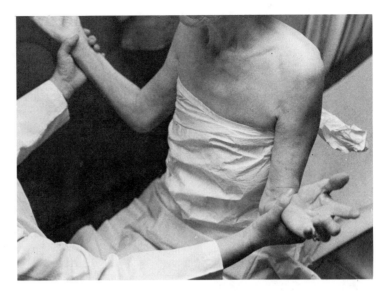

FIGURE 6.38   Examination of the Brachial Arteries.
The nurse grasps the wrists and swings the arms outward. The elbows are moderately flexed. The artery can be seen along the medial aspect of the arm, posterior to the edge of the biceps muscle. This position also permits simultaneous palpation of the radial pulses (see section on assessing the arteries) and inspection of the arms.

Arteries are examined by auscultation as well as by palpation and inspection. Under certain conditions transmission of heart murmurs will be heard. Of greater significance is the presence of a systolic bruit, which is usually caused by an atherosclerotic plaque partly occluding the vessel or by an arterial aneurysm. Bruits that are heard regardless of the position of the body or the limb are significant.

Finally, in hypertensive clients the nurse should simultaneously palpate the femoral and brachial arteries. A delay of femoral pulsation over the brachial pulse is found in coarctation of the aorta and partial occlusion of the aortic bifurcation.

Inspection and Palpation of Veins

The veins are examined by means of inspection and palpation. The nurse notes whether venous filling is bilaterally equal and whether this filling is normal. The right atrium is the point of "0" pressure in the circulatory system. Normally veins lo-

cated above the atrium are collapsed while those below are filled to a degree relative to their distance below that chamber. Since the right atrium roughly corresponds to the manubrium sterni, elevation of a vein to that level should cause it to empty. If emptying does not occur, the pressure is increased. This level of increased pressure is obtained by slowly raising the vein to the point where it empties spontaneously.

When the client is sitting, the internal jugular vein is normally collapsed and should remain so even with the client's head and neck elevated at sixty degrees. At forty-five degrees, the jugulars should not fill more than one or two centimeters above the manubrium. This dilation of the jugular vein may be seen by directing a light obliquely across the vein (see figure 6.39). Such lighting allows the distended vein to cast a shadow and thus outlines it.

Venous pressure is elevated in congestive heart failure, constrictive pericarditis, cardiac tamponade, and in obstruction of the superior vena cava.

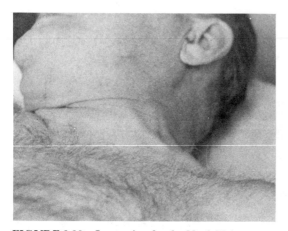

FIGURE 6.39   Inspection for the Neck Veins.
With the client recumbent, the jugular veins are filled. They are outlined by directing a light obliquely across the neck so that the veins cast a shadow.

In normal elderly clients buckling of the left innominate vein can cause an apparent pressure elevation in the left jugular vein and the veins of the left arm. This unilateral elevation disappears with deep inspiration (Sleight 1962).

Local venous obstruction is associated with venous dilation and often with edema below the obstruction. When the obstruction is of long duration and progressive, the veins become tortuous, forming *varicosities* or varicose veins.

Venous pulsation is best seen in the jugular veins of the neck. With the client recumbent, the distended jugular is outlined by an obliquely directed light. If the nurse carefully observes the base of the neck, a pulsation due to the carotid pulse is seen (see figure 6.37). Between these carotid pulsations, a series of smaller waves are noted. These waves are variations in superior vena cava pressure induced by the atrial and ventricular contractions. Those induced by the atrial contraction disappear in atrial fibrillation. Superior vena

cava obstruction totally obliterates venous pulsations in the jugulars.

The direction of venous flow is found by occluding the vein. The index of one hand is placed across the vein to occlude it. The index of the other hand then milks the vein of its contents and remains across the vein so as to occlude it and isolate the collapsed segment. The nurse then lifts one index finger and permits the segment to fill. The procedure is repeated; this time the other finger is lifted. The side of faster filling indicates the direction from which the blood is flowing. Normal flow is toward the heart. This direction is reversed in cases of obstruction and is most commonly seen in clients with obstruction of the portal vein.

Gentle palpation may disclose the presence of a clot. If tenderness is also present, the nurse must consider the possibility of thrombophlebitis.

THE HEART: EXAMINATION AND OBJECTIVE FINDINGS

Inspection

Inspection of the heart is performed in good light. Tangential lighting accentuates movements of the chest wall. Inspection discloses position, character, and rhythm of the point of maximal impulse (PMI) and reveals areas of abnormal pulsation. The client is either recumbent or reclining with the chest elevated at forty-five degrees. While inspecting the chest the nurse also notes other abnormalities, depressions, bulges, and the presence of epigastric pulsations.

Palpation

Palpation is complementary to inspection and serves to verify findings and reveal other conditions that are not visible.

The palm of the hand and fingers are placed lightly over the apex and then over the base of the heart. Next they are systematically passed to the central area of the precordium. Particular attention is paid to the areas of projection of each valve (see figure 6.40). This palpation permits the nurse to appreciate the force of the cardiac thrust and the presence of other pulsations or vibrations (thrills).

Pulsations are localized by lightly palpating with the palmar surface of the index and third finger. The point of apical thrust is the point farthest from the sternum that lifts the fingers. This area, normally less than 2 cm in diameter, is located in the fifth interspace medial to the midclavicular line and 7 to 9 cm from the midsternal line. Thoracic kyphosis in the elderly may displace the point of apical thrust laterally, so that it falls on the anterior axillary line without evidence of cardiomegaly.

Pulsations at the base of the heart are suggestive of an aortic aneurysm. In the elderly such pulsations may be due to a buckled innominate artery. Cardiomegaly or mediastinal shift displace the heart.

Left ventricular hypertrophy displaces the apex downward and to the left; right ventricular hypertrophy moves it upward and toward the axilla. Atelectasis of the right lung moves the apex to the right, and massive right pleural effusion pushes it to the left.

The force of the apical thrust varies in relation to the thickness of the chest wall, the presence of pulmonary emphysema (which places lung tissue between the heart and the chest wall), and the actual force of the ventricular beat. If the apical thrust moves the chest wall and a lateral and downward displacement of the impulse occurs, cardiac hypertrophy is probable.

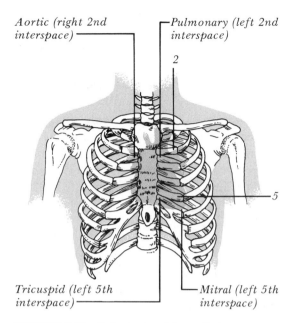

FIGURE 6.40 **Palpatory and Auscultatory Projections of Heart Valves.**

The apical thrust is synchronous with the heart beat; changes in rhythm are felt as variations in regularity and force.

Premature beats occur sooner than expected and have a decreased force. Atrial fibrillation is felt as an irregular pattern of beats of varying force. The arrhythmias will be discussed later.

Thrills are palpable vibrations. They are the palpable equivalents of murmurs and are produced by the passage of blood from one chamber to another through an abnormal orifice. They are similar to the sensation felt when petting a purring cat. Thrills may be systolic or diastolic. They confirm the murmur and indicate that it is organic. They are timed in relation to the apical thrust or carotid pulse, and their location, area of transmission, timing, and intensity should be described.

Auscultation

Because heart sounds are of low intensity and difficult to hear, auscultation is probably the most difficult examination. It requires a relaxed client, absolute silence, and complete concentration by the nurse. Auscultation confirms the rate and rhythm obtained from the pulse and cardiac pulsations and gives information concerning the functioning of the heart valves as well as the state of the myocardium and pericardium.

Nurse and client are in comfortable positions. The nurse is on the client's right side. The room must be warm enough for a client who is undressed to the waist and wearing a gown.

The stethoscope should have both bell and diaphragm. The diaphragm is used for high-pitched sounds; the bell accentuates the low-pitched ones.

The examination proceeds systematically from apex to base and vice versa until the entire precordium is covered. The stethoscope is moved inch by inch so that no area is missed.

Each portion of the cardiac cycle is listened to in turn. Each sound is evaluated for intensity, variations in intensity, and splitting. If splitting is heard, the nurse notes whether it varies, how it varies, and whether it varies with respiration. This evaluation is repeated in each area of auscultation. After listening to and analyzing the first and second heart sounds, the nurse listens between the sounds.

In systole the nurse should listen for systolic clicks or ejection sounds; in diastole the nurse should listen for an opening snap, an atrial or ventricular gallop, or a third or fourth heart sound. Only after each portion of the cardiac cycle is analyzed should the nurse listen for murmurs in systole or in diastole. Through practice this procedure becomes an automatic part of every cardiac examination.

Initially the client is examined while recumbent. Then, during auscultation of the apex with the bell lightly applied to the chest wall, the client is asked to turn to the left lateral position while the nurse listens for low-frequency murmurs over the mitral area. After the client has returned to the supine position and the rest of the heart examination has been performed, the client is asked to sit, lean forward, exhale, and not breathe; then the pulmonic and aortic areas are examined with the diaphragm pressed firmly against the chest.

EVALUATING THE HEART SOUNDS

Classic Heart Sounds

The classic heart sounds are discrete, relatively brief auditory vibrations of varying intensity, frequency, quality, and duration. The *first sound* (S1) corresponds to the onset of ventricular systole. It is produced by the closure of the mitral and tricuspid valves. It is louder at the apex. This sound is often approximated by the soft sound "lub." The *second sound* (S2) corresponds to the onset of diastole and is due to the closure of the aortic and pulmonary semilunar valves. It sounds like "dup" and is louder at the base. Normally a longer pause occurs after the second sound than after the first. (The former is known as the "lub-dup pause.") This relationship is maintained throughout the normal range of heart rates, although careful examination reveals that the period of diastole, after the second sound, is shortened with faster rates. The development of a pendular, or "tic-toc," rhythm is always pathological.

Splitting. The two ventricles may contract simultaneously or one may slightly lag behind the other. The closure of the atrioventricular valves will be asynchronous and will cause a splitting of the first heart sound. Similarly, if the closure of the semilunar valves is not simultaneous, the second heart sound will split. Valve closure is induced by the pressure differences in the chambers on each side of the valve. These pressures are related to the force of contraction of the chamber behind the valve and to the amount of blood ejected by the chamber. Thus the duration of the filling phase directly affects the timing of valve closure. Splitting of the second sound is normally heard in the pulmonic area (P2) during inspiration because the right ventricle empties more slowly at that time.

In bundle-branch block the conduction to the affected side is delayed. The affected ventricle contracts after the unaffected one. In complete right bundle-branch block, the pulmonic valve always closes late, and this delay increases during inspiration. The split either is constant or will increase during inspiration and still be heard during expiration. In complete left bundle-branch block, the order of closure is reversed. Now the split is heard during expiration. During inspiration the normally late-closing pulmonic valve approaches the now delayed aortic valve. The split tends to disappear, causing a "paradoxical" splitting that widens in expiration.

Splitting of the first heart sound is sometimes heard at the apex. Its cause, a delay in closure of the mitral valve, has little sig-nificance. If this split seems unduly widened, it may indicate a complete bundle-branch block, most commonly of the right bundle.

Intensity. The heart sounds may be of increased intensity. This augmentation frequently indicates an increased force of contraction. The loudness of the sounds is related to the force of the contraction (systole) and the position of the leaflets at the onset of their phase of closure. A prolonged and forceful systolic phase causes the leaflets to remain open longer. These leaflets must then spring back a greater distance during the same short period of time. This action increases the sound. Conversely a diminished systolic force will only partially open the valve, and a prolonged diastole will permit the leaflets to float back. Either of these occurrences will decrease the sounds of valve closure.

The first heart sound (S1) is increased at the apex by events that prolong atrial systole, such as mitral stenosis. The second heart sound (S2) is increased by events that prolong ventricular systole, such as systemic or pulmonary hypertension. The combination of an increased apical S1 with a pulmonary S2 should alert the nurse to the possibility of mitral stenosis and should prompt a search for the apical diastolic murmur.

If ventricular diastole is prolonged, S1 is diminished at the apex. This is the sign of a prolonged P-R interval (discussed later in this chapter) and is found in first-degree atrioventricular block.

Other causes of augmented heart sounds are tachycardia, fever, hyperthyroidism, emotional stress, and anemia. Decreased heart sounds may be due to acquired aortic valve stenosis, myocardial infarction, or any obstruction between the heart and the stethoscope, such as pericardial fluid, left pleural effusion, pulmonary emphysema, and thickening of the chest wall due to muscle or fat.

Other Heart Sounds

In addition to the classic first and second heart sounds (S1 and S2), a third (S3) and fourth (S4) sound may be heard (see figure 6.41). The last two sounds are found under special conditions and may be indicative of serious health problems.

The S3 occurs early in ventricular diastolic filling and is commonly heard in mid-diastole very soon after S2. It is related to passive filling of the ventricle. This sound is rarely normal when found in the elderly. The S4 sound occurs in late diastole or pre-systole. It is due to a forceful atrial contraction and is normally heard in the elderly (Perloff 1977). In pathological conditions, these sounds may form one of the *gallop rhythms.* These are cadenced rhythms characterized by a spacing of the heart sounds in a three- or four-timed rhythm resembling the gallop of a horse. A gallop with the extra sound occurring soon after the second heart sound is called a *protodiastolic,* or *S3, gallop;* one with the extra sound occurring just before the first heart sound is called a *presystolic,* or *S4, gallop.* These gallops always indicate a problem related to ventricular filling. Either the ventricle cannot accept all the blood it receives (S3 gallop) or the intraventricular pressure is elevated at the end of diastole (S4 gallop). When both these conditions occur together, the S3 and S4 combine to cause a loud *summation gallop.*

Sounds audible in systole are called *systolic clicks.* In early systole these are called *ejection clicks.* Others occur in middle and late systole. An *opening snap* is a sound heard at the third or fourth intercostal space to the left of the sternum, with the client in the left lateral position. It is a sharp sound heard soon after S2 and is usually associated with mitral stenosis. A pericardial friction rub sounds like creaking leather in both phases of the cycle and is unrelated to respiration.

FIGURE 6.41   Heart Sounds.

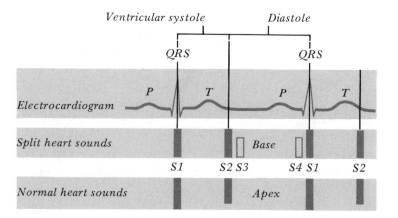

Murmurs

Heart murmurs are abnormal sounds produced when the flow of blood from one chamber to another or from a chamber into a great vessel is associated with increased flow and increased turbulence. This augmentation sets up abnormal vibrations heard as a murmur. Commonly the cause is an abnormality in the region of a valve (see figure 6.42). At that valve the murmur is loudest.

Murmurs may be produced by acquired and congenital defects affecting the heart and the vessels as well as by conditions that increase the rate of blood flow: anemias, fever, hyperthyroidism, and exercise. When these conditions are reversed, the murmur disappears.

Murmurs are described according to their location, timing in the cardiac cycle, quality, pitch, form, and transmission. Only after the murmur has been completely described in these terms can a true assessment be made.

Location. The anatomical location of the murmur is described first. Some murmurs are best heard over the auscultatory projections of the involved valve; others are found along the sternal borders, in the axilla, or at the base of the neck. Murmurs of arterial occlusion (bruits) are heard below the level of occlusion and follow the direction of blood flow. The murmurs of increased venous flow (hums) are localized to the area of increased flow.

Timing. After describing the location of the murmur, the nurse attempts to time the murmur in relation to the cardiac cycle and in particular in relation to the first and

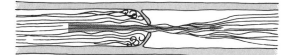

BLOOD FLOW ACROSS A STENOTIC VALVE

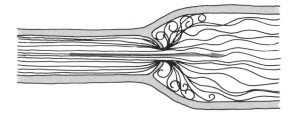

BLOOD FLOW INTO A DIALATED CHAMBER

FIGURE 6.42 Production of Heart Murmurs.

second heart sounds. A murmur that begins with or just after the first sound and ends at the second sound is called *holosystolic* or *pansystolic*. A murmur that begins after the first sound and terminates before the second sound is called *midsystolic*. Murmurs may occur in early, middle, or late systole.

Similar events occur in diastole, which also may be divided into an early, middle, or late portion. A murmur that begins after the second heart sound is called *diastolic* regardless of the phase in which it begins or ends. Early diastole is called *protodiastole* and corresponds to the phase of passive ventricular filling. Late diastole is called *presystole* and corresponds to the time of atrial contraction or active ventricular filling. This period occurs immediately before S1.

A murmur that begins in systole and then continues through S2 into diastole is called *continuous*. Continuous arterial murmurs indicate that a critical obstruction is present.

169

Quality, Intensity, and Pitch. Murmurs may have a soft, blowing quality or they may be harsh, rasping, and rumbling, or even musical, with a whistling quality. As a general rule, murmurs in systole are harsher. A change in quality is associated with a change in the condition causing the murmur.

The murmur should be graded in relation to its intensity or loudness. This classification is done on the basis of six grades. A grade I murmur is very soft. It is often missed if the room is noisy or if the examiner is not listening carefully. Grade II, III, IV, and V murmurs are of increasing intensity. Grade VI murmurs are the loudest and are audible with the stethoscope just off the chest. Murmurs of grade III or louder are usually associated with organic conditions. Those of grade IV or louder are associated with a thrill. An increase in loudness usually indicates an increase in the severity of the condition.

The pitch is related to the speed of blood flow. The faster the flow, the higher the pitch. High-pitched murmurs may sound like a whistle. Murmurs also may be of medium or low pitch.

Form. The form of the murmur is related to the variations of intensity and pitch that the murmur undergoes (see figure 6.43). A *crescendo* murmur progressively increases in intensity from onset to termination. A *decrescendo* murmur decreases in intensity from onset to termination. A *diamond*-shaped murmur increases in intensity during its initial phase and then decreases during the terminal phase (crescendo-decrescendo). A *plateau*-shaped murmur is the same throughout.

In general, the transmission of the murmur is in the direction of the flow of blood. The murmur of aortic stenosis is transmitted into the neck and abdominal aorta. The nurse must attempt to follow the murmur and describe its area of transmission.

Evaluating Murmurs

Systolic. Murmurs occurring between S1 and S2 are systolic and are the most frequently encountered. Two types of murmurs are identified: ejection and regurgitation. These murmurs vary with respiration: those on the right side increase with inspiration, those on the left decrease (Cochrane

FIGURE 6.43   Forms of Murmurs.

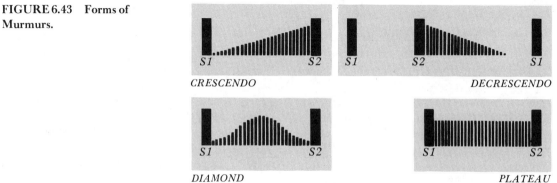

CRESCENDO

DECRESCENDO

DIAMOND

PLATEAU

1978). The evaluation requires assessment of timing, location, and form.

Systolic murmurs associated with *ejection* from the ventricles into the great vessels are usually diamond shaped. Diamond-shaped midsystolic murmurs that start after the first sound and end before the second one are due to semilunar valve stenosis. Those that end before the pulmonary component are due to pulmonic stenosis; they are increased by inspiration, are heard on the left side at the base, and may radiate to the left. If the murmur ends at the aortic component, is heard at the base and the apex, increases with expiration, and radiates into the neck, it is due to aortic stenosis.

Systolic murmurs associated with *regurgitation* are usually holosystolic; they end with and may envelop the second sound. They are usually associated with ventricular septal defect and with atrioventricular valve insufficiency, which permits regurgitation. Systolic murmurs due to tricuspid insufficiency end with the pulmonary component of the second sound and are increased with inspiration. These murmurs are heard over the sternum. If the murmur ends with the aortic component, it is related to a mitral valve insufficiency. These murmurs are heard at the apex and radiate toward the axilla. The murmurs of regurgitation are usually plateau shaped (Perloff 1977).

Diastolic. Diastolic murmurs begin in the pause between S2 and S1. Two types of diastolic murmurs may be recognized by the nurse; regurgitant and ventricular-filling murmurs.

Regurgitant murmurs result from insufficiency of the aortic and pulmonary valves and are usually pandiastolic. They begin with maximal intensity immediately after S2 and then decrease in intensity (decrescendo) during diastole. The murmur of pulmonary insufficiency is accentuated by inspiration and valsalva (Cochrane 1978). It is heard at the third intercostal space at the left sternal border. The aortic murmur of regurgitation is heard at the base and at the apex. It is heard best in expiration and is decreased by inspiration and by valsalva.

Ventricular-filling murmurs are low pitched and occur in middiastole. They are due to stenosis of the atrioventricular valves. Initially these murmurs are decrescendo, but as the condition worsens they extend toward the S1 and develop a terminal crescendo component. They obey the same rules of inspiratory augmentation on the right and expiratory augmentation on the left.

The nurse must recognize the presence of the murmur and describe its location and qualities. An accurate description will lead to appropriate care and permit the nurse to follow the evolution of the condition and the results of treatment.

The Arrhythmias

Many arrhythmias may be assessed by evaluation of the apical and peripheral pulses and by cardiac auscultation. Others may be extremely confusing and require electrocardiography for elucidation. We will discuss here the common disturbances of cardiac rhythm and the clinical findings associated with them.

Normal Sinus Rhythm. The heart possesses an automaticity that comes from the regular, spontaneous depolarization of the sinus node. The spread of the electrical impulse to the atria, to the atrioventricular (A-V) node, and into the bundle of His and its branches is a temporal process that is clearly seen on the electrocardiogram (see figure 6.44). This image is composed of a series of waves and lines induced on the surface of the skin by the sum of electrical activity occurring in the heart from moment to moment in the cardiac cycle. The first wave is called the *P wave* and is the electrical invasion of the atria. The P wave is followed by an isoelectric line, during which time the impulse invades the A-V node. Next follows a small negative wave, the *Q wave*. The interval between the beginning of the P wave and the end of the isoelectric line is called the *P-R interval*. This normally lasts for 0.13 to 0.21 seconds. Some variation of the P-R interval, within the normal range, may occasionally be noted in a phenomenon called *shifting atrial pacemaker* (see figure 6.45).

FIGURE 6.44 Normal Sinus Rhythm at 72 Beats per Minute.
Each small box is 0.04 seconds. The P-R interval is 0.18 seconds; QRS is 0.08; and R-R is 0.81. This tracing is a modified lead II rhythm strip.

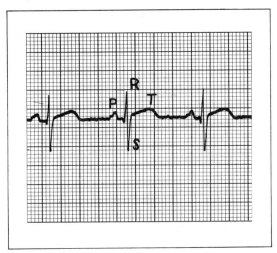

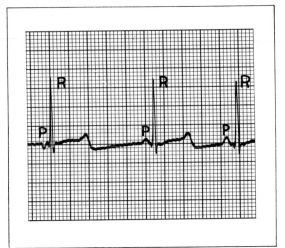

FIGURE 6.45 Shifting Atrial Pacemaker.
Note the change in appearance of the P. The P-R varies from 0.14 to 0.16 seconds; R-R is 1.08 seconds and regular. (Modified lead II rhythm strip.)

The small negative Q wave signals the beginning of the electrical invasion of the ventricles. This wave is followed by a positive wave called *R* and another negative one called *S*. These three waves, the *QRS complex,* are the summation of the electrical activity of ventricular depolarization. The normal QRS interval lasts from 0.05 to 0.11 seconds.

The QRS complex is followed by an isoelectric line, the *S-T interval,* and then by a final wave, the *T,* which may be upright or inverted. Depressions or elevations of the S-T interval and changes of direction of the T wave reflect myocardial nutrition and oxygenation (see figure 6.46). (A discussion of these various changes is beyond the scope of this book.)

Normally, at a given rate the interval from R wave to R wave is fixed from beat to beat. Auscultation confirms that this interval is equal to the interval from S1 to S1. A

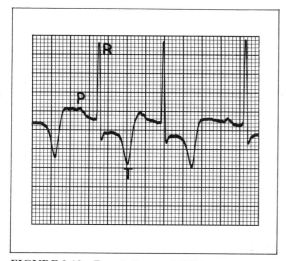

FIGURE 6.46   Deeply Inverted T Wave Associated with S-T Depression. *(Modified lead II rhythm strip.)*

Sinus Tachycardia. In sinus tachycardia, the rhythm is perfectly regular but the rate is greater than 100 beats per minute for at least three successive beats. The electrocardiogram shows a normal P-R interval and a normal QRS complex. Only the rate is increased. Sinus tachycardia rarely occurs at rates above 140 per minute. This condition may be due to exercise, fever, emotional stress, thyrotoxicosis, anemia, or congestive heart failure.

Sinus Bradycardia. In sinus bradycardia the rate is less than 60 beats per minute for at least three successive beats. The rhythm is perfectly regular, with possibly a minor variation related to respiration. The electrocardiogram reveals normal complexes at a slow rate.

Extrasystoles. Extrasystoles, also known as *premature* or *ectopic beats,* are common in the elderly. Two principle varieties of extrasystoles exist: the atrial and the ventricular premature beat. The *atrial premature beat* arises from an abnormal impulse focus in the atrium. This abnormal im-

normal rhythmic variation, called *sinus arrhythmia,* may occur, with slowing on inspiration and speeding up on expiration. Here the P-R interval is fixed from beat to beat and the total number of beats per minute is the same from minute to minute (see figure 6.47).

FIGURE 6.47   Sinus Arrhythmia. *The P-R is 0.21 seconds; the R-R varies from 0.92 seconds to 0.8 seconds in a rhythmical manner with the phases of respiration. Note the inverted T and depressed S-T. (Modified lead II rhythm strip.)*

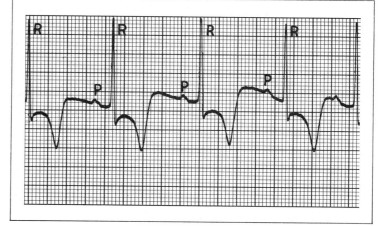

pulse discharges the sinus node and invades the ventricles more quickly than normal. The sinus node then discharges at a normal interval after the premature beat. Auscultation reveals a beat occurring sooner than normal, followed by a normal sequence of beats. This early beat may be louder than normal. The peripheral pulse reveals a premature beat that is weaker than normal; or the beat may not be transmitted at all, giving the appearance of a dropped beat, and is followed by beats in normal sequence. The electrocardiogram shows a small P wave with a P-R interval that is shorter than normal; the QRS complex is normal (see figure 6.48).

The *ventricular premature beat* arises from an abnormal impulse focus in a ventricle. This impulse is not transmitted to the atria and causes the ventricles to contract in an abnormal, uncoordinated fashion. Then, when the sinus node discharges at the normal time, the ventricles are refractory, are not excited, and do not contract until the next sinus discharge. This irregularity gives rise to a long pause after the ventricular premature beat (compensatory pause). Cardiac auscultation reveals that the premature beat occurs close to the preceding normal beat and is often louder than normal. The premature beat is followed by the long compensatory pause and then by the normal sequence of beats. The peripheral pulse examination reveals a weaker than normal beat occurring earlier than expected. This beat is followed first by a long pause and then by a normal sequence of beats. Often the pulse after the pause is stronger because of the delay and the associated increased filling of the ventricle. The electrocardiogram reveals a grossly abnormal QRS complex that is wider than nor-

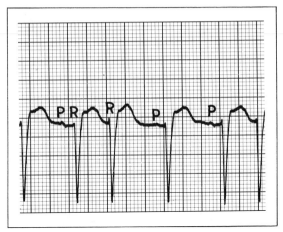

FIGURE 6.48   **Premature Atrial Contractions.**
Normal sinus rhythm is at 100 beats per minute. The third beat is premature. Note that the R-R interval following the premature beat is the same as the interval between two normal beats at 0.59 seconds. (Modified lead II rhythm strip.)

mal (greater than 0.11 seconds), slurred in appearance, and usually followed by a T wave whose deflection is opposite the main deflection of the QRS complex (see figure 6.49). Premature ventricular beats may alternate with normal beats, causing a *bigeminal* (every other beat) or *trigeminal* (every third beat) pulse.

The Tachyarrhythmias

Atrial Tachycardia. Atrial tachycardia is a series of three or more atrial premature contractions occurring in sequence. The pulse and auscultatory findings reveal a rapid, regular rate usually between 150 and 200 beats per minute. The electrocardiographic image is that of a series of premature atrial beats and normal QRS complex (see figure 6.50). Frequently the P wave is difficult to see. If this arrhythmia occurs in bursts that resolve to normal sinus rhythm, it is called *paroxysmal atrial tachycardia.*

174

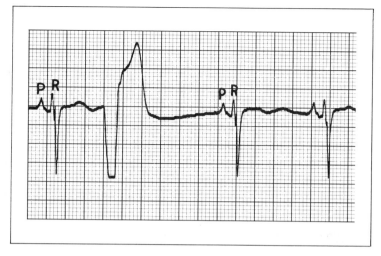

FIGURE 6.49 Premature Ventricular Contractions.

Normal sinus rhythm is at 62 beats per minute. The second beat is premature; the QRS is bizarre, widened, and slurred. The T wave deflection is opposite the main QRS deflection. Following the PVC is a long (compensatory) pause greater than the normal R-R interval (0.99 seconds). The normal P is buried in the abnormal QRS. (Modified lead II rhythm strip.)

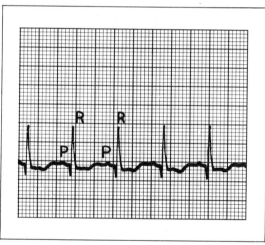

FIGURE 6.50 Atrial Tachycardia at 130 Beats per Minute.

Note the small P with a P-R of 0.12 seconds. (Modified lead II rhythm strip.)

Atrial Flutter. Atrial flutter is a more rapid tachycardia with the atria contracting at a rate above 240 beats per minute. The ventricles cannot follow at this rate, a block is present, and the ventricles beat at a rate of one-half (2:1), one-third (3:1), one-

quarter (4:1), or less. Pulse and auscultation reveal a rapid rate that may appear slightly irregular. The electrocardiogram shows abnormal atrial waves, called *f waves*, which occur in a rapid, regular sawtoothed sequence and upon which are grafted the normal-appearing QRS complexes (see figure 6.51).

Atrial Fibrillation. Atrial fibrillation is an arrhythmia characterized by a very rapid and irregular atrial rhythm at a rate of over 300 beats per minute. The ventricular response to these impulses is equally variable in rate and in rhythm. Thus the ventricular contraction occurs at different moments in the filling cycle. The resultant pulse is variable in force and timing from beat to beat.

Auscultation reveals sounds varying in frequency and loudness. A discrepancy called the *apical-pulse deficit* often occurs between the pulse and the apical beat. This irregularity is the hallmark of atrial fibrillation. Electrocardiographic findings mirror these events. The P wave is absent and is replaced by a wavering line. The normal

175

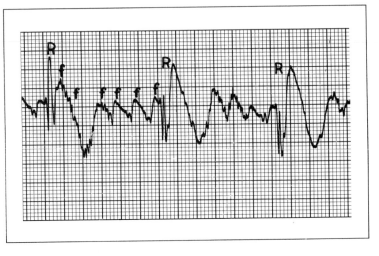

FIGURE 6.51 Atrial Flutter with 6:1 Block.

Note the flutter waves at 270 per minute and the QRS at 45 per minute. The rate of the QRS determines the peripheral and apical pulses. (Modified lead II rhythm strip.)

QRS complexes occur at totally irregular intervals (see figure 6.52).

Other tachyarrhythmias include ventricular fibrillation and ventricular flutter. These conditions require electrocardiography for assessment and are beyond the scope of this book.

The Bradyarrhythmias (Heart Block)

The bradyarrhythmias appear clinically as slow rates and must be separated from

FIGURE 6.52 Atrial Fibrillation.

Note the absence of any discernible P waves and the total irregularity of the R-R intervals. The rate here is at 82 beats per minute. The variations in R-R cause a marked variation in ventricular filling and may cause an apical-pulse deficit. (Modified lead II rhythm strip.)

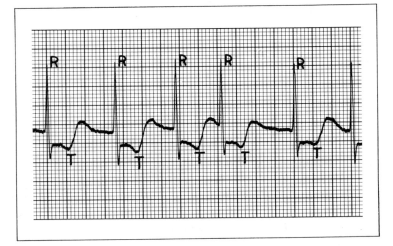

sinus bradycardia. In the heart block situation, the atrial impulse is prevented from passing to the ventricles. Heart blocks are divided into first, second, and third degree atrioventricular (A-V) blocks.

First Degree A-V Block. In first degree block the P-R interval is prolonged beyond 0.20 seconds. This condition is associated with a decreased first heart sound at the apex (see figure 6.53).

Second Degree A-V Block. In classic second degree block the ventricular rate is

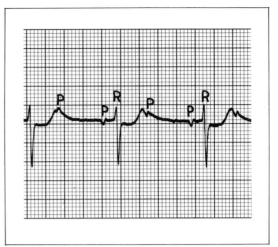

FIGURE 6.54   Second Degree A-V Block.
The regular sinus rhythm is at 130 beats per minute; the ventricular response is at 65 beats per minute. Two regularly spaced P waves precede each QRS. The P-R is 0.17. The first P wave is seen superimposed on the T wave of the preceding complex. The atria are beating at 130 per minute. (Modified lead II rhythm strip.)

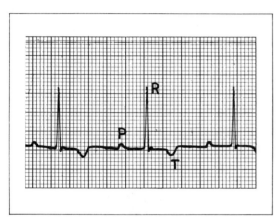

FIGURE 6.53   First Degree A-V Block.
The regular sinus rhythm is at 68 beats per minute. The P-R is 0.28 seconds. (Modified lead II rhythm strip.)

slowed as the ventricle beats for every second, third, or fourth atrial impulse. If the nurse examines the jugular pulse while auscultating the apex, several "a" waves will be noted for each ventricular beat. On the electrocardiogram, several P waves are seen for each ventricular complex (see figure 6.54). The block is classified according to the number of P waves that occur prior to each QRS complex: in a 2:1 block two P waves occur prior to each QRS; in 3:1 and 4:1 blocks three and four waves, respectively, occur prior to each QRS.

A variant of the second degree block is the Winckeback phenomenon, in which the block is irregular—for example, 3:2, 5:4, and so on (see figure 6.55).

Third Degree A-V Block. In third degree block atrial impulse is no longer conducted to the ventricles. The atria beat at their own rate, while the ventricles beat independently, usually at less than 50 beats per minute. Auscultation reveals a slow ventricular rate with a first heart sound of varying intensity. The electrocardiogram reveals that the P waves are progressing

177

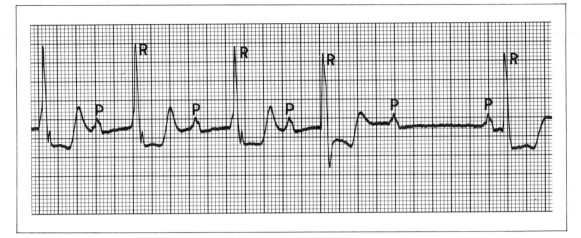

FIGURE 6.55   Winckeback (2°) A-V Block (4:3).
Note the progressive prolongation of the P-R. The fifth P is not followed by QRS. The interval after the sixth P is the shortest P-R. (Modified lead II rhythm strip.)

regularly at their own rate, while the QRS complexes are occurring at their own, usually slower, rate (see figure 6.56).

Other types of heart block, such as the bundle-branch block, may be evaluated by means of the electrocardiogram. Further discussion of electrocardiographic interpretation is beyond the scope of this book.

The clinical importance of the heart blocks lies in their ability to cause a severe bradycardia. This disorder leads to diminished cerebral perfusion, to the development of Stokes-Adams attacks with seizures, or to congestive heart failure because of the inability of the heart to respond to peripheral needs.

FIGURE 6.56   Third Degree A-V Block.
The atria (P waves) are beating at 150, and the ventricles (QRS complexes) at 52 per minute. The lack of relationship between the two is shown by the patternless changes in the P-R. (Modified lead II rhythm strip.)

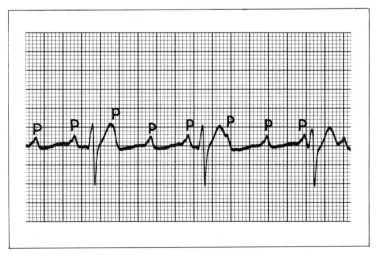

178

Any of the cardiac arrhythmias may be encountered in the elderly. Their detection and proper treatment constitute an important part of the cardiology of old age (Harris 1970). The nurse must be aware of the associated findings and their implications for the treatment and management of the older client.

REFERENCES

COCHRANE, P. T. 1978. "Bedside Aids to Auscultation of the Heart." *Journal of the American Medical Association* 239:54–55.

HARRIS, R. 1970. *The Management of Geriatric Cardiovascular Disease.* Philadelphia: J. B. Lippincott.

KENNEDY, R. D., and F. I. CAIRD. 1972. "Application of the Minnesota Code to Population Studies of the Electrocardiogram in the Elderly." *Gerontological Clinics* 14:5–16.

PERLOFF, J. K. 1977. "A Practical Guide to Revised Auscultatory Terms." *Primary Cardiology* 3:14–19.

RODSTEIN, M. 1956. "The Characteristics of Nonfatal Myocardial Infarction in the Aged." *Archives of Internal Medicine* 98:84–90.

SLEIGHT, P. 1962. "Unilateral Elevation of the Internal Jugular Pulse." *British Heart Journal* 24:726–30.

UNIT 11: THE GASTROINTESTINAL SYSTEM

The gastrointestinal system is composed of the digestive tract and its accessory organs. Apart from the mouth and esophagus, this system is almost entirely within the abdomen. In the older client complaints relating to the gastrointestinal tract become increasingly prominent. Anorexia, heartburn, dyspepsia, gas, and constipation are commonly encountered and present the nurse with the problem of separating the functional from the organic. Frequently the client's fears become so intense that this separation taxes the skills of even the best trained clinician.

Actual aging changes have been documented. In addition to the loss of teeth and diminished taste and smell, diminished secretion, absorption, and motility all play some role in the frequency of digestive problems.

If the nurse is to help clients, a thorough evaluation must be performed so that appropriate decisions regarding management may be made. This unit reviews the subjective and objective findings as they relate to the elderly client.

For descriptive purposes two different ways of dividing the abdomen have been developed (see figure 6.57). The classic method uses two horizontal and two vertical lines to divide the abdomen into nine regions. One horizontal line extends through the lowest point of the tenth costal cartilages, and the other extends through

FIGURE 6.57   Topographical Divisions of the Abdomen.

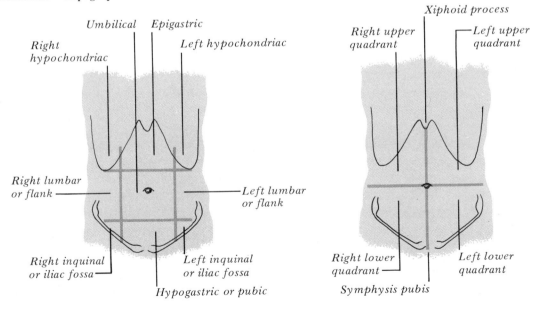

NINE REGIONS   FOUR QUADRANTS

the two iliac tuberosities. The vertical lines are parallel to, and on each side of, the midline groove and halfway from the midline to a line extending upward from the anterior iliac spine. Alternatively a vertical midline and a horizontal line crossing at the umbilicus divide the abdomen into four quadrants (figure 6.57).

HEALTH HISTORY AND SUBJECTIVE FINDINGS

The assessment of the gastrointestinal tract is extremely dependent on a thorough history. Frequently, objective findings are few, and routine x-ray examinations may not provide diagnostic information.

Dysphagia is the inability to swallow easily. Clients complain that food sticks in their throats. The nurse must distinguish this problem from the inability to initiate swallowing, where the bolus remains in the mouth. In true dysphagia food descends to some point in the esophagus where it either sticks or slowly descends. Dysphagia may be *progressive:* at first the difficulty is only with firm solids, such as roast beef, and can be overcome by chewing more thoroughly. This difficulty becomes more severe, until only liquids are tolerated. Clients often indicate that sticking occurs in the distal esophagus by pointing to the xiphoid. Painless, progressive dysphagia is usually due to neoplasm (Edwards 1976).

Dysphagia may be *intermittent*. In the oropharynx intermittent dysphagia is usually associated with dry mouth and the feeling of a lump in the throat. This "globus hystericus," found more commonly in the anxious client, should not be confused with true dysphagia. Distal intermittent dysphagia is more common in elderly than in younger clients. Typically it

occurs when the client eats meat, and long periods of time may pass between episodes. This type of intermittent dysphagia is usually associated with a lower esophageal constriction ring (Pope 1978).

Inability to initiate swallowing may be associated with oropharyngeal conditions such as the pain of a sore throat, a neuromuscular weakness such as pseudobulbar palsy, or Parkinson's disease (Edwards 1976).

Pyrosis, or heartburn, is the most common esophageal complaint. It indicates esophageal irritation and is most commonly due to the reflux of gastric acid. When aggravated by recumbency, it indicates the presence of *chalasia,* an incompetent lower esophageal sphincter (Scheurer and Halter 1976). This condition is frequently associated with obesity and hiatal hernia. Pyrosis is often induced by citrus juices, spicy tomato juice, and carbonated beverages. It frequently indicates *esophagitis,* an esophageal inflammation due to refluxed gastric acid.

Odynophagia is painful swallowing. It is commonly associated with severe esophageal inflammation. The sensation of food sticking and slowly descending is associated with pain.

Regurgitation is the effortless return of material from the esophagus without vomiting. In chalasia the material is sour and may be described as hot. Both in *achalasia,* a neurogenic esophageal obstruction, and in obstructing carcinoma the material is frequently foul. If the client describes the regurgitated food as bland tasting and undigested, some type of esophageal obstruction must be suspected.

Abdominal complaints may be related to any of the functions of the digestive tract, including transport, digestion, and absorp-

181

tion. The complaints consist of abdominal pain or discomfort, nausea and vomiting, belching, loss of appetite, diarrhea or constipation, jaundice, hematemesis, and melena.

Abdominal Pain and Discomfort

Three kinds of abdominal pain may be encountered: somatic, visceral, and viscerosomatic.

Somatic pain is mediated through the cerebrospinal system and is characterized by its precisely localized nature. It is encountered in cases of pain disorders of the abdominal wall and with inflammation of the parietal peritoneum (peritonitis) through the peritoneocutaneous reflex.

Visceral pain is less precisely localized and may be vaguely related to a certain region or to the midline. It is found in the early stages of inflammation or dysfunction of a hollow viscus, early acute appendicitis, the imprecise gnawing of peptic ulcer, and the vague discomfort of inflammatory bowel disease.

Viscerosomatic, or referred, pain is indicative of a worsening intraabdominal inflammation. The inflammation spreads from the viscus to the parietal peritoneum and sensation spreads into the cerebrospinal system. Localization is precise, usually away from the midline, and referred into the dermatome of the nerves of the involved organ. For a more complete discussion of visceral pain, the reader should consult texts of human physiology or gastroenterology.

Assessing Abdominal Pain

The correct assessment of abdominal pain requires a complete description, which will also diminish the number of examinations. All details must be obtained, including the location and character of the pain, aggravating conditions, ameliorating conditions, evolution and duration, and associated phenomena.

Location. The degree of preciseness or vagueness of the pain aids in determining the cause and location. Upper abdominal localization helps exclude the left transverse, descending, and sigmoid colon, as well as the rectum and contiguous structures. Pain in these organs is felt more commonly in the low abdomen.

Character. The severity of the pain may range from a mild discomfort or "indigestion" to the severe, sharply localized point of a perforated appendix. In the elderly pain is usually less precisely felt and localized (Ponka et al. 1963). Cramping usually means an increase in peristaltic activity and may indicate bowel obstruction or irritation of a hollow viscus. Steady pain is more consistent with an inflammatory reaction in an organ, such as a duodenal ulcer.

Aggravating Conditions. Digestive disorders are frequently related to eating. Ascertaining the effect of eating upon the symptomatology is useful. The time between eating and the onset of the discomfort should be noted. In *peptic esophagitis,* heartburn begins immediately after the offending substance is ingested or after the client lies down. In *gastric ulcer* a pain-free period of thirty minutes to one hour precedes the steady gnawing. In *regional enteritis* the cramping pain is frequently relieved by eating but begins again thirty minutes after completion of the meal.

Ameliorating Conditions. The nurse ascertains the effect of fasting. Peptic ulcer is frequently pain free after an eight- to twelve-hour overnight fast. The nurse should ask about the effect of eating, the ingestion of alkali, and the evacuation of bowels and bladder. Relief afforded by alkali or by the ingestion of food usually indicates peptic ulceration, whereas relief afforded by bowel movements points toward the bowel as the source of pain.

Evolution and Duration. An attempt to have the client describe the evolution and duration of pain is extremely important. Biliary colic is epigastric, frequently begins at night, is severe or progressive, and typically resolves with vomiting. Pancreatic pain, also in the epigastrium, is severe, persistent, and unaffected by vomiting. Peptic ulcer is epigastric; usually increases in severity over the course of days, weeks, or months; and is relieved by vomiting. The nurse should determine if the client ever has a pain-free period. Small-bowel disease causes cramping frequently relieved by the bowel movement; the cramping then reappears and remains until the next bowel movement. Pain caused by carcinoma of a viscus occurs with gradually increasing severity. Biliary colic rarely lasts for more than forty-eight hours; pain due to pancreatitis may continue for several days.

Associated Phenomena. The nurse should evaluate the effect of the pain on the client's lifestyle. Pain that awakens the client at night is usually indicative of an organic disorder. An association with diarrhea points toward the bowel. Vomiting may indicate obstruction if associated with severe constipation for both stool and gas.

Nausea and Vomiting

Complaints of nausea and vomiting are nonspecific. They may be due to a disorder of the intestinal tract but are also found with disorders of organic and psychic origin. Pain, bad odors, anxiety, or medications may induce vomiting. To determine if these complaints are related to a disorder of the gut, the nurse looks for other associated findings. Dietary indiscretions, cramping, and diarrhea may indicate acute disorders. Recurrent vomiting in a client with a history of peptic complaints might indicate pyloric obstruction. An association of cramping pain, obstipation, and foul vomitus points toward an intestinal obstruction. The nurse must identify the nature and character of the vomitus, its degree of chronicity, its color, and the presence of undigested food or any particular odor. The nurse must also differentiate vomiting from regurgitation.

Belching and Loss of Appetite

Belching and loss of appetite are extremely nonspecific. When associated with gastrointestinal disorders, they are usually accompanied by other phenomena.

Diarrhea or Constipation

A distinction must be made as to the character of the diarrhea. A client suffering from diarrhea often has a long-standing constipation related to a diet deficient in bulk. Frequently the client uses laxatives that cause loose, watery bowel movements.

Further differentiation requires knowledge of the nature and frequency of the bowel movements. Large, bulky, greasy stools that float are found in malabsorption; the diminished absorption of fats leads to the formation of intestinal soaps and diarrhea. Intestinal inflammation causes irritation with the passage of frequent watery stools. An association of diarrhea and *hematochezia* (blood in the stool) should alert the nurse to the presence of intestinal disease. These situations are commonly indicative of bowel carcinoma and ulcerative colitis. Diarrhea that awakens the client at night is always due to organic disease of the intestine.

Constipation is most commonly functional and due to diminished dietary fiber (Burkitt et al. 1972). When the constipation is of recent onset or is becoming progressively severe, the nurse must be alert to the possibility of a bowel tumor. Constipation alternating with diarrhea is a classic presentation of a cancer of the descending colon.

These findings may be associated with emotional difficulties. Depression is frequently heralded by an association of constipation, anorexia, and insomnia. Diarrhea may be induced by anxiety. It behooves the careful nurse faced with a bowel-habit change to investigate the possibility of a gastrointestinal disorder.

Jaundice

Jaundice, a yellow discoloration of the skin, must be distinguished from carotenemia. In clients who may have jaundice, the nurse attempts to ascertain the presence of other complaints that help in the differentiation. An associated itching often indicates biliary obstruction due to a common duct stone, a carcinoma of the head of the pancreas, or a carcinoma of the common bile duct. Classic carcinomatous obstruction of the bile duct is painless. Biliary colic may indicate the presence of a stone.

Other causes of jaundice include hepatic disorders such as infectious or toxic hepatitis. A history of blood transfusions or the use of drugs or medication should be sought.

Hematemesis and Melena

In all clients with complaints of vomiting, the nurse should determine the color of the vomitus. *Hematemesis* may look like coffee grounds, indicating partially digested blood, or it may be dark or bright red in color, indicating fresh bleeding.

Fresh bleeding may be induced by forceful vomiting. In these cases the vomitus is initially clear, followed by the blood. Hematemesis always indicates that the bleeding source is above the angle of Trietz, at the junction of the duodenum and the jejunum.

Melena is the passage of black stool containing digested blood. It usually indicates that the bleeding has occurred above the descending colon. Bleeding in the descending colon is usually red or dark but rarely black. In the elderly with decreased bowel frequency, blood passed in the descending colon may be quite dark.

Hematemesis and melena may be induced by bleeding from the nose and pharynx or from any point in the gut. Certain drugs, such as acetylsalicylic acid and reserpine, are associated with gastrointestinal bleeding.

EXAMINATION AND OBJECTIVE FINDINGS

The examination of the gastrointestinal system must be systematic. The nurse care-

184

fully examines the mouth and pharynx as well as the supraclavicular area for adenopathy before proceeding to the abdomen.

The esophagus may be directly evaluated by a physician using an esophagoscope or indirectly by means of barium-contrast x-rays. The radiologist must be made aware of the clinical presentation so that special swallowing studies or maneuvers may be performed.

The order of examination of the abdomen is inspection, auscultation, percussion, and palpation. The client is relaxed and recumbent with the head elevated on a pillow and the arms at the sides or across the chest; the abdomen is exposed but dignity is maintained by draping. The abdominal musculature should be relaxed.

Inspection

Inspection is performed in good light. The nurse looks at the condition of the abdominal wall, the contour of the abdomen, movements of the abdominal wall and movements of the abdominal contents seen through the abdominal wall.

Condition of the Abdominal Wall. The nurse observes first the general symmetry of the abdominal wall, the condition of the skin, and the client's general state of nutrition. The presence of any obvious mass is noted. The skin condition should be similar to that of the rest of the body; the presence of silver stria (streaks) in the lower quadrants may be due to ascites or a large weight gain. Color changes such as jaundice or increased pigment are noted.

The skin may be taut and glistening in the presence of large intraabdominal tumors or ascites, and enlarged veins of the abdominal wall may indicate portal or inferior vena caval obstruction. Inferior vena caval obstruction will cause venous distension in the lateral abdominal veins. These veins fill from below. Portal vein obstruction causes the development of dilated veins in the central abdomen. These flow away from the umbilicus. Portal vein obstruction is most commonly associated with cirrhosis. Venous flow may be determined by the technique of milking.

The nurse looks for local herniations along the midline. These are more common near the umbilicus and in the epigastrium.

Abdominal Contour. The nurse looks for swelling and, if it is present, notes whether it is localized or symmetrical. Generalized, symmetrical swelling is found with obesity, simple distension, and ascites. Tumors of internal organs cause swelling localized to the area of the involvement. Large tumors, particularly of the ovary, may appear to cause symmetrical swelling. Localized low abdominal swelling may be seen in clients with overfilled bladders due to prostatic obstruction, pelvic tumors, and tumors of the sigmoid colon.

Movements of the Abdominal Wall and Abdominal Contents. Normally the abdomen participates in the movements of respiration. These motions are blocked with acute peritonitis. If peritonitis is generalized, the entire abdomen is rigid. In localized problems, such as cholecystitis or appendicitis, the rigidity is localized to the involved area. Rarely, in thin clients with long-standing intestinal obstruction, movements of the bowel may be seen.

185

Auscultation

Auscultation is performed next, as palpation of the abdomen may alter the auscultatory findings. The diaphragm is used and is lightly placed against the skin. The nurse listens for bowel sounds, vascular bruits, rubs, and succussion splash. The stethoscope is placed first in the upper left and right quadrants, then in the lower ones, and then on the midline.

Bowel Sounds. Bowel sounds are produced by peristalsis. Changes of importance are the absence of any sounds after several minutes of listening and the presence of increased, loud rushes of a high-pitched, tinkling quality. Sounds are absent in cases of generalized peritonitis; rushes are usually associated with intestinal obstruction.

Vascular Bruits. Vascular bruits are associated with increased turbulence in an artery and indicate partial occlusion.

Rubs. Intraabdominal rubs have the same significance as pleural rubs. In splenic infarction a rub may be heard over the spleen. A rub over the liver indicates malignancy. Rubs are timed to the movements of respiration.

Succussion Splash. Succussion splash may be heard in the epigastrium when the client is shaken. It indicates fluid and air in the stomach and, if present several hours after eating, reveals a delay in gastric emptying. This condition may be due to pyloric obstruction.

Percussion

Though of limited value, percussion can reveal the presence of fluid, distension, tumors, and visceral enlargement. In general, light percussion provides the most information as it yields a clearer note. Distension is revealed by a tympanitic note; solid viscera give one that is dull. Percussion is performed systematically, first on the left and then on the right side. The examination begins in the chest with the pleximeter finger placed parallel to the ribs. The nurse percusses downward toward the abdomen along the left midaxillary line. The normal resonance of the lung should change to a tympanitic one at the diaphragm.

Dullness above the ninth intercostal space raises the possibility of *splenomegaly*. Slight splenic enlargement may be demonstrated by dullness to percussion in the lowest intercostal space, on the anterior axillary line, while the client takes a deep breath. But consolidation of the left lower lung or left pleural effusion invalidates this diagnosis.

The nurse repeats the procedure on the right side. The passage from resonance to dullness indicates the upper limit of the liver, normally near the sixth intercostal space. The lower limit of liver dullness is found normally at the costal margin. The normal liver span should not exceed twelve centimeters.

The rest of the abdomen is percussed. Normally the abdomen is tympanitic. Ascites may be demonstrated by percussion. With the client lying face up, ascitic fluid gravitates to the flanks, causes these to bulge, and creates bilateral flank dullness and a central area of tympany due to the intestinal loops. The nurse percusses from the midline toward the flanks and marks the skin at the point of transition from tympany to dullness. The client is turned onto the right side and percussion is again performed from the midline to the flanks. If ascites is present, the fluid shifts to the dependent right flank while the tympanitic bowel moves up toward the left flank. The line of dullness shifts toward the abdominal midline. This *shifting dullness* indicates free fluid in the peritoneal cavity. The procedure is repeated with the client turned onto the left side.

Another finding in ascites is the *fluid wave*. Again the client lies face up. The nurse places the palm of the left hand on the client's right flank and an assistant or the client places the ulnar edge of the hand lightly on the abdominal midline. The nurse's right hand then sharply strikes the client's left flank. Ascites, if present, induces a wave that strikes the nurse's hand placed on the client's right flank. The hand pressing on the midline prevents transmission of the shock through the tissues of the abdominal wall. Ascites may be due to cirrhosis of the liver, intraabdominal malignancy, vena caval obstruction, and congestive heart failure.

Palpation

Palpation is the most difficult and most rewarding part of the examination. Successful palpation requires good relaxation of the client's abdominal muscles. The client is recumbent with the head on a pillow and the arms at the sides or folded on the chest. The nurse instructs the client to breathe quietly through an open mouth. When the abdomen is moving freely, the nurse begins palpation, using the flat of the hand. The fingertips are used to exert pressure only after palpation with the flat of the hand has been completed. Fingertip pressure may be painful and cause the client to reflexly tense the abdominal muscles, preventing an adequate examination. Light palpation permits an estimation of the de-

gree of persistent muscle tone, reassures the client regarding the production of pain, and affords an initial impression about areas of differing resistance. These areas may indicate the existence of masses, enlarged organs, or localized areas of inflammation. If the abdomen remains tense, the nurse must distinguish between voluntary tensing due to nervousness or fear and reflex rigidity due to peritoneal inflammation. In all cases localized rigidity is more suggestive of an abnormality. Further relaxation may be obtained by having the client flex the thighs and knees. This position may be useful for a client with a very muscular abdomen.

The purposes of palpation are to find painful areas, to determine the presence of rebound tenderness and rigidity, to determine the existence of organomegaly or masses, and to recognize the existence of hernias in the abdominal wall.

Painful Areas. Pain elicited by palpation is called *tenderness*. If the client's history has given clues about the site of expected tenderness, the examination should begin away from this area. Thus if the client complains of right lower quadrant pain, the examination begins in the left lower quadrant. The nurse should compare the findings of the first area with those of the suspected region. Once a tender area is located, the nurse maintains pressure in that area to determine if the tenderness is constant. If the pain disappears with maintained pressure, inflammation is unlikely. Such tenderness probably relates to the contraction or distension of a viscus. Tenderness of inflammation tends to persist or worsen.

Tenderness in the abdominal wall may be distinguished by having the client tense the abdomen during palpation of the tender area. The client is asked to cross arms over the chest and attempt to sit up while the nurse continues to palpate the area. If the pain is located in the abdominal wall, it will remain the same or will worsen. If the pain is due to an intraabdominal disorder, it should lessen or disappear as the tensed muscles protect the viscera. Tenderness associated with localized abdominal rigidity suggests an intraabdominal origin.

A special form of tenderness, called *rebound tenderness,* is highly suggestive of intraabdominal inflammation. To distinguish rebound tenderness, the nurse applies pressure in an area distant from the tender one and then suddenly releases the pressure. If the client complains of a sharp stab of pain in the suspected area, an inflamed viscus and associated peritonitis are indicated. If sharp pain is produced during gentle palpation when the client coughs or strains, widespread peritonitis is evident.

Organ Enlargement or Masses. The nurse palpates for the enlargement of organs—in particular, the liver, spleen, and kidneys. If an organ is found to be enlarged, the nurse must determine its location, degree of enlargement, consistency, form, and degree of tenderness.

Palpation of the liver is performed with the fingers parallel or perpendicular to the edge of the organ. The nurse should begin in the right lower quadrant to avoid missing a massive enlargement. The nurse is on the client's right and palpates with the right hand. The examining fingers are pressed firmly against the abdomen with a slight upward pressure. If no resistance is encountered, the hand is moved upward until the fingers are under the right costal margin. If resistance is felt or if the hand is at the costal margin, the client is asked to take a deep breath. A firm edge will be felt to strike the fingers. If the edge descends more than one centimeter below the costal margin, the liver is abnormally enlarged.

The nurse attempts to palpate the entire edge of the liver and to determine whether it is smooth or irregular. Next the nurse attempts to feel whether the edge is thin and sharp or thick and blunt. Finally the nurse attempts to feel whether the organ is soft, firm, hard, or rock hard. For the enlarged liver, the observation includes a description of the surface smoothness, granularity, or gross irregularity.

Hepatomegaly may be due to congestive heart failure, inflammation, fatty infiltration, cirrhosis, or infiltration with tumor. Each of these conditions will cause a different combination of palpable findings. Tender, soft enlargement is usually associated with inflammation and congestion (e.g., hepatitis and heart failure); painless, soft, smooth enlargement is associated with fat; a hard, thin, granular feeling is produced by cirrhosis; and a hard, grossly irregular liver indicates tumorous enlargement.

Palpation of the spleen is performed with the nurse on the client's right with the left arm extended over the client's abdomen so that the left hand is placed in the left costovertebral angle. This hand will exert pressure to move the spleen anteriorly. The right hand is placed so that the fingers exert pressure into the left hypochondrium and under the left anterior costal margin. The client is then told to take a deep breath. If the spleen is enlarged, it is felt to slide forward and strike the fingers of the right hand. A normal spleen is not palpable. If the spleen is not felt but the nurse suspects

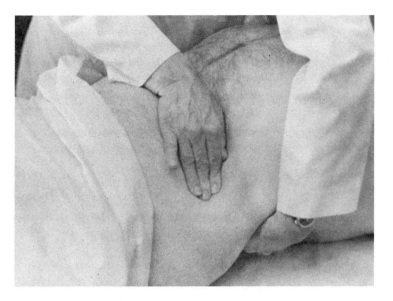

FIGURE 6.58 Palpation of the Left Kidney from the Right Side.
The left hand reaches across the abdomen and is placed with the fingers at the costovertebral angle. The right hand is inserted into the left costal margin. The flank is compressed between the hands as the client is asked to take a deep breath.

enlargement, the client is turned onto the right side while the same palpating procedure is performed. To avoid missing a massively enlarged spleen, the nurse palpates the left lower quadrant and lumbar region prior to these maneuvers.

Palpation of the kidneys may be performed by placing one hand firmly under the loin with the fingertips at the costovertebral angle and the other flat on the abdomen with the fingers pointing outward toward the costal margin. If the nurse is on the client's right, the left hand is placed on the client's loin to examine the right kidney and the right hand is placed on the abdomen. The position is the same for the left kidney, examined from the right side (see figure 6.58). With the hands in position and compressing the flank, the nurse asks the client to take a deep breath. The kidneys are organs that move downward with inspiration. They may normally be palpated in thin clients, particularly the right kidney in

thin women. The lower pole is palpated as a firm mass with a form not unlike the lower half of a kidney bean. A tumor is felt as a distinct enlargement.

Other organs are palpated under special conditions. In the presence of acute inflammation, such as *appendicitis* or *acute cholecystitis,* the omentum wraps itself around the inflamed organ to seal it off from the rest of the abdomen. This omental mass may then be palpated. It is usually tender and is a clue to the condition. The *gall bladder* occasionally may be palpated as a ballotable ball (see figure 6.59). In jaundiced clients this phenomenon is *Courvoisier's sign* and indicates carcinoma of the head of the *pancreas* or the distal *common bile duct.* This conclusion is based on the fact that long-standing cholelithiasis causes fibrosis of the gall bladder, which prevents its dilation; thus if a stone passes into and obstructs the common bile duct, the gall bladder cannot expand and become palpable. Carcinoma

189

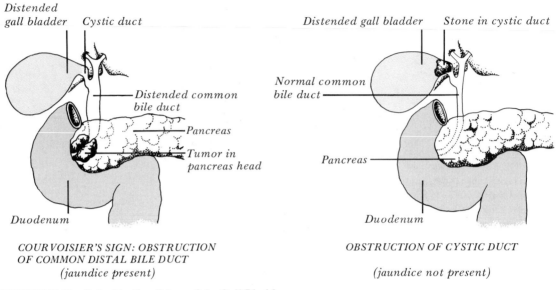

FIGURE 6.59 Palpable Conditions of the Gall Bladder.

of the pancreas is not necessarily associated with stones, and the normal gall bladder can passively expand.

In the nonjaundiced client, a gall bladder stone may become impacted in the *cystic duct* (figure 6.59). This condition causes pain and tenderness in the right upper quadrant, frequently radiating into the back, and the gall bladder may be distended and palpable.

If the nurse detects an abdominal tumor, its position, palpable size, consistency, and mobility are described. This description permits an identification of the source and possibilities of malignancy.

Hernias. The nurse inspects and palpates the anterior abdominal wall for the presence of hernias. The client is asked to cough or bear down while the nurse palpates any apparent weak points. Weaknesses are more common along the midline groove, over surgical scars, and in the region of the umbilicus. If a *ventral or incisional hernia* is present, the nurse attempts to reduce it. This action reveals the presence of the hernia ring, which is palpated by a finger in the orifice. A separation of the recti in the epigastrium is called *diastasis recti* and is of no clinical consequence.

The common hernia is the *inguinal hernia.* An indirect inguinal hernia traverses the internal and external rings of the inguinal canal. The direct one enters the external ring from a weak spot in the abdominal wall. Direct inguinal hernias are more common after a hernia repair.

The technique of examination is to have the client stand and slightly flex the leg on the examined side. The inguinal areas are inspected for a "tell-tale" bulge. Then the fifth finger of the right hand is inserted into the side of the right scrotal sac until the inguinal ring can be felt. The nurse attempts to determine if the ring is tight or large. The client is then asked to bear down and cough. A hernia is felt as a soft mass against the finger.

The rarer *femoral hernia* is seen as a bulge in the femoral triangle, located on the anterior surface of the thigh, just below the groin. The soft mass is palpated and felt to grow larger with coughing and straining.

Examining the Rectum

The rectal examination concludes the examination of the digestive system. Because this examination is the most uncomfortable one, it is usually left to the end of any physical examination. Inspection is limited to the anus. The rest of the examination is by palpation.

The examination may be performed with the client in the left lateral position with the thighs and knees flexed. Other positions include the knee-chest position, in which the client kneels with head and shoulders resting on the table, and the dorsolithotomy position, one commonly used for the pelvic examination in women.

The client is placed in the proper position and the area of the anus is well exposed. Using an adequate light, the nurse inspects the perineum and anus and attempts to spread the anus so as to note the presence of skin masses, hemorrhoids, fissures, or fistulas. The well-lubricated gloved finger is gently and slowly inserted into the anus. The pressure of the finger is directed inwardly and anteriorly, away from the sensitive area of the coccyx. The mucosa of the anal canal and rectum are palpated for any induration and irregularity. Considerable pressure can be brought to bear on the finger in order to reach as high as possible. The client is asked to bear down in order to force any high-lying masses toward the finger. Finally the finger is turned anteriorly to palpate the prostate gland. The finger sweeps to both sides of the entire prostate and the nurse estimates its size, consistency, and shape and notes the presence of any irregularities, tenderness, or hard or nodular areas. The normal prostate has a consistency not unlike that of the end of the nose and has two lobes with a median groove. Any encroachment into the rectum should be considered an enlargement. The finger is then slowly and gently withdrawn and the examination comes to an end.

REFERENCES

BURKITT, D. P., A. R. WALKER, and N. S. PAINTER. 1972. "Effect of Dietary Fiber on Stools and Transit Times and Its Role in the Causation of Disease." *Lancet* 2:1405–15.

EDWARDS, D. A. W. 1976. "Evaluation of Dysphagia." *Clinics in Gastroenterology* 5:49–57.

PONKA, J. L., et al. 1963. "Acute Abdominal Pain in Aged Patients: An Analysis of 200 Cases." *Journal of the American Geriatric Society* 11:993–1007.

POPE, O. E. 1978. "The Esophagus, Rings and Webs." In M. A. Schlesinger and J. S. Fordtran, eds., *Gastrointestinal Disease*. Philadelphia: W. B. Saunders.

SCHEURER, U., and F. HALTER. 1976. "Lower Esophageal Sphincter in Reflux Esophagitis." *Scandinavian Journal of Gastroenterology* 11:629–35.

UNIT 12: THE GENITOURINARY SYSTEM

The cessation of menses and the frequency of symptomatic prostatic hypertrophy are the obvious age-related physical changes that occur in the genitourinary organs. Less well known are the other, more subtle changes that may cause problems related to the system. Some of these changes result in diminished renal function (Rowe et al. 1976), increased frequency of urinary incontinence (Brocklehurst and Dillaine 1966a), and increased susceptibility to urinary infection (Brocklehurst et al. 1968; Staney et al. 1968). The nurse must be aware of such changes in order to correctly assess problems related to the system.

This unit is devoted to the evaluation of the urinary system and the male and female genital organs (see figure 6.60). The examination of the kidneys and prostate was described in the sections on abdominal and rectal examinations in unit 11, on the gastrointestinal system.

HEALTH HISTORY AND SUBJECTIVE FINDINGS

The common complaints suggestive of urinary disorders include difficult or painful urination *(dysuria)*; alteration of normal emptying time, most commonly increased *frequency* and *nocturia;* variation of urine appearance; pain of renal, ureteral, vesical, and urethral origin; incontinence; and systemic complaints such as edema, vomiting, headache, and, in the elderly, confusion, and insomnia.

FIGURE 6.60   **Anatomy of the Male and Female Genital Organs.**

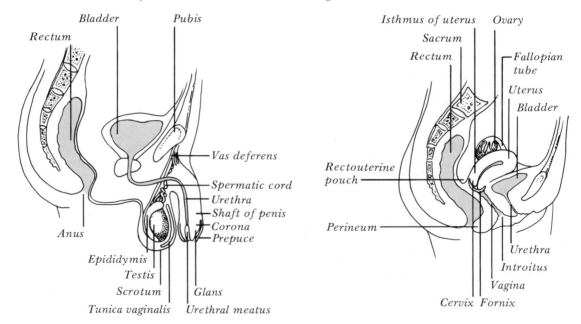

Dysuria

Difficulty in urination may be associated with pain. In such cases the nurse must inquire whether the pain begins with the onset of urination. Onset dysuria indicates inflammation of the tract below the bladder. The passage of urine through the urethra is the irritating factor. In men this condition is associated with urethritis and prostatitis; occasionally a balanitis is found. In women urethritis and vulvovaginitis are the common causes. In clients with vulvovaginitis or balanitis, the nurse also must consider the possibility of diabetes mellitus. Urethritis and vulvovaginitis also may be due to venereal disease or other nonspecific infections. If the pain occurs after the onset of urination and increases toward the end, the nurse should consider the possibility of inflammation above the urethra with involvement of the bladder.

Nonpainful dysuria is often associated with progressive diminution in the size and force of the urine stream, which may culminate in complete retention. Frequent causes are urethral strictures and, in men, prostatic hypertrophy.

Alteration of Emptying Time

Most adults void three or four times daily. Occasionally one voiding at night may be a normal habit. Most significant is a persistent change from the normal habit.

Frequency is an increase in the number of daily voidings and may be caused by an inflammation of the bladder or prostate. The client feels a sensation of *urgency* and a frequent need to urinate; this condition may become painful if ignored. When frequency is associated with thirst and the passage of large volumes of urine, the nurse should consider the possibility of diabetes mellitus. Anxiety and nervousness also increase the frequency of urination.

Increased urinary voiding at night is more significant. This *nocturia* indicates a disorder of the system at any point from the kidneys to the urethra. It also can be caused by ingestion of fluids or alcoholic beverages at bedtime.

Decreased frequency may be associated with a diminished ingestion of fluids or with some type of urinary retention problem.

Variation in Urine Appearance

Urine appearance may change under a variety of conditions. Cloudiness due to the presence of pus or color changes may occur. Darkening may be due to increased concentration. Hematuria causes a deep redness or a smoky appearance, bile gives an appearance not unlike that of a cola drink, and certain medications also color the urine. A urinalysis is helpful in these cases.

Pain

Renal inflammation is usually painless. Usually pain is associated with some kind of ureteral obstruction due to stone, tumor, pus, or blood. The pain is localized to the flank and radiates toward the groin, testicle, or thigh. This *renal colic* is usually steady and severe, aggravated by movement, and accompanied by vomiting and prostration.

Vesical pain is associated with acute obstruction, most commonly because of a stone. This pain is felt in the low abdomen, usually on the midline, and radiates out toward the penis and the perineum.

193

Incontinence

The nurse should attempt to differentiate between the various types of incontinence. Incontinence associated with urgency is often due to inflammation of the bladder or urethra; other forms are related to peripheral and central nervous system disease. Stress incontinence is more common in elderly women with pelvic relaxation (Brocklehurst et al. 1966b) or with urethral narrowing (Moodgoaker 1976). In such cases coughing, sneezing, and straining with a full bladder leads to loss of small quantities of urine.

Systemic Complaints

Certain generalized problems have long been recognized to be caused by urinary tract disease. Such problems may be divided into complaints that are due to renal disease and nonspecific complaints that are manifestations of a uremic state.

Edema is directly related to diminished renal function. It is associated with fluid and sodium retention as well as protein loss and hypoalbuminemia. The result of this combination is a generalized edema, which is most commonly recognized as involving the face as well as the rest of the body.

Complaints related to *uremia* can be insidious and totally overlooked if the nurse is not aware of the relationship. Vomiting, drowsiness, insomnia, and nocturnal confusion are common with this condition. Indeed the picture may resemble that of senility. These symptoms may be caused by an obstruction of the bladder, bilateral ureteral obstruction, or bilateral renal disease.

Male genital disease is most commonly associated with complaints relating to the urinary system. Additional complaints may relate to scrotal swelling or enlargement, testicular pain, and urethral discharge.

The nurse ascertains the length of time that these conditions have been present, the existence of prior illness and treatment, the color of any discharge, and other associated complaints.

EXAMINATION AND OBJECTIVE FINDINGS

The abdominal and rectal examinations were discussed in unit 11. In examining for evidence of genitourinary disorders a general examination is performed. Particular attention is paid to the presence of edema, the funduscopic examination, the cardiovascular examination, and the abdominal and genital examinations.

The examination of the kidneys and bladder by inspection and palpation was discussed in unit 11, and the reader is referred to the abdominal examination described in that unit for those details. In the evaluation of renal pain and infection, the nurse also examines the costovertebral angles, formed by the twelfth rib and the large muscle mass of the back. The nurse presses deeply into this area with the tips of the index and third fingers. Alternatively a light blow may be delivered to this area with the lateral border of the fist. Normally this examination does not reveal any sensitivity. In cases of inflammation of the kidney due to obstruction, stone, or infection, the area may be quite sensitive.

Other areas of tenderness may indicate irritation of the ureters. One of these ureteral points is located in the right lower abdominal quadrant, two or three centimeters medial to the anterior iliac spine. Palpation of the bladder during a rectal or pelvic examination may reveal tenderness in this organ.

THE MALE GENITALIA: EXAMINATION AND OBJECTIVE FINDINGS

Inspection

If the client is not circumcised, the foreskin is retracted to expose all of the *glans* (figure 6.60). The *urethral meatus* is normally at the apex. A deviation toward the ventral side is called *hypospadia;* if the orifice is on the dorsum, it is called *epispadia.*

Meatal discharge is evidenced by crusting or a marked erythema of the urethral orifice. If no discharge is available for culture, the *urethra* is milked from its base distally, between the thumb and index. Any discharge may be placed on a slide for bacterial examination, and if the glans is first prepared with an antiseptic solution, a drop may be swabbed for bacterial culture. The nurse particularly looks for any sores or masses.

Palpation

If the foreskin cannot be retracted behind the glans, the condition is known as *phimosis* and surgical release is necessary. Plaques palpated on the penile *shaft* are found in *Peyronie's disease.* These plaques cause the penis to bend during erection and may render intercourse painful.

The *scrotum* is inspected for sores and tumors. If a *testis* is missing, the nurse palpates for it in the inguinal canal. Undescended testes have a high incidence of malignant degeneration.

The normal testicle is sensitive to compression. An insensitive testicle indicates a central or peripheral nervous system disor-

der. The testes also are palpated for the presence of masses. Any mass found is evaluated by transillumination. In a darkened room a bright penlight is placed behind the mass and the nurse observes whether the light passes through. Fluid-filled masses, such as hydrocele and spermatocele, usually transilluminate. Solid tumors will not transilluminate and must be evaluated for malignancy. Occasionally a solid mass is surrounded by fluid. In these cases the central mass is usually visible. Varicose enlargement of the veins of the scrotum may form a mass that appears when the client stands. This varicocele looks and feels like a bag of worms.

THE FEMALE GENITALIA: HEALTH HISTORY AND SUBJECTIVE FINDINGS

Although many disorders of the pelvic organs may be completely asymptomatic, the following complaints call attention to this region of the body: pelvic or low abdominal pain; vaginal discharge; and pruritus of the vulva and perineum.

Low Abdominal and Pelvic Pain

As in all viscera, pelvic pain is a visceral type of pain. When the cause is sufficiently extensive to involve the peritoneum or the surrounding muscles, a more precise viscerosomatic pain will be described. Clients may have great difficulty distinguishing between pain due to rectal or bladder disorders and pain due to disorders of the genitalia. Often these other organs must be carefully assessed before a correct evaluation can be made. In all cases the nurse obtains a thorough history of the pain, its relation to the menstrual cycle, and the

195

presence of any other helpful factors, such as a discharge or variations of the pain caused by changes in posture or position.

Pelvic pain and backache due to uterine prolapse are eased when the client is recumbent and worsened when the client is erect. The longer the client is erect, the worse the pain. Prolapse, because it changes the position of the bladder, may cause incomplete emptying, straining at urination, and urgency.

Discharge

The nurse obtains a history of the color, character, and quantity of the discharge. Symptomatic *trichomoniasis* usually causes a profuse wetness. However, in postmenopausal women this discharge may be absent or scanty. A purulent discharge may be related to *pelvic inflammatory disease* or *atrophic vaginitis*. A bloody discharge may be due to vaginal, cervical, or uterine *polyps*, cervical, uterine, or vaginal *cancer, inflammation of the cervix,* or *atrophic vaginitis*. The nurse must be particularly careful to examine clients who complain of bleeding after intercourse or the recurrence of menstruation after a prolonged period of amenorrhea.

Vulval or Perineal Pruritus

Pruritus is frequently associated with a discharge. Particularly common with *trichomoniasis,* pruritus is also associated with severe postmenopausal *atrophic vaginitis* and with *Paget's disease* of the vulva, which is a precancerous lesion.

Miscellaneous Complaints

The nurse should also pay careful attention to complaints related to *vaginal odors,* particularly in older women. Advanced cervical carcinoma with necrotic tissue is often attended by a foul odor.

Stress incontinence is usually associated with relaxation of the muscles of the pelvic floor. This condition leads to retroversion of the uterus and a gradual prolapse with an accompanying urethrocele, cystocele, and rectocele.

THE FEMALE GENITALIA: EXAMINATION AND OBJECTIVE FINDINGS

The client is instructed not to douche for at least twenty-four hours before the examination, as this will interfere with a proper evaluation of any smears or cultures that might be obtained. The bladder is emptied before the examination; the examination is best if the rectum is also emptied. The examination is commonly and best performed with the client in the dorsolithotomy position. Other positions such as Sims's and knee-chest may be used, but the exposure of the external genitalia is less adequate. The nurse examines for inguinal hernia, prolapse, and stress incontinence with the client standing erect.

The evaluation begins during the examination of the abdomen with the patient supine. The order of this examination is inspection, auscultation, percussion, and palpation. For specific details, refer to the section in unit 11 on the examination of the gastrointestinal system.

Inspection

The nurse notes the quality of the pubic hair as well as its distribution. The male pubic-hair pattern is diamond shaped, the female escutcheon is shieldlike or triangular, with the apex of the triangle pointing downward. The inguinal area is palpated for masses and lymph nodes. Aging causes a decrease in the fat of the mons and in the amount of hair. The pubic hair may whiten; the labia may be atrophic.

The client is then placed in the dorsolithotomy position, with the knees separated as widely as possible, and suitably draped to preserve dignity. The external genitalia are inspected. The nurse notes the condition of the skin, its color, and the presence of any abnormal bulges or masses.

A variety of skin changes may be noted. In atrophy the skin takes on a thin and shiny appearance. Inflammation causes an erythema, and linear excoriations due to scratching may be evident. The nurse notes the presence of any white plaques consistent with leukoplakia; ulcerations and tumors also are noted and appropriate cultures and smears taken.

With the gloved hand the nurse then separates the labia and exposes the vestibule and the inner surface of the labia. Ulcerations of the inner labia are checked for syphilitic chancre. Inflammation of the Bartholin gland appears as a reddened bulge on the labia, which may be quite tender. Skene's glands are on the inner surface of the labia; any purulent discharge should be smeared and cultured for gonorrhea. In the inspection of the vestibule, the slitlike orifice of the *vagina* will be apparent (figure 6.60). The nurse evaluates the integrity of the pelvic muscles by asking the client to bear down. Posterior wall bulging is due to a *rectocele;* anterior wall bulge is caused by a *cystocele* or *urethrocele.* In severe prolapse the *cervix* may appear at the *introitus.* Loss of urine during this maneuver is consistent with stress incontinence and should be evaluated further. The nurse also inspects the urinary meatus; abnormal red-

ness indicates urethritis. The meatus may be milked and any discharge taken for culture and smear.

Any bulges in and around the labia should be palpated. The nurse should note their exact location, size, shape, tenderness, degree of firmness, and degree of fixation to surrounding tissue.

With the thumb and index finger of the gloved hand separating the labia, the nurse gently inserts the speculum into the posterior portion of the vestibule (see figure 6.61). The largest bivalve speculum that can be comfortably inserted is used. The speculum is held so that the blades are closed and their wide part fits the configuration of the introitus. The insertion is in a downward and backward direction so that no pressure is exerted on the *urethra* and the sensitive anterior structures. The gentle pressure of insertion is maintained until the speculum is at the top of the vagina. At that point the nurse slightly elevates the handle of the speculum and gently rotates the speculum to bring the axis back to the midline. Then the nurse gently depresses the handle while opening the blades. The cervix should now be visible at the top of the vagina.

The nurse inspects the cervix and the visible portions of the vagina. The color and texture of the mucosa are noted; increased redness indicates inflammation (vaginitis). The normal vaginal mucosa is pink and shining. The absence of folds indicates decreased estrogen levels. If this condition is associated with pallor and thinning of the mucosa, atrophy exists. An associated erythema is due to a condition of atrophic vaginitis.

The presence of secretion is noted. Normal secretion is clear and mucoid. Purulent secretions may be creamy or frankly

197

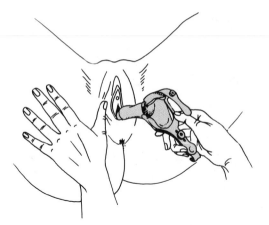

INSERTION INTO POSTERIOR VESTIBULE
(blades closed)

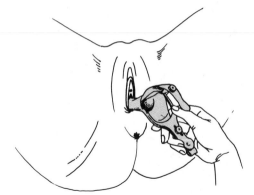

DOWNWARD AND BACKWARD INSERTION
(blades closed)

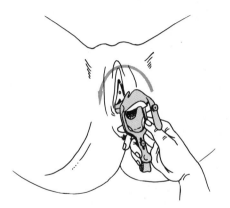

ROTATION OF SPECULUM
(blades closed)

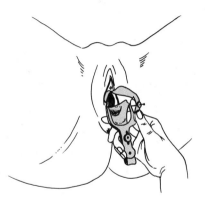

SLIGHT ELEVATION OF SPECULUM HANDLE
(blades opened)

FIGURE 6.61   Speculum Insertion.

purulent; these are swabbed for appropriate smears and cultures.

The cervix is wiped clean and then examined for abnormalities of color or appearance. The external os may have a variable form in women who have borne children. Any healed lacerations have no significance if the overlying mucosa is intact. Any abnormal-appearing areas of increased whiteness are described. A cotton-tipped swab, previously moistened in normal saline, is inserted into the external os and gently rotated. The swab is removed and smeared on a slide. A wooden spatula is then placed against the posterior vaginal vault. This area is gently scraped and the spatula is then removed and scraped on another clean slide. The two slides are then fixed and sent for Papanicolaou cytological examination (Pap smear). The slides must be fixed quickly to prevent drying of the sampled cells.

A variety of cervical problems may be visible. A beefy redness extending from the cervical os may be an erosion. A benign erosion has regular borders, whereas a carcinoma has irregular edges. The endocervical mucosa may be visible. This eversion may become infected, giving rise to a mucopurulent discharge. This condition is usually associated with an enlarged edematous cervix with multiple cysts on its surface (Nabothian cysts). Cervical carcinoma often has a granular and friable appearance. A dark cherry-red mass protruding from the cervix is usually a cervical polyp, but it may also be an endometrial polyp or a prolapsed intrauterine tumor. These conditions should be sampled for Papanicolaou examination.

Upon completion of the inspection, the nurse removes the speculum slowly and gently, with the blades open until they clear the cervix. The speculum is then permitted to close partially. The nurse inspects the mucosa of the vagina during the phase of withdrawing the speculum. As the tips of the blades arrive at the introitus, they are allowed to close completely prior to withdrawal. If the nurse sees any lesion, the speculum is not withdrawn until an inspection is made and a sample taken for culture and smears.

Vaginal Palpation—The Bimanual Examination

The nurse explains the procedure to the client before beginning and reassures the client that the examination, although un-comfortable, is not painful. The client should be relaxed with the arms at the sides or crossed on the chest. The nurse stands before the client and begins the examination by palpation of the abdomen. The gloved hand may be either the right or the left. Use of the left hand permits the right one to manipulate instruments and to palpate the abdomen. This arrangement may be advantageous if the examiner is right-handed. The index and third finger of the gloved hand are lubricated and inserted into the introitus with gentle posterior pressure (see figure 6.62). The fingers are kept extended in a straight line with the hand and the forearm. The fourth and fifth fingers are flexed; the thumb is hyperextended. The ulnar surface of the hand al-

FIGURE 6.62 Bimanual Examination.

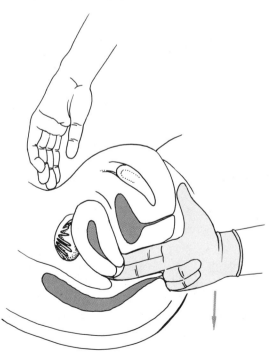

ways points toward the floor. The wrist is kept stiff, and pressure is directed inward toward the *perineum* (figure 6.60).

As the examiner's fingers palpate the vaginal walls, all abnormalities are noted, including tumors, cysts, and scars of old lacerations. Any relaxation or weakness of the walls is noted. The other hand maintains gentle abdominal pressure.

Cervix. The fingers of the inserted hand encounter the cervix. They are placed anteriorly to palpate the region of the *bladder* for tenderness and tumors. Performing the palpation between the two hands permits the nurse to differentiate abdominal-wall pain or tenderness from tenderness in the deeper lying organs. Tenderness may be found in cystitis. Occasionally stones or tumors are palpated.

The nurse then evaluates the cervix, noting its size, shape, position, mobility, consistency, and regularity. The nurse also notes whether the cervix points anteriorly or posteriorly or is deviated laterally. Change of position may be due to a tumor in the parametrium or to pelvic inflammatory disease. The normally mobile cervix may be fixed by inflammation or cancer. Tenderness induced by mobilizing the cervix may be due to an inflammatory process. Cancerous invasion of the cervix hardens it and often gives it a granular consistency. The nurse estimates the length of the cervix. The cervix becomes quite small in the elderly; because it retreats with aging and lies flush with the vaginal vault, it may be only barely palpable.

The parametria, which are lateral and posterior to the uterus, are also palpated. They become small and less mobile with age. Induration and tenderness are found with inflammatory disorders, induration, nodularity, and immobility with cancer. Inflammation of the parametria is unusual in the elderly but can occur after surgery on the genital tract.

Uterus. The *uterus* (figure 6.60) is then examined bimanually to determine its size, position, shape, consistency, and mobility. The abdominal hand is placed on the abdomen so that the fingers are half the distance from the pubic symphysis to the umbilicus. The vaginal hand perceives the pressure of the abdominal palpation as the abdominal fingers make contact with a pelvic mass or the uterine fundus. If the abdominal hand is unable to make contact with the uterus, the nurse begins again by starting farther up in the abdomen and then slowly descending until a mass or the fundus is encountered. Once contact is established, a thorough examination is made. The vaginal fingers explore the anterior *fornix* first; if the uterus cannot be palpated, the posterior and lateral fornices are each examined.

In premenopausal women the uterus is normally the size of a small fist. After menopause it becomes smaller. It is usually twice the size of the cervix. The position of the uterus determines in which fornix the uterus is palpable. Anteroversion is normal; posteroversion is frequent and is commonly associated with prolapse. Lateral displacement is usually associated with a parametric pelvic tumor.

As the uterus is palpated, the nurse attempts to outline its shape and regularity. Fibroids are felt as smooth, hard masses that give an irregular outline; uterine hyperplasia and carcinoma cause a smooth enlargement. Tenderness frequently indi-

200

cates inflammation, but it is also found with necrosis, cystic degeneration, or hemorrhage into a fibroid or a tumor. Another cause of tenderness is endometrial infection (endometritis).

Finally the nurse checks for mobility. If the uterus lies in retroversion, an attempt is made to lift it. If the uterus is immobile, the examiner should immediately suspect a pelvic tumor or extensive pelvic adhesions.

Tubes and Ovaries. After completing the examination of the uterus, the nurse examines the *fallopian tubes* and *ovaries* (figure 6.60). Normally the tubes are not palpable. If palpated, they are assessed for size, form, consistency, and sensitivity. If the tube is cystic and hard, the examiner should consider the probability of carcinoma; if it is sausage shaped, the probability of pelvic inflammation. In these cases the client usually has a history of genital surgery (Heaton and Lodger 1976).

The ovaries are approximately 3 by 4 cm in size and are tender prior to menopause; afterward they tend to become smaller. They are normally palpated laterally to the uterus, with the vaginal fingers deeply inserted in the fornix, and the abdominal fingers deeply exploring from a point above the medial third of the inguinal ligament and pointing toward the midline. Occasionally the ovary may be palpated in the *rectouterine pouch.*

Perineal Body. The perineal body may be evaluated by removing the third finger from the vagina and inserting it into the *rectum* (figure 6.60). This rectovaginal examination can also give considerable information about the posterior aspect of the pelvis. The nurse must maintain the pres-

sure on the rectovaginal hand to ride well back into the rectum. In cases where the vaginal examination is impractical, a bimanual abdominorectal examination should be performed. The cervix is easily palpated from the rectum and should not be confused with an anteriorly lying tumor.

REFERENCES

BROCKLEHURST, J. C., and J. B. DILLANE. 1966a. "Studies of the Female Bladder in Old Age: I. Cystometrograms in Nonincontinent Women." *Gerontological Clinics* 8:285–305.

————. 1966b. "Studies of the Female Bladder in Old Age: II. Cystometrograms in 100 Incontinent Women." *Gerontological Clinics* 8:306–19.

————et al. 1968. "The Prevalence and Symptomatology of Urinary Infection in an Aged Population." *Gerontological Clinics* 10:242–53.

HEATON, F. C., and W. J. LODGER. 1976. "Postmenopausal Tubo-ovarian Abscess." *Obstetrics and Gynecology* 47:90–96.

MOODGOAKER, A. S. 1976. "Management of Stress Incontinence in Women." *Geriatrics* 31 (6):60–64.

ROWE, J. W., et al. 1976. "The Effect of Age on Creatinine Clearance in Man: A Cross-Sectional and Longitudinal Study." *Journal of Gerontology* 31:155–63.

STANEY, T. A., et al. 1968. "Antibacterial Nature of Prostate Fluid." *Nature* 218:444–47.

In the course of normal aging, muscles, bones, and articulations (see figure 6.63) undergo changes that affect their physiological function and physical appearance. Muscle mass, strength, and coordination diminish (Shock and Norris 1970; Timaris 1971) in association with regressive changes in cartilage and joints (Nikityuk 1966) and long-bone density (Garn 1975). These degenerative and osteoporotic changes may predispose the older person to develop problems that vary from simple aches and pains to an increased incidence of degenerative hip disorders (Danielsson 1964), hip fractures (Alffram 1964; Voose and Lockwood 1965), and loss of vibratory and position sensation due to cervical spondylosis (Valergakis 1976). Osteoporosis affects fifteen million people in the United States; in five million it is severe and causes painful vertebral fractures (Lutwak and Whedon 1963). Furthermore, the elderly are not immune to rheumatoid disorders, gout, and a variety of musculoskeletal conditions that they share with the young.

Studies have shown that sustained physical conditioning may prevent some of these changes as well as those occurring in other systems (Webb et al. 1977). Others (Hartung and Farge 1977; Suominen et al. 1977) have described reversal of these changes through physical conditioning programs. The nurse caring for the elderly must accurately assess musculoskeletal function not only to try to prevent further deterioration but also to help the client plan a program of preservation and rehabilitation of the capacity for independent motor activity.

It is beyond the scope of this unit to analyze every muscle, bone, and articulation. Rather, the unit covers the general techniques of the assessment and, in particular, their application to the evaluation of the more common problems found in older adults.

FIGURE 6.63   Movable Joints.

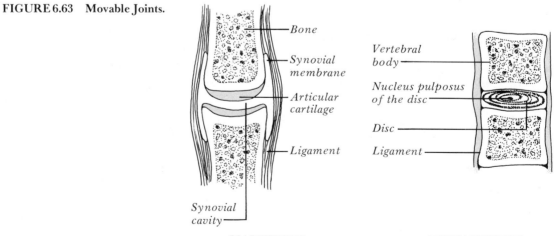

DIARTHROSIS   AMPHIARTHROSIS

HEALTH HISTORY AND SUBJECTIVE FINDINGS

Since the musculoskeletal system is composed of muscles, bones, and articulations, and since disorders of one part affect the other parts, complaints may relate to one of the parts or to the entirety. Furthermore, disorders may appear as anatomically localized lesions or as generalized ones. A further problem is that disorders of the neurological system may appear superficially as musculoskeletal ones, and disorders of the musculoskeletal system may be due to local lesions or systemic disease. The role of the examiner is to determine the source of the disorder and the extent of damage. This analysis permits an accurate assessment and the formulation of a realistic plan of management.

Complaints relating to the system are characterized by pain or stiffness associated with movement, limitation of movement, weakness or paralysis, and articular swelling or bodily deformity.

Pain or Stiffness with Movement

The nurse determines the manner of onset, the duration, the progression, and the existence of any precipitating event related to the onset of pain or stiffness. Severe trauma occurring years prior to the onset of problems may cause the development of articular degeneration and the onset of complaints at a later time. Structural deformity or amputation may place excessive strain on an articulation and lead to premature degeneration. Overextension or an increase in activity may lead to muscle soreness, followed by disuse, atrophy, and chronic pain.

The history of the progression may help distinguish local from systemic problems.

Recurrent bouts of acute articular tenderness and swelling, passing to various joints with increasing frequency, help distinguish gout from rheumatoid arthritis. Rheumatoid disorders are usually associated with muscular complaints and frequent recurrence in the same articulation while they progress to another articulation.

Stiffness, usually occurring after rest and eased by activity, is found with most forms of arthropathy. Muscle pain is usually less precisely localizable than stiffness. Deep muscle pain resembles viscerosomatic pain, which was described in unit 11, on the gastrointestinal system. Deep muscle pain is usually associated with muscle spasm, and the client frequently has great difficulty localizing the exact site of the pain. The examiner should ascertain which muscle groups are involved by determining which movements heighten the pain.

Frequently muscle pain is due to an inappropriate use of a group of muscles. Injury or inflammation of a muscle limits its use and provokes a disuse atrophy. Later the client is unable to use the atrophied muscle and is forced to rely on other secondary muscle groups to move the joint. The use of secondary muscles results in persistent pain and limitation of movement. This condition is most commonly found in the shoulder after a bout of acute bursitis and can eventually lead to adhesive capsulitis, or frozen shoulder. Musculoskeletal pain in the elderly is rarely due to a psychosomatic disorder.

Weakness and Paralysis

Weakness or paralysis may be local or generalized. *Local weakness* or *paralysis* may be due to disuse because of pain, trauma, or a neurological problem. *Generalized weakness*

203

may be due to a systemic disorder. It may be constant in thyroid disease or intermittent in rheumatoid arthritis. The nurse should inquire about the effect of rest and exercise and whether the activities of daily living have been curtailed. Myopathies are usually intermittent. Depression may cause generalized fatigue that may be worsened by rest, whereas true muscular disorders are usually helped by rest.

Articular Swelling and Bodily Deformity

The process of aging gives rise to certain changes in bodily appearance. A thoracic kyphosis creates a stooped appearance, which often obliges the client to compensate by a backward tilt of the head. These gradual changes are not usually cause for concern. Accentuation of this kyphosis with the appearance of a gibbous may be the first indication of osteoporosis and vertebral collapse. Massive skull enlargement and curvature of a long bone may indicate Paget's disease.

Articular swelling due to fluid is fluctuant; swelling due to joint deformity is firm. The nurse should inquire about the duration of the swelling, presence of pain, limitation of movement, warmth and redness, and whether the joint locks or buckles. If the swelling has persisted for more than three days, it usually indicates the presence of an arthritis. Arthritis may be due to other conditions, including blood-borne infections such as gonorrhea or bacterial endocarditis as well as drug hypersensitivity. These conditions are usually associated with other systemic findings such as fever, lymphadenopathy, or, in the case of endocarditis, the presence of a heart murmur. Locking and buckling are good evidence

for intraarticular problems involving the joint surfaces and capsule.

EXAMINATION AND OBJECTIVE FINDINGS

A significant amount of information is obtained as the client performs the movements of the physical assessment. Observation of the manner in which the client rises from the chair, walks to the examining table, sits on the table, lies down, and then sits up provides a wealth of information concerning symmetry and fluidity of movement.

The actual examination requires maximal exposure so that the body can be examined completely. The examination proceeds from the head downward. Muscles, bones, and joints are compared with those on the opposite side of the body. Muscles are evaluated for appearance, consistency, tenderness, and range of motion; bones, for appearance and tenderness. The techniques used are inspection and palpation.

Inspection

All articulations are inspected in their relaxed positions and in flexion and extension. The nurse looks for abnormalities of position or carrying angle, joint deformity, erythema, swelling and nodularity, the presence of spinal curvature, and muscle changes.

Carrying Angle. Abnormalities of the carrying angle are readily seen in the elbow, knee, wrists, and fingers; in the ankle; in the small articulations of the feet; and in the neck. These changes of carrying angle or deformities are usually associated with limitations in the range of motion. The changes may be due to trauma or associated with an acute flare of arthritis; or they may be long-standing chronic changes. All deviations are measured in degrees from the neutral or 0° position. Measurement is most easily accomplished by using a goniometer or large protractor (see figure 6.64).

Erythema, Nodularity, and Swelling. *Erythema* is usually associated with active inflammation and swelling. Joint *nodularity* is found in the interphalangeal joints in os-

FIGURE 6.64   Measurement of Carrying Angle Deviation.
The goniometer is placed to correspond to the long axes above and below the joint. Deviations from normal are read directly in degrees. Note that decreased subcutaneous fat renders muscle tendons and veins more prominent (see section on inspection of articulations).

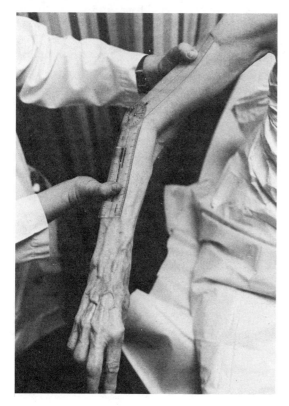

teoarthritis. The nodules of the distal articulations are called *Heberden's nodes;* those of the proximal articulations are known as *Bouchard's nodes.* A firm nodule on the dorsum of the wrist, associated with an extensor tendon, is often a rheumatoid nodule. Fluctuant nodules are usually articular cysts or ganglions. Masses are measured across their greatest diameter.

Spinal Curvatures. Spinal curvatures are best examined with the client erect. In the elderly, kyphosis of the thoracic spine is accentuated (figure 6.24). This condition throws the head forward; the client frequently compensates by arching the neck. Viewed from the side, the client's spine appears to form the figure 3. Accentuation of this curve into a sharp angle, called a *gibbous,* may indicate a vertebral fracture. This gibbous may be the first evidence of osteoporosis. Deviation of the spine may be seen by marking the palpable spinal epiphyses on the skin. These scolioses may cause a deformity of the thorax, creating a condition in which one side is larger than the other. Such deformities may lead to pulmonary stasis and unequal aeration and eventually lead to a chronic restrictive disorder. Flexibility and spinal curvature are appreciated by having the client bend forward while the nurse examines the back.

Muscle Changes. The nurse must inspect for changes in muscles. Muscles and tendons are more easily seen in the elderly than in the young. Guttering in the intercarpal grooves is prominent. Loss of a muscle or a muscle group is usually observable. The limb or portion of the body appears thinner or atrophic when compared with the other side and it contracts weakly.

Diminished muscle tone in the limb causes the extremity to appear oval, with the flattened portions in the anterior and posterior position when the limb is in a horizontal position. In the normal limb the flattened aspect of the oval is found on the sides. Confirmation of thinning may be recorded by measuring the circumference of the limb and comparing it with the other side.

Bone Changes. The bones are inspected for appearance and symmetry. Enlargement, excessive curvature, and irregularity may indicate sequelae of childhood rickets or fracture as well as Paget's disease or bone tumors.

Movements of Joints. The nurse asks the client to perform movements that are proper to the articulations. These *active* movements are observed for ease of action as well as for limits of performance. Joint motion is measured from the neutral position to the extreme limit to which the client can perform. The neutral position is considered as 0°, and the range is measured in degrees from the 0. Thus the wrist passes from 0° to 90° in flexion or to 70° in extension (see figure 6.65). Limitation is considered an inability to reach these limits. The nurse compares the range of motion exhibited by the client with the symmetrical articulation. The range of the client's joint can also be compared with the examiner's joint, used as a reference. Pure joint movements include flexion, extension, abduction, adduction, and external rotation. Circumduction is a circular movement performed by combining the other movements.

Active range of motion should be performed smoothly and with little effort. Dif-

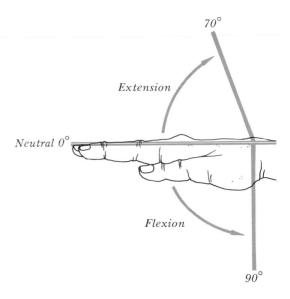

FIGURE 6.65   Movements of the Wrist.

ficulty may be caused by pain in muscles or joints, neurological disorders, or myopathies. Limitation may be due to articular deformity or to muscle weakness.

Upon completion of active motion, the nurse performs *passive* motion. The moving portion of the limb is grasped in one hand while the other hand grasps and fixes the limb on the other side of the articulation. Then, while gently moving the mobile portion, the nurse notes the extent of the induced range of motion (ROM) and the presence of any resistance. To move the elbow passively (see figure 6.66), the nurse fixes the upper arm with one hand while the other hand moves the lower arm in flexion, extension, and rotation. Upon completion of the normal movements, the nurse gently attempts to impart abnormal movements to the joint. In so doing, the nurse explores the integrity of the articular capsule and ligaments. The limits of motion are measured in degrees attained. If the

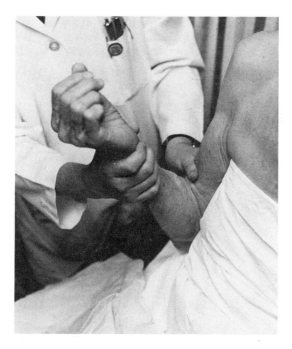

extend both arms and to keep them extended. Weakness causes the affected limb to be slowly lowered. Specific muscles or groups of muscles are tested by having the client perform against a resistance and then by comparing one side with the other. Thus, to test the flexor muscles of the forearm (see figure 6.67), the nurse asks the

FIGURE 6.67   Testing Muscle Strength, Left Biceps.
The client is asked to bend the elbow and resist attempts to straighten it. The nurse's left hand is placed on the client's shoulder. The nurse's right hand grasps the client's wrist and attempts to straighten the arm. The degree of resistance is assessed. If the client's wrist is released suddenly, the fist should not strike the hand on the shoulder. This overshooting response will occur in cerebellar disease (see examination of the cerebellar system in unit 14).

FIGURE 6.66   Passive Range of Motion of the Elbow.
The nurse grasps the upper arm and fixes it with one hand. The other hand grasps the client's wrist and gently moves it. The limits of motion are read directly with the goniometer (see figure 6.65).

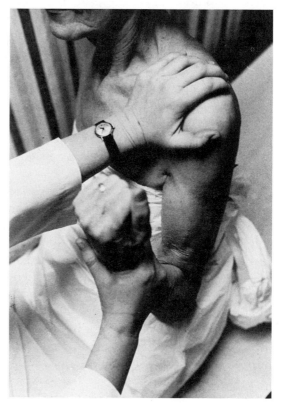

passive range is greater than the active one, the limitation is due to muscular weakness.

Resistance to passive motion may be due to fear, neurological disorder, or joint abnormality. The nurse should note whether the resistance is maintained throughout, lifts suddenly, or is jerky or cogwheellike. Resistance that abruptly ceases (jackknife rigidity) is found in pyramidal disorders, whereas the cogwheel phenomenon is particular to parkinsonism.

Muscle Weakness. Muscle weakness is explored by having the client perform a sustained effort. The nurse asks the client to

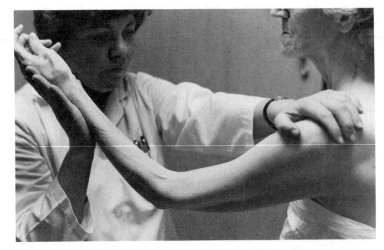

FIGURE 6.68 Testing Muscle Strength, Left Triceps.
The client holds the left arm bent at the elbow. The nurse's left hand is placed on the client's shoulder. The right hand supports the client's wrist. The client is asked to straighten the elbow against the resistance of the nurse's right hand.

client to bend the arm at the elbow. The nurse grasps the client's wrist with one hand and places the other hand on the client's shoulder. The client is then asked to pull the forearm toward the shoulder while the nurse resists the pull. The strength of the extensor muscles is tested by asking the client to straighten the arm while the nurse resists (see figure 6.68). These techniques can be applied to the other muscle groups of the limbs. Strength should be evaluated and graded as paralysis, severe weakness, weakness, minimal weakness, and normal.

Gait Changes. Abnormalities of gait are inspected as part of the evaluation of the musculoskeletal and nervous systems. The client should be asked to walk forward, backward, forward on the toes, and then on the heels. For best observation the client should be barefoot and both lower limbs should be completely visible. The nurse should observe the client from in front, behind, and the side. Abnormalities of the hip and gluteal muscle weakness cause the pelvis to drop on the affected side when that side is weight bearing (Trendelen-

berg's sign). This shift will give the appearance of a lurching limp. Weakness of muscle groups become apparent in the heel or toe walk. Pain due to weight bearing causes a shortened antalgic step. These gait abnormalities alert the nurse to the need for an extensive evaluation of the affected joints and muscles.

Palpation

Articulations are palpated to determine the presence of deformity, laxity, tenderness, nodules, and swelling.

In examining the joint the nurse palpates in both the neutral position and the position that best accentuates the prominent skeletal parts. Palpation is performed between the thumb and index finger of one hand; if the limb must be supported, the thumbs of both hands palpate the articulation while the hands support the extremity.

One palpating digit is placed on the medial side and the other on the lateral side of the articulation. In this way the nurse determines the presence of swelling, bogginess, or tenderness. Thickening of the articular ligaments should be noted. While palpating, the nurse should ask the client to move the joint so that grating may be felt. Grating indicates abnormality of the joint or its capsule and, in the elderly, it may be the first indication of osteoarthritis.

Joint Deformity. The presence of a joint effusion is ascertained by observing one side of an interarticular space while pressing on the other. This pressure will cause an

FIGURE 6.69   Palpation of the Knee.
With the client seated and the leg allowed to hang loosely, the articulation is palpated between the thumb and index of the right hand. To test for effusion, compression is applied above the patella by the left hand. If fluid is present, it is forced down and causes a bulge below and on either side of the patella.

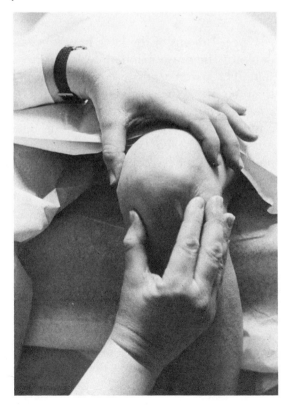

outward bulging of the fluid that is being compressed from the other side. In an articulation such as the knee (see figure 6.69), pressure on the upper portion of the articulation will push the fluid behind the patella. If this pressure is maintained and the nurse taps the patella briskly with the plexor finger, a click will be heard.

Any joint swelling should be palpated to determine whether it is fluctuant and due to fluid or firm and due to thickening or enlargement. Fluctuation may be caused by recent trauma, inflammation, or joint infection. The articular enlargement of rheumatoid arthritis is commonly soft, whereas that due to degenerative joint disease is commonly firm.

Joint Tenderness. Mechanical disorders can be caused by meniscus detachment or by intraarticular cartilaginous or calcific particles or bodies. These conditions are complications of degenerative disease.

Tenderness is tested by compressing the joint along the articular line. Tenderness will be elicited if intraarticular inflammation is present. Joint laxity is found by fixing the proximal bones of the articulation between the thumb and index finger of one hand and the distal bones between the thumb and index finger of the other. The nurse then attempts to move the distal bones in an abnormal direction. When resistance or pain is encountered, the nurse desists. Joint laxity indicates an abnormality in the articular capsule and its intrinsic ligaments.

Nodularity and Swelling. The bursal areas around and near the joints are palpated for swelling, tenderness, ganglions, and nodularity. Ganglions are soft cystic swellings often found near joints. Bursal swelling is usually associated with tenderness. Nodules are firm.

A frequent finding in the elderly is *Dupuytren's contracture*—a progressive contracture of the superficial fascia of the hand, causing a flexion deformity of the affected fingers, which cannot be extended. In these cases fibrotic, hard, thickened plaques may be palpated over the affected tendons.

Muscle Weakness. Muscles may be palpated during contraction and at rest. The nurse notes the presence of fluttering (fasciculations). These patternless, tiny muscle tremors indicate degeneration in the anterior motor horn of the spinal cord and an intact motor nerve.

Specific Musculoskeletal Testing

A large number of specific tests and signs are used in evaluating the musculoskeletal system. This unit concludes with a description of some of the more useful ones.

Lesions of the back may be assessed by straight leg raising. Kernig's, Brudzinski's, and Patrick's sign. These are described in the next unit, as they usually indicate irritation of the neurological system.

Neck. The neck may be evaluated by *Spurling's neck compression test.* In this test the nurse presses the head downward, backward, and laterally. Compression of nerve roots due to foraminal narrowing or a posteriorly protruding cervical disk produces or intensifies the presenting pain.

Hip. Hip lesions may be demonstrated by Patrick's sign, Thomas's hip flexion test, and Trendelenberg's test. Patrick's sign is

described in the next unit. *Thomas's hip flexion test* compares hip flexion in both legs. With the client supine, the healthy extremity is flexed at the hip and knee until the knee rests on the chest. The spine and pelvis are then brought flat on the table. The degree of extension of the affected hip measures the degree of flexion deformity. The hip lesion may be intra- or extra-articular.

Trendelenberg's test is performed by asking the client to stand on the affected side. The other foot is raised off the floor by flexing the hip and knee. The nurse observes the pelvis from behind the client. Normally the unsupported side of the pelvis will rise. In a positive test this side will be seen to drop. The test is positive with hip subluxation, congenital dislocation, pelvic-trochanter shortening, and paralysis or paresis of the gluteus medius muscle.

Knee. Lesions of the knee may be evaluated by the drawer sign and McMurray's sign. The *drawer sign* is used in examining the integrity of the cruciate ligaments. The client is seated with the foot and leg dangling. The knee is bent at a right angle. The nurse grasps the foot between the knees and manipulates the leg backward and forward by grasping it with both hands. Excessive forward mobility indicates a lax or torn anterior cruciate ligament. Excessive posterior mobility is found with lesions of the posterior cruciate ligament.

McMurray's sign is used in examining the integrity of the internal cartilage. The client is asked to flex the knee completely. The nurse grasps the ankle with one hand and rotates the leg. The other hand palpates the knee behind the collateral ligaments. If a click is felt by the palpating hand, a lesion of the anterior or posterior internal cartilage is present.

Further evaluation of the knee may be obtained by abduction with the knee in extension. Normally no lateral movement occurs in this position. If abduction occurs, the collateral ligament is lax.

Elbow. Tendonitis of the elbow may be demonstrated by asking the client to actively extend and supinate the arm while the nurse resists the motion. This resistance will cause pain in the outer elbow in cases of external epicondylitis (tennis elbow).

Hand and Wrist. *Finklestein's test* is positive in tenosynovitis of the abductor pollicis brevis (DeQuervain's disease): pain is elicited over the radial styloid process when the wrist is forcibly moved into ulnar deviation with the thumb folded in the palm of the hand.

REFERENCES

ALFFRAM, P. A. 1964. "An Epidemiologic Study of Cervical Trochanteric Fractures of the Femur in an Urban Population." *Acta Orthopedica Scandinavica, Supplement* 65:1–109.

DANIELSSON, L. G. 1964. "Incidence and Prognosis of Coxarthrosis." *Acta Orthopedica Scandinavica, Supplement* 66:11–114.

GARN, S. M. 1975. "Bone Loss and Aging." In R. Goldman and M. Rockstein, eds., *The Physiology and Pathology of Human Aging.* New York: Academic Press.

HARTUNG, G. H., and E. J. FARGE. 1977. "Personality and Physiologic Traits in Middle Aged Runners and Joggers." *Journal of Gerontology* 32:541–48.

LUTWAK, L., and G. D. WHEDON. 1963. "Osteoporosis." In H. F. Dowling, ed., *Disease-A-Month,* Yearbook. Chicago, April.

NIKITYUK, B. A. 1966. "Skeleton Senescence." Abstract 270 in *Proceedings, Seventh International Congress of Gerontology.* Vienna, June 26–July 2.

SHOCK, N. W., and A. H. NORRIS. 1970. "Neuromuscular Coordination as a Factor in Age Changes in Muscular Exercise." In E. Jakl and D. Brunner, eds., *Physical Activity and Aging,* vol 4. Basel: S. Karger.

SUOMINEN, H., H. HEIKINEN, and T. PARK-ATTI. 1977. "Effect of Eight Weeks of Physical Training on Muscle and Connective Tissue of the Vastus Lateralis in 69-Year-Old Men and Women." *Journal of Gerontology* 32:33–37.

TIMARIS, P. S. 1971. *Developmental Physiology and Aging.* New York: Macmillan.

VALERGAKIS, F. E. G. 1976. "Cervical Spondylosis: Most Common Cause of Position and Vibratory Sense Loss." *Geriatrics* 31(7):51–56.

VOOSE, G. P., and R. N. LOCKWOOD. 1965. "Femoral Neck Fracturing: Its Relationship to Radiographic Bone Density." *Journal of Gerontology* 20:300–12.

WEBB, S., S. C. URNER, and J. McDANIELS. 1977. "Physiologic Characteristics of a Champion Runner: Age 72." *Journal of Gerontology* 32:286–90.

UNIT 14: THE NEUROLOGICAL SYSTEM

Neurological problems have a profound effect on the client's health status. Such problems impact on the activities of daily living, modify the quality of life, and affect the lives of the client's family and friends. The incidence of stroke is approximately 300,000 cases per year in the United States (Stamler 1966); stroke is the third leading cause of death (Kart et al. 1978). In addition, 6 of every 100 persons suffer a stroke in their lifetime (Kottke 1974), and the vast majority of these are over the age of 60 (Wilder 1975).

In spite of morphological and physiological age-related changes (Timaris and Vernadahis 1971) and associated changes seen in the examination (Carter 1971), recent studies reveal that intellectual ability is maintained well into normal old age (see figure 6.70). The changes that do occur are smaller in magnitude and include fewer functions than was previously thought (Ford and Roth 1977).

Hence the nurse must be prepared to assess neurological function in the elderly client. The findings of the neurological assessment can be classified into a series of phenomena.

Neurological Phenomena

Deficiency Phenomena: loss of conducting pathways, as in paralysis and anesthesia

Irritation Phenomena: irritation of a motor area, as seen with convulsions

Release Phenomena: loss of superior center inhibition, as seen with the uninhibited neurogenic bladder or the Babinski sign

FIGURE 6.70 **Major Cerebral Systems Related to Mental Functions.**

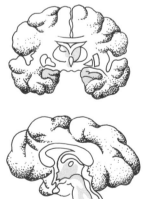
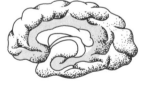
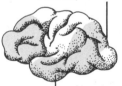
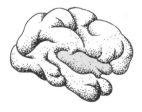
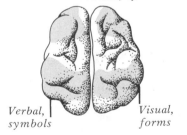

Visual, forms

Verbal, symbols

Verbal, symbols

Visual, forms

CENTRAL CORE—HIPPOCAMPUS
(memory)

LIMBIC CORTEX
(emotions)

NEOCORTEX
(intellectual activities and perceptions)

Compensating Phenomena: overreaction by the normal intact structures, as with steppage in clients with foot drop

A thorough assessment provides a baseline for future reference, helps the nurse understand the client's strengths and weaknesses, and thus permits the nurse and client to form realistic management goals.

HEALTH HISTORY AND SUBJECTIVE FINDINGS

The complaints discussed below should alert the nurse to the possible existence of a neurological problem. These complaints include headache, vomiting and vertigo, visual disturbances, pains and paresthesias, disturbances of consciousness, and sleep disorders.

Headache

The evaluation of headache, one of the most common complaints in primary care, requires a thorough history. The nurse must inquire about the location, character, duration, and intensity of the episodes. The frequency of recurrence, progression, and associated disorders are essential information. A new kind of headache after age 55 is rare and must be carefully assessed (Ziegler et al. 1977). The nurse must remember that the cause of a headache lies outside the skull at least as often as inside.

Headache may be due to cranial or extracranial disorders. Vascular headaches due to dilation of the scalp vessels, such as migraine, are rare in the elderly. Arteritis, a subacute inflammation of the artery and the perivascular tissues, is more common in persons over 55. This headache pain is usually dull and severe. It begins at the af-

fected vessel and then spreads over the head. Involvement of the retinal or ophthalmic arteries causes visual disturbances or permanent blindness. The affected vessel is palpable, tender, and pulseless.

Muscle contraction may cause headache. Many elderly complain of vague neck discomfort radiating to the temples and forehead. These muscle-tension headaches are common in the elderly (Posner 1976). Tension headache may be due to cervical muscle strain or trauma as well as psychological problems such as anxiety or depression. These headaches rarely awaken the client but are frequently present in the morning.

Inflammatory disorders of the ears, nose, and throat may cause headache. Acute and subacute sinusitis is typically painful on awakening and relieved by getting up. The skin and bone overlying the sinus are tender. Temperomandibular arthritis causes headache referred to the ear and temples.

Glaucoma may cause headache. This kind of headache is described with the disorders of the eye in chapter 13.

Intracranial disorders causing headache may be due to vasodilation, as with fever and histamine cephalalgia. Increased intracranial pressure, subarachnoid bleeding, meningitis, and cerebral tumor may all be associated with headache and all require a thorough neurological examination. Papilledema and Kernig's and Brudzinski's signs, discussed with the objective findings, are useful in examining the client for these disorders.

Vomiting and Vertigo

In addition to vascular and digestive problems, vomiting and particularly ver-

213

tigo may be due to disorders of the central nervous system and the inner ear. The nurse must distinguish among unsteadiness; subjective vertigo, in which the client has the impression of rotation; and true objective vertigo, in which the client sees the surroundings rotate like water leaving a sink.

Unsteadiness may have a variety of causes ranging from anxiety to vascular problems. Subjective vertigo is a common complaint and may be related to alcohol intoxication or the effect of medication. Objective vertigo is associated with disorders of the inner ear, the midbrain, and the cerebellum.

Visual Disturbances

Binocular diplopia in adults is a neurological disorder. It is abolished by closing one eye. It may be found in association with encephalitis, intracranial tumors, multiple sclerosis, meningitis, and diabetes mellitus.

Monocular diplopia is an ophthalmological disorder. It is usually related to displacement of the lens or to a torn retina.

Pain and Paresthesias

Osteoporotic vertebral collapse and medullary tumors may cause typical root pain, which has the distribution of the dermatomes. This pain is exacerbated by anything that increases pressure in the vertebral canal, such as a cough, sneeze, or strain. Similar pain is associated with an extruded intervertebral disc.

Paresthesias are sensory changes in which sensation is perceived abnormally. Light touch may be perceived as a painful stimulus. This disorder may be due to irritation of a peripheral nerve or of the spinal sensory pathways. Hypoesthesia and anesthesia are the diminishment and absence of sensation, respectively, due to destruction of these nerves or pathways. Normal aging is associated with diminished sensation (Rockstein 1975).

Disturbances of Consciousness

A variety of consciousness-related problems may occur, including loss of consciousness, déjà vu, amnesia, automatism, dream states, and true convulsions. In convulsive seizures the condition may be generalized or it may begin in one part of the body and spread outward (Jacksonian seizures). An aura may precede the episodes, amnesia may or may not be present, and the nurse may find other associated findings, such as tongue biting and loss of sphincter control.

Disorders of Sleep

Sleep disorders include problems of insomnia and hypersomnia. In cases of insomnia the client may have difficulty falling asleep or remaining asleep. This condition may be provoked by psychic problems, pain, or other complaints. Hypersomnia may be due to neurological disorders or to disorders of other systems. Aging is associated with an alteration in the pattern of sleep and a decrease in time spent sleeping (Timaris and Vernadahis 1971).

THE BRAIN: EXAMINATION AND OBJECTIVE FINDINGS

The nervous system must be examined systematically. The usual order is to begin with the brain and proceed from the head downward. The brain integrates and correlates. The formal mental status assessment will be discussed in chapter 7. Crude consciousness is determined by the pathways that link the thalamus, cortex, and mesencephalon (Guyton 1976). Crude consciousness may be described in terms of six levels.

Levels of Crude Consciousness

Semiconsciousness: The client is excessively drowsy, which may often be associated with hypothalamic injury.

Obtundation: The client is lethargic and mental processes are slowed.

Stupor: The client is spontaneously unconscious and may be easily aroused.

Subcoma: No longer rousable, the client responds to stimuli with movement.

Coma: The client responds only to deep stimuli, such as pain.

Deep Coma: The client does not respond to stimuli; sphincter control is lost.

Coma may be due to increased intracranial pressure (edema, tumors), anoxia, excessive sedation, and metabolic disorders.

THE CRANIAL NERVES: EXAMINATION AND OBJECTIVE FINDINGS

Cranial nerves differ from spinal nerves in that they may be purely motor or purely sensory, and some of the cranial nerves receive a bilateral cortical innervation. Cranial motor nerves that receive the single, contralateral innervation are the trigeminal (V), the glossopharyngeal (IX), the spinal accessory (XI), and the hypoglossal (XII). The facial nerve (VII) has bilateral innervation in the portion that controls movements of the forehead. The portion that controls lower facial movements has only the single source of innervation from the contralateral side.

The Olfactory Nerve (Nerve I)

The sense of smell is diminished in the elderly apparently because of the diminished numbers of nerve fibers (Rockstein 1975). Anosmia and hyposmia may also be due to intracranial tumors, nasal problems, or psychological problems such as depression. The technique for testing the sense of smell was described in unit 5.

The Optic Nerve (Nerve II)

Changes that occur in the eye were described in unit 3 in the sections on the examination of that organ. Disorders affecting the intracranial portion of the optic nerve and its tracts are found by means of field testing, as described in unit 3. Accurate mapping requires special equipment.

To understand and localize lesions of the optic nerve, the nurse must recall that light entering the eye crosses to strike the retina on the opposite side. Thus everything perceived from the client's right side strikes the left side of the retina (see figure 6.71). These images are transmitted through the optic nerve to the chiasma. A portion of the fibers of the nerve crosses over to the contralateral side: the right optic tract contains fibers from the right side of each retina, the left from the left side. These fibers are carried to the respective sides of the occipital lobe.

Thus a homonymous hemianopsia must be due to lesions occurring behind the chiasma, whereas bitemporal and binasal field defects indicate lesions at the chiasma and in the pituitary fossa. Lesions involving one eye are located either in the optic nerve in front of the chiasma or in the eye itself. These uniocular lesions cause blindness and are distinguished by the pupillary reflexes described in the assessment of the

215

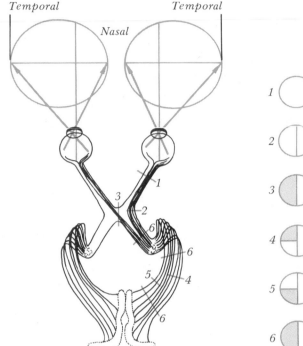

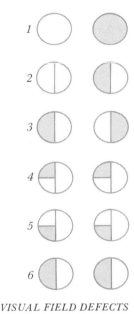

FIGURE 6.71 Location of
Lesions of the Optic Nerve.

VISUAL FIELD DEFECTS

eye (unit 3). Preservation of the consensual reflex places the lesion in the optic nerve.

The Oculomotor, Trochlear, and Abducent Nerves (Nerves III, IV, and VI)

The third, fourth, and sixth nerves serve the extrinsic muscles of the eye. The third nerve also innervates the intrinsic ocular muscles and the levator palpabrae superioris. The assessment of these nerves was described in unit 3. They have a bilateral innervation from the supranuclear pathways.

Lesions involving the oculomotor nerve force the client to wrinkle the forehead when looking upward. This phenomenon is usually associated with ptosis and may also be noted in elderly clients without any apparent oculomotor disorder (Rossman

1971). If ptosis is associated with miosis, ipsilateral anhidrosis and vasodilation, and enophthalmos, the client has *Horner's syndrome.* This disorder is due to destruction of the ipsilateral cervical sympathetic ganglion. Localized at the apex of the lung, it may be invaded and destroyed by a pancoast tumor of that lung.

The Trigeminal Nerve (Nerve V)

The trigeminal nerve has one motor and three sensory divisions.

Motor Division. The motor division is served by the contralateral upper pathways and innervates the muscles of mastication: temporals, masseters, and pterygoids. The nurse asks the client to clench the jaws as tightly as possible and palpates the temporal and masseter muscles on each side; weakness, if present, is apparent. The nurse then asks the client to open the mouth. Deviation of the jaw indicates pterygoid weakness on the side of the deviation.

Facial asymmetry that gives the appearance of weakness can be checked by asking the client to move the jaw from side to side. In the presence of pterygoid weakness, no movement occurs toward the affected side.

Sensory Divisions. The trigeminal nerve has three sensory divisions (see figure 6.72). The opthalmic division serves the forehead, the maxillary division serves the portion of the face above the mouth, and the mandibular division serves the portion below the mouth. These divisions receive sensation from the vortex to the jaw. The angle of the jaw is innervated by the second cervical nerve. Peripheral lesions may affect only part of the trigeminal nerve or its entirety. Central lesions involve all three sensory divisions.

The nurse tests for light touch by stroking the face with paper or cotton, for pain by pricking with a pin, and for temperature sensation by touching with tubes of cold and warm water. Each portion of the face is tested and compared with the opposite side. The client's eyes must be closed during sensory testing. The nurse must avoid leading questions such as "Did you feel that?" or "Was that sharp?" The nurse only asks the client to describe what, if anything, was felt.

After testing the three areas of the face corresponding to the three sensory divisions, the corneal reflex is tested. The client

FIGURE 6.72 Sensory Divisions of the Trigeminal Nerve (Nerve V).

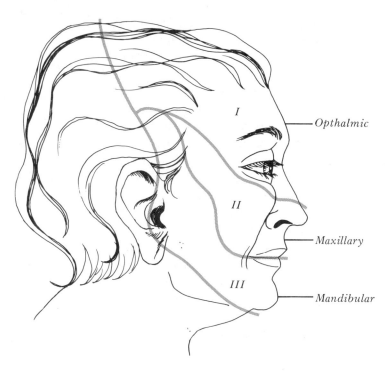

Opthalmic

Maxillary

Mandibular

is asked to look to the side with the eyes open. The nurse touches the temporal side of the cornea on the client's blind side with a wisp of clean cotton and then repeats this procedure for the other eye. The nurse must avoid touching the lashes. The normal response is a brisk closure of the eyes, which tests the integrity of sensation mediated by the trigeminal nerve (V) and the motor response mediated by the facial nerve (VII).

The Facial Nerve (Nerve VII)

The seventh cranial nerve is the major motor nerve of the face. It commands the facial mimic and also contains a small sensory portion that receives sensation from the taste buds of the anterior portion of the tongue.

Motor Division. Observation of the face during the interview and physical assessment provides clues about the presence of any asymmetry. Asymmetry appears as paralysis, contracture, or muscle atrophy and flattening.

The portion of the face above the eyebrows has a bilateral supranuclear innervation and is tested separately. Weakness or paralysis of both upper and lower facial muscles are found in peripheral neuropathies (Bell's palsy). Supranuclear disorders cause only lower facial palsies.

Upper Facial Tests. The nurse asks the client to wrinkle the forehead, frown, and raise the eyebrows. Loss of movement is evident on the affected, paralyzed side. Then the client is asked to close the eyes tightly. If weakness is only slight, the client may be able to close the affected lid. The degree of weakness may be demonstrated by at-

tempting to separate the lids while the client resists. In the event of a peripheral paralysis, the client is unable to close the affected lid and the eye is seen to roll upward (Bell's sign).

Lower Facial Test. Deficiencies of the muscles of the lower face are demonstrated by asking the client to smile and show teeth with a forced grimace. Each side is compared with the other. In the presence of a palsy, movement on the affected side is diminished or absent.

Sensory Division. Testing for taste perception was described in unit 6, on the mouth and throat. A decrease in taste perception is a normal progressive phenomenon of aging (Rockstein 1975).

The Acoustic Nerve (Nerve VIII)

The acoustic, or eighth cranial, nerve is a sensory nerve and has two divisions: the *cochlear* portion, responsible for hearing, and the *vestibular* portion, responsible for balance and orientation in space. The procedures for gross evaluation of these divisions were described in unit 4 in the section on examination of auditory acuity.

The Glossopharyngeal and Vagus Nerves (Nerves IX and X)

The glossopharyngeal and vagus nerves are mixed motor and sensory nerves and are tested together. The sensory portion of the glossopharyngeal nerve innervates the posterior taste buds of the tongue. Testing this area is difficult and requires special equipment.

The motor areas are tested by having the client hold the mouth open and say "Ah!" The normal palate contracts and lifts. Unilateral paralysis causes the palate and the uvula to deviate toward the normal side. Touching the posterior palate or the pillars of the pharynx causes the client to gag. Contraction of the pharyngeal muscles lifts the palate. Unilateral paralysis causes the palate to draw toward the normal side (signe de rideau). If the client is asked to swallow water and regurgitates it through the nose, the client has paralysis of the ninth nerve. Clients with this disorder cannot puff their cheeks outward unless the nose is held closed.

The Spinal Accessory Nerve (Nerve XI)

The spinal accessory nerve is the motor nerve of the sternomastoid and cervical portion of the trapezius. The client is asked to turn the head toward one side while the nurse resists this motion with one hand against the chin. With the other hand the nurse palpates the sternomastoid muscle on the contralateral side of the neck. This procedure is repeated on the other side. Weakness or paralysis is evidenced by inability to turn the head and absence of sternomastoid contraction. Next the client is asked to raise or shrug the shoulders while the nurse resists the movement. Again, weakness or paralysis is the inability to raise the affected shoulder.

The Hypoglossal Nerve (Nerve XII)

Because the hypoglossal nerve is the motor nerve of the tongue, the nurse has only to ask the client to protrude this organ. Muscle atrophy or fasciculations may be present. Fasciculations indicate involvement of the nucleus of the nerve. In case of paralysis deviation is toward the affected side. Minimal paralysis is identified by ask-ing the client to press the tip of the tongue against the cheek while the nurse presses a finger against the client's cheek. Each side is examined in turn and the force of the tongue may be compared.

THE CEREBELLAR SYSTEM: EXAMINATION AND OBJECTIVE FINDINGS

The cerebellar system regulates body tonus and with the neostriatal system is responsible for coordinated movements requiring positional judgment.

Evidence of cerebellar dysfunction is found in syndromes of disequilibrium. These syndromes cause an abnormal gait with pitches and falls, not unlike that of a drunkard. The finger-to-nose test reveals *dysmetria* with overshooting but eventual success. The dysmetria is not worsened by closing the eyes.

A constant sign of cerebellar dysfunction is *dysdiadochokinesis* when the client is asked to perform a repetitive and alternating movement. The nurse asks the client to sit and place a hand on the knee, first with the palmar surface up, next with the dorsal surface up. This alternating supination and pronation is markedly slowed and disjointed with cerebellar disorders. Other signs include a deviation of the client toward the affected side when walking a straight line with the eyes closed and, to be sure, the presence of nystagmus.

THE PERIPHERAL MOTOR SYSTEM: EXAMINATION AND OBJECTIVE FINDINGS

The techniques involved in examining the peripheral motor system are inspection and palpation.

219

Inspection

A large portion of this examination was described in unit 13 in the section on the physical examination of the musculoskeletal system. The nurse looks for abnormal posture, positions, and movements and analyzes the client's gait.

Gait changes may be due to musculoskeletal disorders or to problems of the peripheral or central nervous systems. Clients with parkinsonism develop stiffness and walk with short, shuffling steps, leaning slightly into the direction in which they are walking. Their arms are carried stiffly at their sides. In earlier unilateral stages the body tends to lean toward the affected side.

Clients with hemiparesis have a scissors gait: they swing the affected leg in a semicircle from the hip, with the knee held in extension. If the arm is affected, it is held close to the body with the elbow bent.

Cerebellar disorders cause the gait to be jerky and uncoordinated. The client tends to lose balance and lurches from side to side as though intoxicated.

Palpation

Palpation of muscles and evaluation of range of motion were described in the previous unit.

Testing the Peripheral Motor System

After completing these examinations, the nurse should test for Kernig's, Lasègue's, Patrick's, and Brudzinski's signs (see figure 6.73).

Kernig's Sign. The client is recumbent; one leg is held flat on the table and the other is raised from the hip with the knee bent. The knee is then straightened. Kernig's sign is the inability of the calf to straighten beyond 135° from the thigh. This sign reveals meningeal and posterior root irritation. The client should be asked to trace the path of radiation of the pain with the finger. This path should be described, as it helps to isolate the affected dorsal root.

Lasègue's Sign. The client is recumbent; one leg is held down and the other is raised by the nurse, from the hip with the knee straight. Lasègue's sign is the inability to raise the leg beyond 70° from the horizontal. This sign is often positive in the presence of a herniated intervertebral disc. It also indicates meningeal and posterior root irritation.

Patrick's Sign. Patrick's sign distinguishes between disease of the hip and dis-

FIGURE 6.73   Motor System Tests.

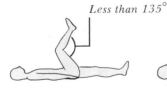   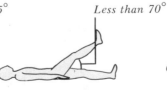

Less than 135°   *Less than 70°*

KERNIG'S SIGN   LASÈGUE'S SIGN   PATRICK'S SIGN   BRUDZINSKI'S SIGN

ease of the spinal column. With the client supine, the nurse flexes one of the client's thighs and places the ankle of that limb above the patella of the extended one. The knee is then pressed down and out, causing abduction and lateral rotation in the hip. Pain appearing before the knee reaches the table top indicates a disorder of the hip or sacroiliac articulations.

Brudzinski's Sign. With the client supine, the nurse flexes the client's head on the neck. Brudzinski's sign is a spontaneous flexion of the hip and knee joints. If the sign is positive, it indicates meningeal irritation.

Testing the Extrapyramidal System

Coordinated movements designed to demonstrate problems in the extrapyramidal system include the finger-to-nose test, the thumb-to-finger test, and the Romberg test. These tests are done first with the eyes open and then with the eyes closed.

Finger-to-Nose Test. The client is asked to extend the forearm and the index finger and to slowly place the index tip on the nose. The nurse observes for the presence of tremor and for a difference between performances with eyes opened and then closed. Abnormalities that occur with the eyes open indicate extrapyramidal and cerebellar lesions. These lesions do not affect performance with closed eyes. Abnormalities that occur only with the eyes closed indicate posterior-column spinal cord disorders.

Thumb-to-Finger Test. The client is asked to place the tip of the thumb against the tip of each finger of the same hand. This test is done with gradually increasing speed, first with eyes open and then with eyes closed. In central motor disorders the client's performance is abnormally slow.

The Romberg Test. The client is asked to stand with arms at the sides, feet together, and eyes open. If this posture can be maintained, the client is asked to close the eyes. The client must be reassured that the nurse will not allow a fall. The nurse places both hands at shoulder level and on each side of the client to prevent a fall. A slight sway is normal. The nurse must not touch the client during the test. A positive test is an inability to maintain this position for any length of time.

THE PERIPHERAL SENSORY SYSTEM: EXAMINATION AND OBJECTIVE FINDINGS

Testing the peripheral sensory system is purely subjective, and fatigue will diminish the accuracy of the results. The techniques are those described in the examination of the fifth nerve.

Thalamic lesions cause pain on the contralateral side. Spinal cord lesions cause sensory changes on the opposite side below the level of the lesion. Lesions involving the spinal nerve roots have a dermatome distribution (see figure 6.74). Peripheral nerve lesions cause sensory changes in the distribution of the peripheral nerve (see figures 6.75a and 6.75b).

Each area of the body is tested and compared with the opposite side. The responses may indicate normal sensation, hypoesthesia, anesthesia, hyperesthesia, and paresthesia.

Deep sensation (bathyesthesia), or position sense, is tested by asking the client to

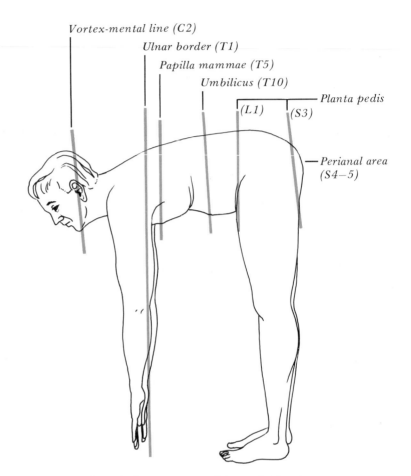

Vortex-mental line (C2)

Ulnar border (T1)

Papilla mammae (T5)

Umbilicus (T10)

Planta pedis

(L1)   *(S3)*

Perianal area (S4—5)

FIGURE 6.74 Landmarks for Dermatome Distribution.

C2	= 2nd cervical nerve	L1	= 1st lumbar nerve
T1	= 1st thoracic nerve	S3	= 3rd sacral nerve
T5	= 5th thoracic nerve	S4–5	= 4th and 5th sacral nerves
T10	= 10th thoracic nerve		

imitate the position of one limb with the other. The nurse places the client's limb in a certain position and asks the client, whose eyes are closed, to imitate the new position. Position sense is also tested by the Romberg test and by asking the client to walk with eyes closed. Failure indicates ataxia.

Other tests for deep sensation include pressing on long tendons, which normally causes pain; testing for vibration sense; and testing for stereognosis. *Achilles tendon ten-*

derness is lost in tabes. *Vibration sense* is another form of deep sensation that is lost in posterior column disease. Vibration sense is tested by placing a vibrating tuning fork (c128) in contact with a bone. *Stereognosis* is the ability to recognize familiar objects by the way they feel, with the eyes closed. The nurse places an object in the client's hand and asks for its identification. Unilateral astereognosis is found in parietal lobe lesions of the cortex.

ANTERIOR

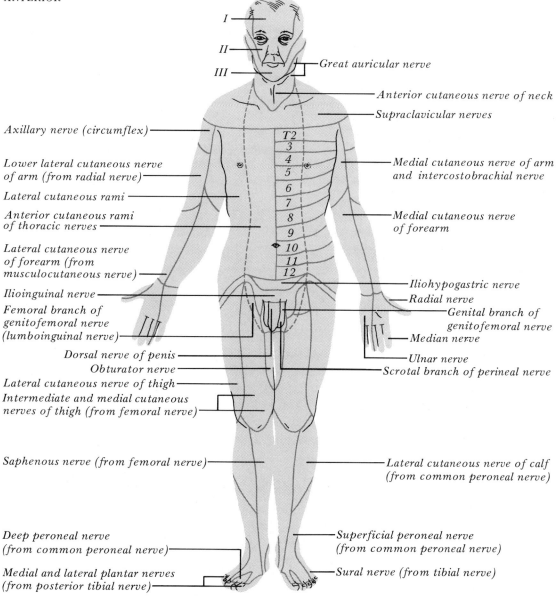

I

II

III — Great auricular nerve

Anterior cutaneous nerve of neck

Supraclavicular nerves

Axillary nerve (circumflex)

Lower lateral cutaneous nerve
of arm (from radial nerve)

Lateral cutaneous rami

Anterior cutaneous rami
of thoracic nerves

Lateral cutaneous nerve
of forearm (from
musculocutaneous nerve)

Ilioinguinal nerve

Femoral branch of
genitofemoral nerve
(lumboinguinal nerve)

Dorsal nerve of penis

Obturator nerve

Lateral cutaneous nerve of thigh

Intermediate and medial cutaneous
nerves of thigh (from femoral nerve)

Saphenous nerve (from femoral nerve)

Deep peroneal nerve
(from common peroneal nerve)

Medial and lateral plantar nerves
(from posterior tibial nerve)

T2
3
4
5
6
7
8
9
10
11
12

Medial cutaneous nerve of arm
and intercostobrachial nerve

Medial cutaneous nerve
of forearm

Iliohypogastric nerve

Radial nerve

Genital branch of
genitofemoral nerve

Median nerve

Ulnar nerve

Scrotal branch of perineal nerve

Lateral cutaneous nerve of calf
(from common peroneal nerve)

Superficial peroneal nerve
(from common peroneal nerve)

Sural nerve (from tibial nerve)

FIGURE 6.75a Distribution of Peripheral Nerves (Anterior).

223

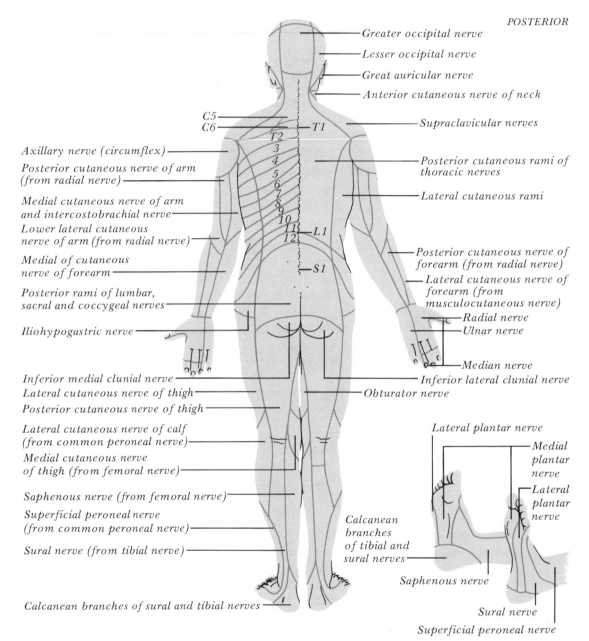

Greater occipital nerve

Lesser occipital nerve

Great auricular nerve

Anterior cutaneous nerve of neck

Supraclavicular nerves

C5
C6
T1

T2
3
4
5
6
7
8
9
10
11
12
L1

S1

Axillary nerve (circumflex)

Posterior cutaneous nerve of arm
(from radial nerve)

Medial cutaneous nerve of arm
and intercostobrachial nerve

Lower lateral cutaneous
nerve of arm (from radial nerve)

Medial of cutaneous
nerve of forearm

Posterior rami of lumbar,
sacral and coccygeal nerves

Iliohypogastric nerve

Posterior cutaneous rami of
thoracic nerves

Lateral cutaneous rami

Posterior cutaneous nerve of
forearm (from radial nerve)

Lateral cutaneous nerve of
forearm (from
musculocutaneous nerve)

Radial nerve
Ulnar nerve

Median nerve

Inferior medial clunial nerve
Lateral cutaneous nerve of thigh
Posterior cutaneous nerve of thigh

Inferior lateral clunial nerve
Obturator nerve

Lateral cutaneous nerve of calf
(from common peroneal nerve)
Medial cutaneous nerve
of thigh (from femoral nerve)

Saphenous nerve (from femoral nerve)

Superficial peroneal nerve
(from common peroneal nerve)

Sural nerve (from tibial nerve)

Calcanean
branches
of tibial and
sural nerves

Lateral plantar nerve

Medial
plantar
nerve

Lateral
plantar
nerve

Saphenous nerve

Calcanean branches of sural and tibial nerves

Sural nerve

Superficial peroneal nerve

FIGURE 6.75b   Distribution of Peripheral Nerves (Posterior).

REFLEXES: EXAMINATION AND OBJECTIVE FINDINGS

Because of their objectivity, reflexes are the most important part of the examination. They consist of the deep reflexes, the cutaneous reflexes, reflexes of spinal automatism, postural reflexes, reflexes elicited through distant receptors, and organic reflexes.

Deep Reflexes

The deep reflexes include the stretch, tendon, and periostial reflexes. They are named after the zone of provocation and are elicited by a brisk tap on a tendon or bony prominence. In lesions involving the pyramidal tracts, the reflex response is heightened and clonus may appear.

The *glabella reflex* is elicited by tapping the glabella to cause a brisk blink. In the normal client the reflex is suppressed after repeated tapping; in clients with extrapyramidal disease the reflex is not suppressed.

The *jaw jerk,* also mediated by the pons, is absent or minimal in the normal client. To elicit this reflex, the nurse asks the client to allow the jaw to sag open, places a finger on the client's chin, and then strikes the finger briskly with a reflex hammer. With hyperactivity due to a pyramidal lesion, the jaw snaps shut.

The *brachioradialis or supinator jerk* is elicited with the client's arm partially flexed and supported on the nurse's hand (see figure 6.76). The nurse then briskly strikes the distal radius with a reflex hammer. The contraction of the brachioradialis muscle causes the elbow to flex.

To elicit the *biceps muscle reflex,* the nurse supports the client's elbow on the hand; the client's forearm rests on the nurse's forearm. The nurse's thumb passes forward and presses on the client's biceps tendon. The hammer briskly strikes the thumb overlying the tendon, which causes the biceps to contract and flexes the forearm.

To elicit the triceps reflex, the nurse supports the client's arm with the elbow bent and the forearm dangling freely. A blow delivered to the distal triceps aponeurosis causes the muscle to contract and extends the forearm. The brachioradialis and biceps are mediated by cervical segment five and six, the triceps by cervical segment seven.

FIGURE 6.76   Brachioradialis or Supinator Jerk.

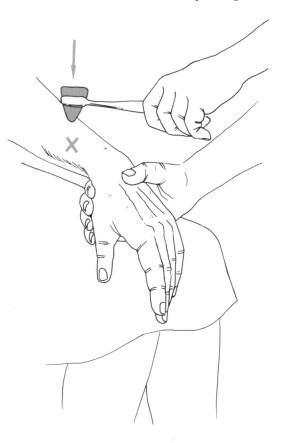

225

If the nurse flicks the client's fingernail, normally no contraction of the finger occurs. In pyramidal lesions with hyperreflexia, this contraction does appear and extends to a flexion of the thumb called *Hoffman's sign.*

In the lower extremities, the *knee jerk,* or quadriceps reflex, is an action of homolateral extension due to contraction of the quadriceps muscle. The knee is placed and supported in flexion, with the muscles relaxed. The nurse strikes briskly against the quadriceps tendon below the patella. The normal response is an extension of the leg and is mediated by the third and fourth lumbar segments. The *ankle jerk,* or achilles reflex, is due to a contraction of the gastrocnemius and soleus muscles when the achilles tendon is tapped. The client may have to kneel on a chair with the feet hanging down to be adequately relaxed. If the client is recumbent, the examiner should hold the client's leg with the hip and knee flexed and the foot at right angle to the leg. The hammer strikes the tendon briskly and causes a sharp jerk of the foot. This reflex is mediated by the first and second sacral segments. It is diminished by ankle edema and is frequently decreased or absent in the elderly (Carter 1971). *Ankle clonus* may be provoked by holding the leg as for eliciting the achilles tendon reflex and then sharply bending the foot upward and holding it there. This sudden stretch of the achilles tendon may elicit a prolonged series of recurrent jerking while the nurse holds the position of tension on the tendon. This clonus is an abnormal hyperreaction and indicates a supranuclear lesion.

The nurse rates all tendon and periostial reflexes. These reflexes are increased in supranuclear lesions. In sudden transection of the cord or immediately after a cerebrovascular catastrophe, these reflexes may be diminished or abolished, but as soon as the phase of spinal shock is passed, they return with heightened force. In cerebellar lesions these reflexes often have a pendular quality due to the diminished muscle tonus. The usual rating system is: $1+$, feeble; $2+$, normal; $3+$, increased; and $4+$, clonic. The rating of each reflex tested permits a baseline comparison of both sides of the body.

Superficial or Cutaneous Reflexes

Superficial reflexes are elicited by stroking the skin of specific areas with a pin or other tapered object.

The *plantar reflex* is elicited by stroking the sole of the foot from the heel toward the fifth toe and then passing medially along the ball of the foot. The normal response is a plantar flexion of all the toes. *Babinski's sign* is a fanlike spreading of the toes and an upward movement of the big toe. This fanning is abnormal in adults and is found with lesions of the pyramidal tract. In peripheral nerve lesions no response occurs. This reflex is recorded as Babinski present, absent, or no response. Cold feet may interfere with this reflex.

The *abdominal reflex* is elicited by a long firm stroke downward along the lateral abdominal wall. This stroke causes a contraction of the rectus muscle and pulls the umbilicus toward the contracting side. It is abolished by pyramidal lesions and interfered with by obesity.

The *cremaster reflex* is an upward contraction of testicle. It is elicited by stroking downward on the inner aspect of the thigh while observing the ipsilateral testicle.

Reflexes of Spinal Automatism

Reflexes of spinal automatism are normally absent. In lesions of the cord they are easily elicited.

Flexion reflex of the lower limbs is elicited by pinching the achilles tendon, which causes flexion of the hip, knee, and ankle on the ipsilateral side. This reflex indicates a pyramidal lesion. Occasionally an extension of the contralateral limb is seen.

The mass reflex is elicited when a painful stimulus is applied to the lower limb, resulting in flexion of that limb and evacuation of the bladder. This reflex has been used to retrain the bladder.

Organic Reflexes

One of the organic reflexes is the cardiac slowing induced by *carotid sinus pressure.* This reflex is mediated by the glossopharyngeal and vagus nerves. A *gooseflesh response* to cold is another organic reflex.

Neurological Assessment

Through sensory, motor, and reflex testing, the nurse can differentiate between a peripheral nerve injury and a supranuclear injury.

Peripheral Nerve Injury. Peripheral nerve injuries are characterized by *flaccid paralysis* with *areflexia, muscle atrophy,* and *sensory loss.* An electromyography can confirm such an injury.

Supranuclear (Pyramidal Tract) Injury. Supranuclear injuries are characterized by hypertonicity or spastic paralysis with *hyperreflexia,* demonstrated by *inferior cutaneous reflex* signs (Babinski), and little or no atrophy or sensory loss. An electromyography, if performed, will be normal.

The *electromyogram* is helpful in assessing lesions of the motor nucleus. It confirms the presence of fasciculations, which are the hallmark of such lesions, by showing the abnormal discharge pattern of the motor nucleus.

Once a lesion is discovered, the nurse should attempt to localize it anatomically. The anatomical localization, combined with the history of onset and progression, will provide much information concerning the possible etiology and will determine the kinds of tests needed for complete assessment and treatment.

REFERENCES

CARTER, A. B. 1971. "The Neurologic Aspects of Aging." In I. Rossman, ed., *Clinical Geriatrics.* Philadelphia: J. B. Lippincott.

FORD, J. M., and W. T. ROTH. 1977. "Do Cognitive Abilities Decline with Age?" *Geriatrics* 32(9):59–62.

GUYTON, A. C. 1976. *Textbook of Medical Physiology.* Philadelphia: W. B. Saunders.

KART, C. S., E. S. METRESS, and J. F. METRESS. 1978. *Aging and Health: Biologic and Social Perspectives.* Reading, Mass.: Addison-Wesley.

KOTTKE, F. J. 1974. "Historia Obscura Hemiplegie." *Archives of Physical Medicine and Rehabilitation* 55:4–13.

POSNER, C. M. 1976. "The Types of Headaches That Affect the Elderly." *Geriatrics* 31(9):103–06.

ROCKSTEIN, M. 1975. "The Biology of Aging in Humans." In R. Goldman and M. Rockstein, eds., *The Physiology and Pathology of Human Aging.* New York: Academic Press.

ROSSMAN, I. 1971. "The Anatomy of Aging." In I. Rossman, ed., *Clinical Geriatrics.* Philadelphia: J. B. Lippincott.

STAMLER, J. 1966. "Epidemiology of Cerebro-vascular Disease." In R. E. DeForest, ed., *Proceedings of the National Stroke Congress, 1964, Chicago, Illinois.* Springfield, Ill.: Charles C. Thomas.

TIMARIS, P. S., and A. VERNADAHIS. 1971. "Structural, Biochemical, and Functional Aging of the Nervous System." In P. S. Timaris, ed., *Developmental Physiology and Aging.* New York: Macmillan.

WILDER, C. S. 1975. "Prevalence of Selected Impairments: United States—1971." *Department of Health Education and Welfare,* Publication no. (HRA) 75–1526. Rockville, Md.

ZIEGLER, D. K., R. S. HASSANEIN, and J. R. COUCH, 1977. "Characteristics of Life Headache Histories in a Nonclinic Population." *Neurology* 27:265–69.

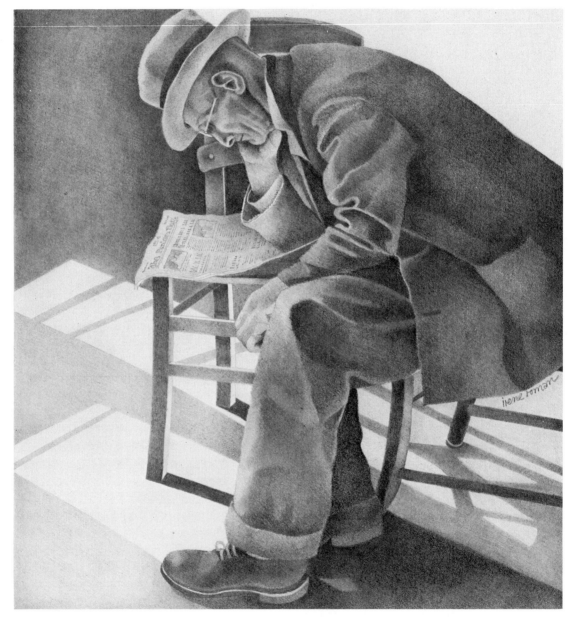

William O'Rourke

Chapter 7

THE MENTAL HEALTH
ASSESSMENT

Simone de Beauvoir (1972) reminds us of Prince Siddhartha's first venture away from the protection of his father's palace. On that afternoon he chanced to see an old, old man for the very first time. The man was bald, gray haired, and bent as he shuffled along with the help of a cane. Puzzled, Siddhartha asked his carriage driver what or who this was. Informed that this was a man grown old, he was saddened and asked to return to the palace with this comment: "What is the use of pleasure and delights since I myself am the future dwelling place of old age?" (de Beauvoir 1972, p.1).

We can assume that Siddhartha was appalled at the physical or biological effects of growing old. Insightful as he was, he was immediately aware that he, too, might suffer a like fate and he became saddened. This of course was the *young* Buddha. He had not yet learned to look more deeply beyond the biological or physical to the other dimensions of human aging. Accordingly Siddhartha may have been like people today who still tend to think of growing old in terms of biological change—that is, in terms of physical loss or decline.

Experience, however, tells us that understanding growing old only in terms of the body and its decline is to misunderstand the heart of the aging process itself. Humans cannot be explained or understood merely in terms of their bodies. Consider the example of a 97-year-old woman who was fully alert but confined (because of broken hips) to a wheelchair. She was peaceful and acceptant and a delight to everyone. When asked how she managed to smile and stay relatively content, she replied gently, "It's my legs that are paralyzed, not my heart." Or consider this conversation between two 80-year-old women who were sharing the difficulties of being wheelchair-bound and almost totally de-

231

pendent. One woman said with a sigh, "It's a long trek"; the other with empathy added, "And we've got to be strong to stand it." An observer would know that she was referring to a strength other than physical and would sense that these two physically weak elderly women were actually great and strong people. Their bodies were indeed in decline but their courage and patience had grown and developed in spite of physical loss. How can we become more aware of or even begin to understand this very beautiful growth so common among the elderly? Perhaps we could begin by shifting from a largely biological to a more holistic, or body-and-spirit, perspective that emphasizes aging as *development* rather than decline. The life-course developmental model for human aging exemplifies such a perspective. It shows aging as a forward and upward movement characterized by continued growth and adaption until death.

Figure 7.1 depicts the life-course developmental model with the difficult period of the younger years marked by incline. The long period of adulthood is depicted with a more gradual ascent; here one solidifies and maintains trends developed in adolescence. Somewhere around age 60 to 65, the period of later maturity and old age begins. Note the steep incline, indicating that the developmental tasks of this period are again difficult, though the slope is always upward, indicating continued growth.

The biological model of aging shown in figure 7.2 looks very different. From birth to early adulthood, the body grows and develops. Then, after reaching its peak, it slowly begins to decline. Indisputably, biological aging, or senescence, is decline. The problem arises when we come to understand human aging only in terms of this decline. If the biological model of aging is superimposed on the developmental model (see figure 7.3), one can see how vastly different the two perspectives are.

Perhaps up to now students of aging have focused too narrowly on the research of the early gerontologists, who were generally biological and clinical medical researchers. We do indeed owe a huge debt to

FIGURE 7.1   Developmental Model of Aging.

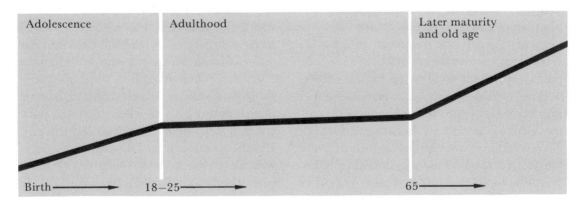

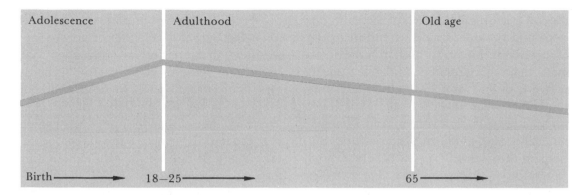

FIGURE 7.2   Biological Model of Aging.

these pioneers, but the nature of the total person demands that we widen our perspective. The study of aging must be multidisciplinary. The humanities—literature, philosophy, theology, art, and law—must join with biology, psychology, and sociology in helping us understand and appreciate human aging.

With the help of the sciences and the humanities we can begin to understand how many older persons continue to adjust and thrive, revealing a strength, courage, and wisdom that demand the admiration and emulation of all.

AGING AS DEVELOPMENT

We can conceptualize aging as development rather than simply decline by using a model that is sensitive to the social, psychological, and spiritual dimensions of the individual while we continue to attend to the very important fact of gradual physical decline. In this effort we are aided by Eric Erikson (1976), who conceived the human life course as an eight-stage developmental process. Erikson's theory, as modified by Peck (Kimmel 1974), is presented in these pages because it suggests specific develop-

FIGURE 7.3   Comparison of Developmental and Biological Models of Aging.

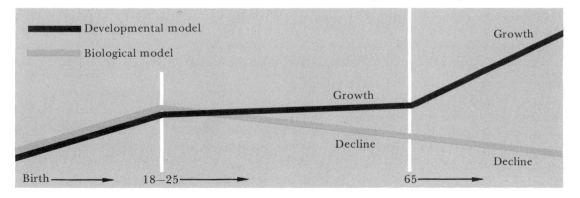

mental tasks involving each of these dimensions and because it calls attention to the close relationship and interaction between one's inner development and one's social network or environment. However, note that other stage theorists, such as Havighurst, Levinson, Loevinger, and Neugarten, have also made important contributions to this growing specialty. For a brief comparative discussion of stage theories and some comments on their tentative nature, see the standard texts.

Each of Erikson's stages is marked by a turning point in which a challenge for continued growth is offered by the circumstances of life itself. If the challenge is accepted and mastered, growth occurs; if the challenge is refused, one remains stunted and fixated and less capable of mastering the challenge of the next stage. Some have likened Erikson's model to a journey on the "river of life," with eight critical turns. As we approach each turn, we experience tension and uncertainty. If we make the turn safely, we grow and gain new strength. If we do not make it safely, we emerge bruised and less prepared for the turns ahead. In the model as in life itself, we must keep moving while carrying, for better or worse, the results of each earlier stage.

Erikson calls each stage a crisis because at each turn we are torn or pulled by opposing forces: the invitation to stretch and grow conflicts with the desire to remain secure with the familiar or status quo. For example, during the seventh stage, which covers the midlife or working years, the challenge is to generate or contribute to the upbuilding of life itself. If we choose not to generate through child rearing, work, or community development, then we inevitably settle for a kind of impotency that Erikson calls *stagnation.* Whether or not we successfully navigate the seventh stage and become at least to some extent "generators" is important both in itself and as a preparation for the challenge of the next and final stage of the life course. Most agree that the middle years are formative for the later years. What we are throughout this long developmental period will deeply influence the kind of persons we will become in old age. However, in no way is the die cast in midlife! All of life is developmental; even if we cannot rise to the challenges of the earlier stages, we can change and accept long-denied or rejected possibilities and realities in the final stage of life. In fact, the specific task of the eighth and last stage is to pull all of life together into a finished wholeness.

THE EIGHTH STAGE: INTEGRITY VERSUS DISGUST AND DESPAIR

Erikson's final stage, integrity versus disgust and despair, is so named because the task at this time of life is to "integrate"— that is, to gather together our whole life, to come to terms with our personal past, present, and future. Integration implies a wholeness suggesting that those who are successful at this stage are comfortably able to be what they are: individuals with a history of both success and failure; individuals who must here and now accept multiple-role loss together with an aging and often chronically ill body; and finally, individuals nearing the end of the life course who cannot realistically expect more than a few months or years of life. Failure to integrate past, present, and future leaves one in disgust or despair—disgusted about the past, despairing and hopeless about the present and future.

Although these tasks or challenges are read or spoken about rather easily, they are the most formidable and most deeply personal of all life's challenges. They demand a strength and a courage that we tend to take for granted in the old. The remainder of this section describes the tasks of integrating the past, present, and future and includes some elaboration of the strategies through which the tasks are accomplished.

Integrating the Past

Integrating the past is often accomplished through reminiscing and life review. In a weekly therapy group of nursing home residents age 80 and older, the conversation frequently moves to the good and not-so-good old days. Personal memories are explored and exchanged. The group sometimes shares feelings of regret about the past, but most often they share, with contentment, stories about the good old days. The group members, all of whom are physically disabled but mentally alert, seem to leave these sessions cheerful, light hearted, and satisfied with themselves. Even the sad feelings sometimes generated seem to be accepted and worked through.

An 88-year-old resident at the nursing home once stated that he was kept very busy thinking. When asked what he thought about, he replied, "All the things I've ever done." He was looking back over his life to gather it together, fitting pieces that would not join before, coming at last to "own" all of his past, good and bad inseparably bound together. Butler (1963) has called this process *life review,* or *reminiscing.*

A student described the life-review process as being similar to going back over slag discarded from a coal mine with modern coal-reclaiming machinery. With the more refined or sensitive equipment, much that has been lost can be reclaimed and used. This is a beautiful way to describe reminiscing. The new equipment is, of course, a more mature perspective on life. From this vantage point some things and events that before seemed important are not so anymore, and others that were unimportant seem to be precious now.

Integrating the past also means dealing with guilt and regrets—forgiving oneself for past mistakes and coming to terms with memories that cannot be changed. This difficult developmental task can be facilitated by family, friends, or a "significant person" (Federal Council on Aging 1976) from the community who will listen to these feelings and offer empathetic understanding. In such a climate the process of life review can and will lead to self-forgiveness and acceptance.

Ebersole (1976) states that reminiscing can be enriching whether done alone, in pairs, or in groups. The elderly need to be encouraged and helped in this effort. The story may be an old one, told and retold, but each telling has a purpose. We must learn simply to listen with attention, for perhaps in each retelling there is something new and different to the story teller himself.

Integrating the Present and Future

Integrating the present and future is perhaps as difficult a task as learning to live

235

with the past. As Butler and Lewis (1973) note, older people live with a keen sense of the present. For many elderly people, waking up to one more day of life is a gift. An 89-year-old man explained to a class of younger people that he was on borrowed time. The class heard something negative or pessimistic in this remark and pressed him for an explanation. He laughingly reminded them that according to statistics he should have died fifteen years earlier, so every day was an "extra" for him. They then understood that he was not negative but was simply realistically surprised and grateful to be alive at that moment.

INTEGRATION THROUGH TRANSCENDENCE

Clearly, the realness of the present may be a source of great stress to the older person. Feelings of uselessness and uncertainty associated with the loss or change of life-long roles, such as spouse, provider, parent, homeowner, and community worker, must be dealt with on a daily basis. Every day also brings renewed struggles with a weakening and sometimes frail body as well as a sense of being one day closer to the very end of the life course itself. Peck (1968) has suggested that these losses may be integrated by transcending, or rising above, them. To transcend the losses does not mean to deny them, but rather to endeavor to put them in a different and more positive perspective. Specifically Peck suggests that to adapt successfully to these later years, we must transcend in three areas: our roles, our bodies, and the end of the life course.

Transcending One's Role

In a society that promotes and expects excellence in doing and having, the experience of merely *being* seems empty and even boring. Modern technological society tends to see and value individuals according to their function or role—that is, according to what they *do,* rather than who they *are.* Keen (1968) notes that the existential philosopher Gabriel Marcel called this attitude the "dis-ease" of modern society. When roles become all-important, they cannot be dropped or switched without experiencing the loss of a sense of self. At the final stage in the life course, however, one must come to value oneself outside the role of spouse, parent, tradesperson, club member, or athlete, because often these roles are stripped away by the circumstances of life. In terms of transcendence, therefore, the task is to rise above these roles, to discard them as external and superficial to the real self, and to find in the process that the roles are not the real "me." In essence we are not any of these roles: we are more. A felt sense of freedom develops in this experience—a feeling associated with integrity. For example, an 80-year-old widow whose arthritis has forced her into a wheelchair can still smile and hope and pray. She can still be a warm, loving human being without the roles she exercised throughout her earlier life.

Transcending One's Body

Transcending the frailty, discomfort, and even the looks of one's body is the task suggested in the example mentioned earlier of the 97-year-old woman who said that she kept reasonably content despite being wheelchair-bound, because only her legs were paralyzed, not her heart. How does one arrive at this state of mind? When the question was put to a group of frail elderly, they answered by saying that there are no secret methods. One simply "makes up one's mind" that he or she will keep doing as much as possible despite aches and pains. This challenging and difficult task requires support and encouragement from significant others. At its roots, however, transcending one's body is a personal decision based on one's philosophy of life and demands the special courage that seems available to men and women at this stage of the life course.

Transcending the End of the Life Course

Robert Lifton (1972) suggested that at least three types of transcendence tend to allay the very basic fear or uncertainty associated with death: *biosocial* transcendence, which is a sense of living on in one's children or in the society one has helped to build; *natural* transcendence, which is a sense of being a part of all life and thus continuing to exist as part of the universe; and *religious* transcendence, which is a sense that life on earth is but a preparation for eternal life with God.

These tasks, like the others proposed earlier, pose formidable challenges to the older adult. Family, friends, and neighbors are most important at this time, as is a working religious belief or philosophy of life. Erikson suggests that " . . . every human being's Integrity may be said to be religious (whether explicitly or not), namely, in an inner search for, and a wish to communicate with, that mysterious, that Ultimate Other: for there can be no 'I' without an 'Other,' no 'We' without a shared 'Other' " (Erikson 1976, p. 11). Continuing spiritual or religious experiences are important to the elderly, as is the opportunity to share and deepen a personal philosophy of life.

Tragically, however, many older people must meet these challenges alone. During the earlier life crises, familial and institutional support are available. Parents, siblings, school, and church offer assistance throughout infancy, childhood, adolescence, and adulthood. But in old age frequently no spouse is present, children are busy or removed, relatives and old friends are dead or far away, and even the churches tend to withdraw, leaving many older people to go this last developmental mile alone.

THE DEVELOPMENT OF WISDOM

According to Erikson, a specific virtue or strength is born of the struggles to meet the challenge or task of each stage. For example, the challenge of the final stage is to develop integrity rather than disgust or despair. In the personal battle to integrate one's past and present in late life, a dynamic interchange occurs between feelings of acceptance (integrity) and feelings of disgust and despair. This interchange is a personal struggle, and at any given moment one may be winning or losing. If one is successful, the result is not a complete victory over disgust and despair, but rather what Erikson calls "a dynamic balance in integrity's favor" (Erikson 1976, p. 23). The decision is to accept and carry on despite continuous awareness of loss and change. This decision gives rise to the new strength or virtue that emerges from the conflict. This late-life strength Erikson called *wisdom,* which is "the detached and yet active concern with life itself in the face of death itself, and [which] maintains and conveys the integrity of experience, in spite of the decline of bodily and mental functions" (Erikson 1976, p. 23).

With this new strength—this wisdom— the elderly can stand back from life and cri-

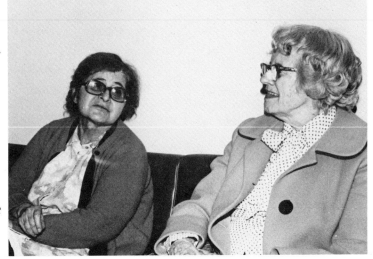

The gerontological nurse can help the elderly adapt to the aging process by encouraging relationships with significant others; elderly clients need to share their feelings about the past and present with someone who understands and cares.

tique it from a new and positive perspective. For example, the values that tended to predominate throughout the earlier phases of the life course may now be revealed as wanting; this new perspective allows better, more authentically human values to emerge as important. In practice, elderly individuals with the strength called wisdom may now feel that though they are no longer spouses or parents or workers, they are still persons. In effect they are *who* they *are* rather than *what* they *do*. They can also feel that though physical health and strength are of great value, the body is, in fact, not the total person, and even in the face of serious disabilities and loss one can love and be loved, trust and be trusted; one can still smile, be kind, forgive, and offer comfort to those around. Such elderly are truly survivors with a message for those who will listen. To attempt to present the message here may be presumptuous, but it might be something like this: Do not put all your stock in physical strength or health

because such qualities will not last, and do not act as if you own anything forever, even your life, because you do not. There comes a time when health, strength, and possessions may be taken, and then you will learn that these are only accessories to authentic human existence, which is typified by love, concern for others, and mutual kindness and support. To philosophize a bit further, our technological society, which has prolonged life for millions through better food and health care, may have actually produced a group of wise elders who will challenge the depersonalizing aspects of technology and will transcend them by adapting to higher values. If so, then we must be grateful for the large number of the very old in our society. They are not our problem, but our solution. We need the wisdom of the aged today, much as it was needed in the preindustrial era.

Clark and Anderson (1967) found in their large community sample of San Franciscans that the majority of older people do in fact adapt to higher values. According to Clark and Anderson, most aging people face five adaptive tasks:

1. Recognition of aging and definition of instrumental limitation,
2. Redefinition of physical and social life space,
3. Substitution of alternate sources of need satisfaction,
4. Reassessment of criteria for evaluation of the self,
5. Reintegration of values and life goals.

Their study indicated that 61 percent of those sampled were adapting to these tasks and 39 percent were not. Clark and Anderson concluded:

> Those in our sample whom we found to be adapted in their old age have suggested the answer to this problem [of maladaptation and alienation in old age]. These are the elderly who have successfully developed personal codes of values which have eased their resolution of the adaptive tasks of aging . . . . These codes are not alien to American culture—they are the secondary values—and those who survive best in their later years are simply those who have been able to drop their pursuits of primary values . . . and to go on to pick up, as workable substitutes, the alternative values which have been around all along: conservation instead of acquisition and exploitation; self-acceptance instead of continuous struggles for self-advancement; being rather than doing; congeniality, cooperation, love, and concern for others instead of control of others. These are the values the aged in our society have been forced to embrace. [Clark and Anderson 1967, p. 429]

Those who are adapting seem to be transcending or integrating in the Eriksonian sense, giving birth in the process to wisdom—to a new and better perspective on life itself.

LEARNING TO LET GO— ADAPTATION

Aging understood as development implies adapting to change as we move through the life course—accepting new roles and responsibilities and discarding or losing others. This adaptation is facilitated when we develop a certain skill in the letting go of roles, persons, places, and things that must be relinquished through circumstances often beyond our control. For example, choosing a job in another state involves many "leavings," including house, neighborhood, and often friends. Entering high school or college, getting married, having a first child, and sending the last child off to school all involve a leaving behind or a letting go in the process of adjustment.

The process of letting go may offer some clues to successful aging. It has been said that we spend the first part of our lives collecting things and the remainder slowly giving them up. In this context collecting refers to the process of involving ourselves with persons, places, and things in such a way that they almost become part of us. As an analogy, consider two plants growing in the same pot—their roots, though always separate, become intertwined. If one plant dies or must be moved, it must be gradually worked loose from the other. So it is that when an individual must separate from a loved person or place, the disentanglement must be done carefully, over time. One does not merely pull loose and walk away. Letting go is a process.

239

This process of disentangling or separating has been called *grieving*. In some ways this term is unfortunate, because most people associate it only with loss through death. In a larger sense, however, it refers to the natural and gradual process by which we separate ourselves from any loved person, place, or object. The process is natural in the sense that we have a native ability to work through the separations; it is gradual in that separation almost never happens instantly but takes place over time; and the process is undergone whether the loved object is a person, place, or thing—we grieve over lost jobs, neighborhoods, pets, and even jewelry and furniture.

Several obstacles to the process of good grieving exist, the most common being the learned inability of some persons to cry and express their feelings. In American society tears are often regarded as unmanly, a sign of weakness; guilt or anger, as unjustified; and a feeling of depression or isolation, as a sign of self-pity. These cultural prohibitions deprive the organism of its natural and healthy expression of grief. Another obstacle to good grieving for some older persons is the reduction of their social network. People need people. It has been said that a joy shared is a joy extended, a grief shared is a grief diminished. Grieving is almost impossible when one has nobody to grieve with. For example, an 80-year-old woman whose last relative was dead related that she cried only at night and alone. Although she cried often, she seemingly could not adjust to her loss. In reality she needed someone to cry with, someone to share and *affirm* her feelings as she reflected on her situation.

In summary, grieving is considered a natural and organismic process by which a person disentangles from any loved object. Good grieving means letting go, or adjusting to loss and change. Good grieving, therefore, facilitates adaptation and successful aging. And, finally, a person can work through loss (grieve) most easily by sharing feelings with others.

GRIEF AND GRIEF WORK

The landmark study on grief was done by Erich Lindeman (1944). Working with survivors of the famous Coconut Grove nightclub fire, which took many lives, he found remarkable similarities among their symptoms, which he described as signs of acute grieving:

> . . . common to all is the following syndrome: Sensations of somatic distress occurring in waves lasting from twenty minutes to one hour at a time, a feeling of tightness in the throat, choking with shortness of breath, need for sighing, and an empty feeling in the abdomen, lack of muscular power and an intense subjective distress described as tension or mental pain.
> . . . The patient soon learns that these waves of discomfort can be precipitated by visits, by mentioning the deceased, and by receiving sympathy. There is a tendency to avoid the syndrome at any cost. [Lindeman 1944, p. 142]

Because these "waves of discomfort" are so painful, the grieving person learns to avoid thinking of the loss and to avoid anyone or any place that may recall the loss. A small-town funeral director relates that he often feels he is deliberately avoided by the families of recently deceased persons. The bereaved may also avoid restaurants, theaters, stores, and even familiar streets if these remind them of their loss. One widow could not listen to the radio for months because if one of her and her husband's favorite songs was aired, she felt too badly. She also avoided their bedroom, raking leaves, and shoveling snow because these were powerful reminders of her spouse. The situations are numerous, but the underlying cause is the same—the griever tends to avoid anything that awakens the felt experiences of the loss.

Lindeman found that the survivors who worked through the grief reaction best were those who did not avoid the painful memories and the resultant terrible feelings of loss. Accepting and dealing with these he called *grief work*. Such work is painful and lonely, for one must simply allow the loss and its consequences to seep into awareness. It follows that to grieve well oneself and to help others grieve properly, one should encourage and facilitate what seems to be the natural organismic response to loss. Tears, anger, guilt, and feelings of isolation should not be denied or explained away, but accepted as normal and healthy. This response is good grieving and, as Lindeman suggests, it facilitates letting go of the lost object and moving toward new beginnings.

Grief work needs to be encouraged in modern American society (Nichols and Nichols 1975). Religious and cultural rituals such as the wake, the funeral, and the Jewish memorial custom of Shivah need to be reevaluated and strengthened. Here again it must be emphasized that grieving or grief work must be undergone for every loss of any consequence. Leaving school, a job, and good friends or sending a daughter off to college are occasions for grieving. The head says, "I'll get used to the new job" or, "She'll be home at Christmas," but the heart, "the gut," is very lonely. We must learn to listen to our "gut" and own our feeling of loss with tears, anger, or depression. For it is only by so doing that we let go.

THE PROCESS OF GRIEF

To understand grief as a process,* it is useful to relate the stages in grieving to Kübler-Ross's (1972) stages in dying. They are very similar, probably because both find their origin in the clinical experiences of loss.

Stages in the Process of Grieving or Dying
Shock and denial
Guilt
Anger
Isolation and depression
Acceptance

Shock and Denial

Shock and denial are the first reaction to loss *or* gain. Getting the job you really wanted often comes as a shock. It takes time to really believe it happened to you. In the process of "learning" that it has indeed happened, you perhaps will cry and others may cry with you. You will have the urge to tell the good news to as many of your friends as will listen. Generally they rejoice with you, allowing you to grow to the realization that you truly got the job. The same process takes place with loss. At first you feel that this can't be happening to you. Only gradually does the meaning of the loss come to your awareness. Telling

---

* I am indebted here to Dr. George F. Jackson of Springfield, Ohio, an experienced grief counselor and friend whose insights I have freely borrowed.

and retelling, often with tears, serves the purpose of bringing it into awareness, of learning this painful news. Good friends will facilitate those tears, often crying with the bereaved. Unfortunately, at this stage some discourage tears or suggest medication, denying the organism its normal expression.

From shock one moves in and out of denial, which can last for days or months. A man forced into retirement may continue to awaken at work time; a widow will hear familiar footsteps, hear "his" car door slam, even hear "his" voice during the night. This experience is frightening at first, and the griever needs to be reminded that it is normal. Perhaps the explanation for the widow's illusions is that part of her still insists that her husband is not really gone, for to become aware of this awful truth all at once is too painful. She becomes fully aware only over time.

Guilt

As the denial fades and the reality of the loss becomes clearer, feelings of guilt develop: "What did I neglect to do?" "Could I have done more?" Past disagreements flood back into memory, causing untold anguish. The caregiver must learn to listen and empathize. Responses like "But you did all you could" are really not to the point. We must learn simply to listen to the feelings and facilitate their honest expression. After they have been expressed, the inner or deeper self can take over and work through the process.

Anger

Grieving persons often find it difficult to admit to the feeling of anger. Only the very open recognize its presence. More often people are surprised at themselves for feeling angry and tend to discount or hide their feelings of resentment toward the deceased and toward God or anyone who may in some way be responsible. Family and friends reinforce this denial of anger by generally not allowing its expression. On the face of it, to be resentful toward the spouse who has died is illogical. But feelings are not logical. And the spouse clearly did leave many responsibilities to be borne alone by the survivor. It is also true that "If doctors knew more, perhaps my husband would have been cured," and "If God had made the world differently, perhaps I would not be alone." To reason with the griever in the anger stage does not help. We must simply listen and facilitate the expression of this honest feeling without judging it in order to help.

Isolation and Depression

The growing realization that the loss is permanent leads us to a sense of felt aloneness or isolation. At the deepest level of ourselves, we *are* alone, though we seldom face that reality. When we must face it, the feeling is so frightening that we tend to run. We get busy, take a drink, or swallow a pill; but most people realize that these solutions are easy ones. We cannot run from so basic a reality. Rather we must simply stand our ground and let the "alone" feelings in. We need to own them. When we do, the terror is relieved and we pass to a more mature acceptance of life as it is. To help someone through this stage, the counselor or friend simply listens and communicates that he or she understands. Perhaps the most powerful assistance comes through merely being willing to be "with" the griever in his or her aloneness. No explanations or reassurances of "not aloneness" are useful. In essence, grievers must learn not only that they are indeed radically alone, but also that they can endure and survive.

Acceptance

Acceptance, the final stage, is the fruit of a long journey through the process of grief. Acceptance occurs when the griever comes to terms with the loss and begins to open up to new possibilities and relationships. It is not resignation or acceptance of defeat, but an awareness that new beginnings are possible and that one can and will carry on.

In summary, the stages in the process of grief do not always follow in sequence as described above, nor is there any time line that applies to everyone. In real life individuals may move rapidly or slowly. Some get stuck at a stage and need time and help to keep growing. Others move back and forth from one stage to another; they may appear to have worked it through and then relapse on the occasion of an anniversary or some significant moment, like the first snowfall. Many people need at least a year to accept a major loss. They must experience each of the seasons, each holiday, each birthday, in the changed situation. Finally, many grievers feel a terrible loss of hope in the future. They need to be comforted with the hope that the painful feelings associated with the grieving process (anger, guilt, isolation) will pass and they can and will find new meaning in life.

Thus far we have discussed development through the life course with emphasis on adaptation and have suggested that this adaptation is accomplished through a process of letting go called grieving. Griev-

ing is learning "in the heart" to surrender those persons, places, and things lost through the circumstances of life in the later years and to move ahead to new possibilities for happiness and fulfillment. We will consider now the problem of failing to adapt. How can we understand this problem and how can we assist those who do not seem to be adapting?

UNDERSTANDING THE DYNAMICS OF LOSS

"Grow old along with me; the best is yet to be." Robert Browning's words, so familiar to the student of gerontology, seem to be an invitation to experience aging as maturing, ripening, a time of fulfillment and integrity.

Every experienced clinician knows numerous older people who are experiencing old age in this way, a testimony perhaps to the resourcefulness and endurance of the human spirit. Tragically, however, we also know other older persons who are discouraged, resentful, and sometimes depressed because the later years are marked by loneliness and boredom rather than by fulfillment. How many people fall into this latter category? Exact figures are almost impossible to get. In their study on successful aging, Clark and Anderson (1967) found that the majority (61%) did adapt. However, a full 39 percent were not adapting, which indicates that these older persons were not successfully aging and might indeed be called an "at risk" group. Such persons are "at risk" in the sense that as the stress of normal aging increases, they are more likely to need help. Busse and Pfeiffer (1977) suggest that of the total U.S. population age 65 and older, at least 15 percent suffer from significant (not just occasional) functional psychiatric illness. They carefully point out that much of this disturbance arises for the first time in late life and can be attributed to the failure to accept or tolerate the many losses experienced at this stage of the life course.

This insight into understanding mental illness in late life is important. We suggest in these pages that the emotionally disturbed elderly person is most often struggling to regain a sense of mastery or control in the face of devastating loss and change. Alvin Goldfarb (1974a), a pioneer in geriatric psychiatry who devoted a lifetime of service to the elderly and their families, developed an excellent explanatory schema for understanding these dynamics (see figure 7.4). This simple and brief schema is useful for the practitioner because it provides both a clear explanation of why emotional disturbance may occur in late life and some directions for therapeutic intervention.

GOLDFARB'S SCHEMA

Goldfarb suggests that due to multiple causes a person may experience a loss of physical, mental, social, or economic resources. In this context such conditions as good vision, the ability to walk, the presence of a spouse, or the holding of a job are considered resources. If one or several of these resources are lost or diminished, the result is often a reduced ability to control one's own life and an increased dependency on others. Goldfarb calls this situation a *loss of mastery*. He argues that when one loses a significant degree of mastery over one's life, feelings of helplessness and powerlessness flood the consciousness.

THE RISE OF ANXIETY, FEAR, AND ANGER

Anxiety, fear, and anger surface as normal organismic responses to feelings of helplessness. These emergency or survival emotions are triggered by the situation itself. Most of us can relate personally to this experience. Frequently we get into temporary situations that seem beyond our control and we generally respond with fear or anger—such as when we have an important appointment and the car will not start. Atchley (1977) points out that older people have a very negative attitude toward dependency; he cites Clark and Anderson's finding that this situation is a primary cause of low morale. We should therefore expect feelings of helplessness to give rise to these emergency emotions.

Paradoxically, anxiety, fear, and anger make it more difficult to organize our remaining resources in a constructive way. These powerful emotions, though basically mobilized for survival, often have a disorganizing effect that leaves us less able to cope with life crises.

We must emphasize that anxiety, fear, and anger are normal, healthy responses to an overpowering situation. In this context they are purposive, goal-directed emotions. The caring person needs to be sensitive to this issue. Anger, for example, on the part of the old, the ill, or the discriminated against is not well tolerated by our culture. Perhaps an angry person makes us feel responsible, guilty, or powerless to change an oppressing situation. When caregivers experience powerlessness, many also respond with fear and anger, which may be used to retaliate against the already frightened and angry client. And so the frustrated caregiver or family strikes back with reprimands, lectures, or, worse, avoidance. A better approach, of course, would be to rec-

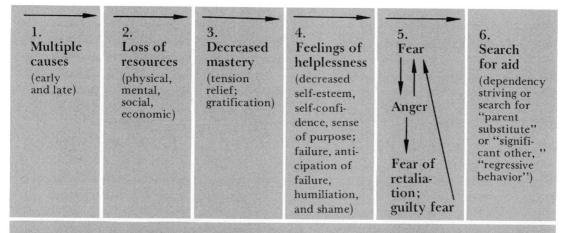

| 1. Multiple causes (early and late) | 2. Loss of resources (physical, mental, social, economic) | 3. Decreased mastery (tension relief; gratification) | 4. Feelings of helplessness (decreased self-esteem, self-confidence, sense of purpose; failure, anticipation of failure, humiliation, and shame) | 5. Fear → Anger → Fear of retaliation; guilty fear | 6. Search for aid (dependency striving or search for "parent substitute" or "significant other," "regressive behavior") |

1. Multiple causes or initiating factors, which occur either early in life and are reinforced or modified with aging, or occur late in life and are peculiar to old age, several of which may combine forces and some of which may be necessary but insufficient alone, result in

2. an absence or loss of resources for minimally adequate functioning, so that

3. there is decreased mastery of problems, challenges, and need for adjustments posed by internal changes (biologically determined drives or acquired needs) and external changes and threats, with resulting

4. feelings of helplessness or actual powerlessness, and consequent

5. fear with accompanying or subsequent anger, with consequent

6. "rationally" or "irrationally" aimed and elaborate search for aid expressed in patterns acceptable to the individual in terms of his personality organization based upon his past, his present, and his expectations; these patterns are also contingent on his perception of what is acceptable to and likely to work in "his world," as well as on the social response he receives. In this search there are observable constellations of motivated personal actions which range from apathy through pseudoanhedonia, display of helplessness, somatization, hypochondriasis, depression, and paranoid states to the most open and manipulative behavior. In predisposed persons there may be a physiologic shift to a new and relatively inefficient homeostatic level with depressive states, which are then revealed by alterations in appetite, bowel function, sleep, and other vegetative signs.

FIGURE 7.4   Components of Disorder: Psychodynamic Sequence.
Source: *A. I. Goldfarb, "Clinical Perspectives,"* Psychiatric Research Report 23 *(February 1968). Reprinted by permission of the American Psychiatric Association.*

ognize that anger is a healthy response to feelings of powerlessness; it is a cry for help or, as Goldfarb puts it, a search for aid. The angry person is looking for someone to assist in regaining a measure of control. Most of us tend to do precisely that in times of crisis: we seek help from a parent, spouse, relative, or friend.

THE SEARCH FOR AID

If the helpless and therefore frightened and angry person can find someone strong and supportive to depend on, some sense of mastery is regained, diminishing helplessness and the accompanying fear and anger. In effect, this dependable or trusted person, whom Goldfarb calls a *surrogate parent,* offers security in the sense that he or she would be available for assistance in an emergency. With this sense of security, a feeling of mastery or control gradually returns. With fear and anger in check, the helpless can reorganize their remaining resources and begin to cope more effectively with their problems. Goldfarb calls this sense of regained control an *illusion of mastery.* Total mastery or complete independence may no longer be possible for the frail elderly, but as long as they can depend on someone in an emergency, they will have a sense of being in control again. They will consequently make more efforts at self-care and will continue to manage their own affairs without a great deal of outside help.

Who will this strong, dependable helper be? According to Goldfarb it may be anyone who is willing to act in this capacity. Doctors and nurses are especially powerful in this role because medical professionals are perceived as acceptable persons to depend on. Many older people remain independent in the community because of help from such professionals: "My doctor knows how I am and he feels I'm doing well." A social worker, pastor, grandchild, or neighbor may also serve as this trusted friend. Recall the research of Lowenthal and Haven (1968): in their careful study of 289 San Franciscans, they found that the presence of a confidant was a most important variable in helping a person continue to adapt despite great stress, because the confidant served as a "buffer" against loss. Note, too, the Federal Council on Aging's call for the provision of a "significant person" who would act as a confidant and trusted friend to an otherwise isolated and lonely elderly individual. This suggestion is a cornerstone of the council's 1976 report to the president.

For caregivers the role of confidant often means allowing frail older persons to depend on them. This role raises questions such as: How many people can I have depending on me? or Is it fair to allow this dependency to develop when I might change jobs or leave the area for some reason? Goldfarb himself entered such relationships without feeling overwhelmed; he suggested that the illusion of mastery could be maintained with infrequent and brief but regular contact.

Sometimes the frail elderly person is comforted simply in knowing that the doctor, nurse, or helper-friend is available by telephone. For example, a rather isolated and paranoid older man began to improve dramatically after several months of regular weekly visits by an outreach counselor. On one of these visits, the counselor told his client that he was planning a vacation and would be out of town for several weeks. The old man looked at him and said in a quiet way, "You know, it's strange but I feel better when I know you are around town. Even if I don't see you, it's a comfort to know you are there." The counselor had become for him a strong and dependable support. Through brief but regular visits, the old man felt more secure. The paranoid behavior disappeared and he became better able to manage the ordinary details of daily living.

Some individuals, however, are irrational in their search for aid. Because of personality organization or lifestyle patterns developed through the earlier years, they seemingly cannot accept a dependency relationship and cannot ask for aid in an appropriate manner. For them the search for aid is elaborated as apathy, displays of helplessness, somatization (overconcern with bodily ailments), hypochondriasis, paranoia, or depression.

Recognizing these behaviors as a search for aid and therefore as purposive and goal directed does offer the caregiver some direction in preparing a treatment plan. Most important, we can understand the individual's behavior. We can make special efforts to develop a trusting and stable relationship with this emotionally isolated person in the hope that at some point the maladaptive defense will be dropped and a more appropriate response developed. We can also look for opportunities to restore some control by facilitating personal decision making on the part of the elderly. In these efforts we need to remember that all of the symptoms mentioned do respond in varying degrees to supportive counseling (Busse and Pfeiffer 1977).

Further discussion of emotional disturbance in late life is beyond the scope of this book. For more information see Goldfarb's chapter in the *American Handbook of Psychiatry,* Busse and Pfeiffer's *Mental Illness in Late Life,* and Daniel Blazer's excellent monograph on *Psychopathology of Aging.*

ASSESSMENT OF THE ELDERLY CLIENT

MULTIDIMENSIONAL ASSESSMENT

Clinical work with elderly persons has demonstrated that understanding a client's problem requires a multidisciplinary perspective that takes into account each area of a person's life. For example, a person who appears to be emotionally stable but has physical, social, or financial problems may, unless some of these problems are resolved, also begin to experience emotional impairment. Each area of functioning influences other areas of functioning. Financial hardship can lead to impaired physical status through poor diet and lack of medical care. This impairment, in turn, leads to a loss of social roles. The resultant isolation and helplessness are or become emotional problems. Abundant research justifies each of these conclusions (Lowenthal and

Haven 1968; Pfeiffer 1975a; Butler 1963).

To assist the practitioner who wants to approach assessment from this multidimensional perspective, the so-called OARS (Older Americans Resources and Services) methodology was developed at Duke University's Center for the Study of Aging under the direction of Eric Pfeiffer (1975a). The actual instrument is called the "Multidimensional Functional Assessment Questionnaire" (MFAQ).* This rather complete questionnaire measures the client's present level of functioning in each of five areas: social resources, economic resources, mental health, physical health, and activities of daily living. For each of these dimensions a score of 1 to 6 is produced, ranging from outstanding functioning to complete impairment. Dimensions in which the client is impaired stand out clearly. Most important, other problems that contribute to the total picture also come into focus, allowing the caregiver to plan for the wide range of services that may be needed. The instrument also yields a cumulative impairment score on all five dimensions, which predicts the need for long-term care. It yields valid and reliable data and can be administered by nonprofessionals after a brief training.

Time for administration is an hour to an hour and a half, depending on the skill of the interviewer and the cooperativeness of the client. The busy practitioner may have to spread the administration of the MFAQ over two visits. The time, however, is well spent, for the questionnaire keeps the in-

---

* The MFAQ (OARS methodology) is available from the Center for the Study of Aging and Human Development, Duke University, Durham, N.C. 27710.

terviewer's perspective broad and multidimensional and offers some assurance that a physical or social need will not be treated in isolation from the total picture. Most important, the actual test taking itself is therapeutic, for it gives elderly clients a chance to tell how they feel about themselves to a person who really wants to know. For isolated or otherwise impaired older persons, this extended interview might be the first time anyone has really asked about their problems.

The questionnaire does not mention sexuality, so the interviewer is cautioned to remain sensitive to this issue. Sometimes older persons are fearful of discussing sexual problems because they feel these problems are abnormal. Gentle questioning, when one senses that problems may exist in this area, can open the door to a frank and open discussion and a calming of fear and anxiety.

ASSESSING MENTAL HEALTH

The nurse or social service worker needs to have at hand an easy to use, easy to understand, reliable instrument suitable for a mental health assessment in the office or during a home visit. Pfeiffer and the OARS team have gone a long way toward providing this tool with the mental health resource section of the OARS methodology. This part of the questionnaire yields a gross measurement of two factors: cognitive impairment and nonorganic, or functional, impairment.

Assessing Cognitive Impairment

Intellectual impairment may range from a slight memory loss to a total inability to remember. When cognitive dysfunction is associated with the loss of brain tissue function and a consequent inability to learn or assimilate new information, it is called *organic brain syndrome* (OBS). To understand what the OBS patient feels, we need only to realize how much we depend on our ability to learn. As you enter a room, for example, you "learn it" so that you can recognize it again another time. As you eat your breakfast, you learn what you are eating so that, if you care to, you can tell another about it later. Organically impaired persons, in contrast, have great difficulty learning or integrating their daily experiences. You may have visited and talked with such a person yesterday, but she could not register and learn that event, so she will not remember it. As she had her breakfast, she was not registering it, so she does not remember what she ate or even that she ate. From a behavioral point of view, this experience is frightening. The sense of familiarity and continuity tends to disappear. Every place and every face is new and strange. With no anchors in time and place, disorientation follows. Clients with severe OBS may even forget familiar persons and thus feel that they are always among strangers. We can easily understand why the loss of such an important resource as memory can lead to fear, anger, and often psychiatric symptoms such as depression and paranoia, which often overlie the basic problem of memory loss and disorientation.

OBS can be *acute,* or reversible—the result of a temporary condition such as fever, drug intoxication, or malnutrition; or it can be *chronic*—the result of permanent neuronal damage. Distinguishing between these two conditions (see figure 7.5) is very

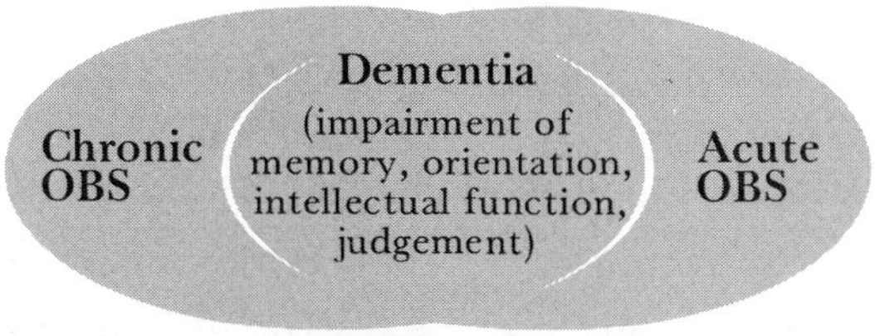

Dementia
(impairment of memory, orientation, intellectual function, judgement)

Chronic OBS   Acute OBS

	Chronic OBS	Acute OBS
Onset	Insidious; no definable starting point	Usually recent; noticeable by marked changes in mental capacity
Affect	Fluctuates from sadness to happiness but within moderate range; anxiety lacking except at onset	More sustained (usually depressive) but associated with anxiety, restlessness, and aggressiveness
Mental aberrations (hallucinations, delusions of persecution)	Uncommon	Common
Level of awareness	Fairly stable but may slowly decline with time	Fluctuates acutely (from confusion to stupor to delirium)
Adjustment to deficit	Relatively good; patient functions within his limitations and remains fairly active in familiar environment	Poor; patient is distressed and unable to adapt to any environment
Duration	Chronic and irreversible	Varies according to cause (e.g., stroke) and effectiveness of treatment; reversible except in permanent brain damage; can become chronic if untreated

FIGURE 7.5   Differential Diagnosis: Chronic OBS vs. Acute OBS.
Source: *Dan G. Blazer,* Psychopathology of Aging *3, monograph series of the American Academy of Family Physicians, Kansas City, June 1977, p. 14. Reprinted by permission of the publisher.*

important. Acute OBS is reversible when the underlying medical cause is detected and treated. If left untreated, the acute condition may become chronic (Blazer 1977).

Screening for OBS is relatively simple and straightforward and can be done as part of a routine office examination. The diagnosis is based on four criteria: disorientation to time, place, person, and situation; memory loss, both recent and remote; inability to recall, learn, and retain general information; and inability to do calculations of the simplest type (Goldfarb 1974a).

The Mental Status Questionnaire. Cognitive impairment can be measured by a brief and simply administered ten-item screening tool called a "Mental Status Questionnaire" (MSQ). Ample evidence shows that despite its simplicity of administration and interpretation, it yields valid results (Goldfarb 1974a; Pfeiffer 1975b; Haglund and Schuckit 1976). Eisdorfer (1975) has noted that frequently the problem in diagnosing OBS is simply that the interviewer fails to ask these brief questions, perhaps under the assumption that diagnosis would require sophisticated laboratory techniques. Pfeiffer's (1975b) "Short Portable Mental Status Questionnaire" (SPMSQ) shown in figure 7.6 is the most reliable version of the MSQ and is published as part of the OARS methodology mentioned above. Ideally the nurse or practitioner should commit the ten questions to memory and be prepared to ask them whenever some memory loss is apparent in the client. Scoring is simple: 0 to 2 errors indicate intact intellectual functioning; 3 to 7 errors, mild-to-moderate intellectual impairment; 8 to 10 errors, severe impairment. Blazer (1977) offers several other diagnostic suggestions that bear summarizing here:

1. To confirm the diagnosis of OBS, look for characteristic findings in the patient's history, clinical profile, and behavior patterns.
2. Because signs of memory loss and disorientation are mimicked by patients in deep depression, repeating the SPMSQ over a period of time (hours, days, or even weeks) is useful.
3. Chronic OBS is usually slow and insidious; acute OBS tends to be rapid and immediately noticeable to observers.
4. The level of adjustment to the deficit is well developed in chronic OBS clients. These clients may continue to cope despite moderate impairment; they will have learned strategies to hide their impairment and will deny any cognitive loss. Acute OBS clients will generally not have had time to develop these defenses.

The Face-Hand Test. An added backup to the SPMSQ and routine history taking in the diagnosis of organic brain syndrome is Goldfarb's (1974a) face-hand test (FHT), an easy-to-use series of simultaneous touching of the client's cheek and hand. Failure to report the touches to the hand is indicative of cognitive impairment. For a description and directions for administration, see Goldfarb's (1974) monograph. The face-hand test is highly correlated with the MSQ and psychiatric evaluation. When one test indicates a more severe OBS than the other, Goldfarb suggests that cognitive functioning can be improved to the level of the best test performance.

Goldfarb's claim that the "Mental Status Questionnaire" and the face-hand test may be used together as a rapid and reliable mental status assessment tool was validated by Haglund and Schuckit (1976). They compared several measures and found that the "SPMSQ most effectively singled out the OBS cases" (p. 657) and "the FHT produces an increment of improvement in the identification of the organic group, thus serving as a useful second test" (p. 658). In practice the nurse or clinician must gently prepare the client for

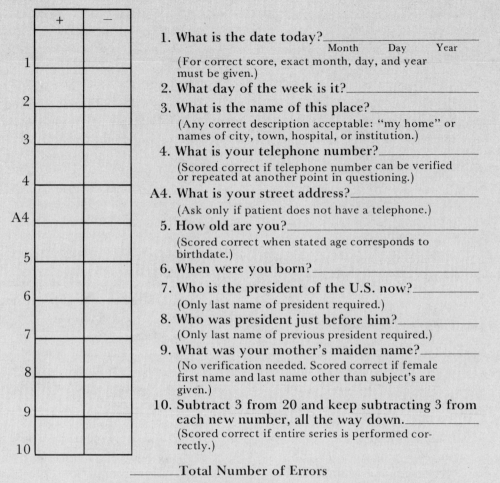

INSTRUCTIONS: Ask subject to answer all questions without reference to calendar, newspaper or other memory aids. Record and evaluate subject's response according to *Scoring Criteria* below.

	+	−
1		
2		
3		
4		
A4		
5		
6		
7		
8		
9		
10		

1. What is the date today?_____
   Month   Day   Year
   (For correct score, exact month, day, and year must be given.)

2. What day of the week is it?_____

3. What is the name of this place?_____
   (Any correct description acceptable: "my home" or names of city, town, hospital, or institution.)

4. What is your telephone number?_____
   (Scored correct if telephone number can be verified or repeated at another point in questioning.)

A4. What is your street address?_____
   (Ask only if patient does not have a telephone.)

5. How old are you?_____
   (Scored correct when stated age corresponds to birthdate.)

6. When were you born?_____

7. Who is the president of the U.S. now?_____
   (Only last name of president required.)

8. Who was president just before him?_____
   (Only last name of previous president required.)

9. What was your mother's maiden name?_____
   (No verification needed. Scored correct if female first name and last name other than subject's are given.)

10. Subtract 3 from 20 and keep subtracting 3 from each new number, all the way down._____
   (Scored correct if entire series is performed correctly.)

_____Total Number of Errors

Scoring Criteria: Severe intellectual impairment is indicated by eight or more errors, mild-to-moderate impairment by three to seven errors and intact intellectual functioning by up to two errors.

These are gross criteria applying to white subjects who have had partial or complete high school education. One more error should be allowed for subjects who have gone only through grade school or whose learning has been retarded by socioeconomic, environmental or discriminatory factors. One less error should be allowed for subjects who have gone beyond high school.

FIGURE 7.6   Short Portable Mental Status Questionnaire (SPMSQ).

Source: *Eric Pfeiffer,* Journal of the American Geriatric Society, *vol. 23 (October 1975). © 1974 by Eric Pfeiffer. Reprinted by permission of the author and publisher.*

these examinations. A question such as Who is the president of the United States? immediately signals that the interviewer is testing memory loss and may cause anxiety. Butler and Lewis (1973) remind us of the Goldstein catastrophic reaction—that is, the tendency of brain-damaged subjects to become flooded with anxiety and irritability when confronted with a task they cannot handle. Saying something like "I have to ask you some routine questions as part of our interview. I know they sound silly but please bear with me" is helpful to an anxious patient. Note, too, that the client may fail to answer because of obvious inattentiveness due to nervousness, worry, or depression. Physical defects such as deafness or even poor eyesight (Blazer 1977) may also reduce physical cues from the interviewer, leading to errors by the client.

Assessing Functional Impairment

The second factor to consider in a general mental health assessment is functional impairment. To assist in this task, the nurse needs a brief but valid and reliable screening tool. With this need in mind Pfeiffer (1975c) designed and tested a "Short Psychiatric Evaluation Schedule" (SPES), a fifteen-item yes-or-no questionnaire. The interviewer asks simply worded questions, circling the yes or no answer. Answers that point to psychopathology are written in capitals. To score the test, the examiner simply adds the number of capitalized yeses or nos. A score of 0 to 4 indicates healthy psychological functioning. A score of 5 or more indicates probable psychiatric problems—the higher the score the greater the probability of disturbance. Note that the test is a screening tool. It does not offer a

differential diagnosis of the specific problem, but it alerts the practitioner to its presence. The SPES is part of the OARS "Multidimensional Assessment Questionnaire."

The OARS methodology is highly recommended even to the busy practitioner who needs to know the overall functioning of the older client. When administering the OARS methodology is not possible, the routine use of the SPMSQ learned by memory would be a wise diagnostic procedure. When some doubt remains, the face-hand test should be administered. This test should be followed by a SPES, which is scored immediately.

SUMMARY

Normal aging is a process of growth or development rather than decline. Erikson's stage theory, with an elaboration by Peck, suggests the tasks appropriate to the stage of later maturity. Successful completion of these tasks yields wisdom—a strength or virtue special to the aged, since it is born of the struggle to integrate.

Moving or growing through the life course is facilitated by the process of letting go or grieving, which is a normal, healthy way of separating from persons, places, and things lost through the normal course of growing old.

Mental illness in late life is, in Goldfarb's view, purposeful, goal-directed behavior. But it is an *inappropriate* way of reducing the fear and anger arising from feelings of helplessness caused by an increasing loss of mastery. A more appropriate response to this loss is to find a strong, trusted "other" to depend on. When such a person is found, fear and anger are reduced, allowing the elderly to focus their remaining powers on regaining some degree of mastery.

Assessment of the older person can best be accomplished by using a multidimensional technique such as the OARS methodology. Screening for organic brain syndrome can be done in the office by using the "Short Portable Mental Status Questionnaire." Goldfarb's face-hand test gives an added degree of security in the diagnosis. Pfeiffer's "Short Psychiatric Evaluation Schedule" is suggested for office screening of psychiatric problems.

REFERENCES

ATCHLEY, R. 1977. *Social Forces in Later Life.* Belmont, Calif.: Wadsworth.

BLAZER, D. G. 1977. *Psychopathology of Aging.* A monograph. Kansas City, Mo.: American Academy of Family Physicians.

BUSSE, E. W., and E. PFEIFFER. 1977. *Mental Illness in Late Life.* Washington, D.C.: American Psychiatric Association.

BUTLER, R. N. 1963. "The Life Review: An Interpretation of Reminiscence in the Aged." *Psychiatry* 26:65–76.

———, and M. I. LEWIS. 1973. *Aging and Mental Health.* St. Louis: C. V. Mosby.

CLARK, M., and B. G. ANDERSON. 1967. *Culture and Aging.* Springfield, Ill.: Charles C. Thomas.

DE BEAUVOIR, S. 1972. *The Coming of Age.* New York: G. P. Putnam.

EBERSOLE, P. E. 1976. "Reminiscing and Group Psychotherapy with the Aged." In I. M. Burnside, ed., *Nursing and the Aged.* New York: McGraw-Hill.

EISDORFER, C. 1975. "Organic Brain Syndromes: Reversible and Irreversible." Unpublished lecture at workshop—"Psychiatric Problems of the Aged." Louisville, Ky.: Gerontological Society Meeting.

ERIKSON, E. H. 1976. "Reflections on Dr. Borg's Life Cycle." *Daedalus* 105:1–28.

Federal Council on Aging. 1976. *Annual Report to the President.* Washington, D.C.: U.S. Government Printing Office.

GOLDFARB, A. I. 1974a. *Aging and Organic Brain Syndrome.* A monograph. Bloomfield, N.J.: Health Learning Systems.

———. 1974b. "Minor Maladjustments of the Aged." In A. Silano and G. Chrzanowski, eds., *American Handbook of Psychiatry,* 2d ed., vol. 3. New York: Basic Books.

HAGLUND, R. M. J., and M. A. SCHUCKIT. 1976. "A Clinical Comparison of Tests of Organicity in Elderly Patients." *Journal of Gerontology* 31:654–59.

KEEN, S. 1968. *Garbriel Marcel.* Richmond, Va.: John Knox Press.

KIMMEL, D. 1974. *Adulthood and Aging.* New York: Wiley.

KÜBLER-ROSS, E. 1972. *On Death and Dying.* New York: Macmillan.

LIFTON, R. J. 1972. "Protean Youth Grows Older." Address delivered at 25th Annual Scientific Meeting of Gerontological Society. San Juan, Puerto Rico, December 17–21.

LINDEMAN, E. 1944. "Symptomology and Management of Acute Grief." *American Journal of Psychiatry* 101:140–48.

LOWENTHAL, M. F., and C. HAVEN. 1968. "Interaction and Adaptation: Intimacy as a Clinical Variable." *American Sociological Review* 33:20–30.

NICHOLS, R., and J. NICHOLS. 1975. "Funerals: A Time for Grief and Growth." In E. Kübler-Ross, ed., *Death the Final Stage of Growth.* Englewood Cliffs, N.J.: Prentice-Hall.

PECK, R.C. 1968. "Psychological Development in the Second Half of Life." In B. Neugarten, ed., *Middle Age and Aging.* Chicago: University of Chicago Press.

PFEIFFER, E. 1975a. *Multidimensional Functional Assessment: The OARS Methodology.* Durham, N.C.: Center for the Study of Aging and Human Development.

———. 1975b. "A Short Portable Mental Status Questionnaire for the Assessment of Organic Brain Deficit in Elderly Patients." *Journal of the American Geriatric Society* 23:433–441.

———. 1975c. "A Short Psychiatric Evaluation Schedule (SPES)." Paper presented at the Annual Scientific Meeting of the Gerontological Society, Louisville, Ky.

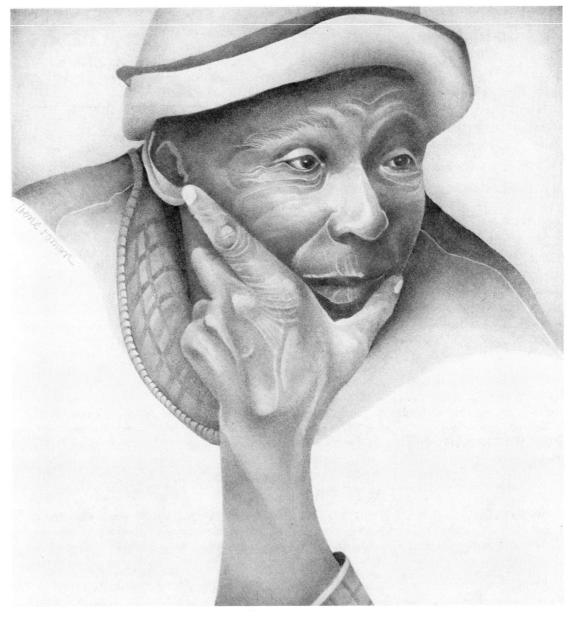

Susan Crocker Houde

Chapter 8

RECORDING THE DATA

The ultimate goal of the gerontological nurse providing care to the elderly client is the provision of holistic, continuous health care. The problem-oriented record system provides a means to achieve this goal. The system helps the nurse and other members of the health care team (1) to avoid fragmentation of care, (2) to accurately and comprehensively identify health needs in an organized manner, and (3) to assess the quality of care administered to the client.

As a coordinator and provider of care, the gerontological nurse understands the importance of viewing the elderly client as a bio-psycho-social being who frequently has a multitude of interrelated problems. In order for the nurse and other members of the health team to effectively intervene in the management of these problems, each member must be able to view the patient holistically and to recognize interrelationships between the problems.

The problem-oriented record system is an essential component of coordinated and effective management of an individual client's health problems. Because all members of the health team utilize the same portion of the record, each can analyze the data recorded by the others. The traditional approach to recording data is inadequate because it does not allow for a systematic, holistic approach to health care. Traditional records have a separate section of the chart for each member of the multidisciplinary health team, thereby making communication between team members difficult.

Another deficit of the traditional record system is that it does not readily allow audits to be performed because of the lack of standardization in the format for recording data. Gerontological nurses who are concerned about the quality of their nursing assessments, diagnoses, and interventions have identified the need for evaluation of their actions by their peers. With proper utilization of the problem-oriented record system, which consists of a standardized format that illustrates the nursing process of assessment, planning, implementation, and evaluation, gerontological nurses and their peers have access to a tool for quality care audits. Nurses who are aware that self-evaluation is important to promote professional growth can utilize the problem-oriented record for the purpose of analyzing their decision-making ability and nursing actions to determine whether they are providing quality care.

PROBLEM-ORIENTED RECORD SYSTEM

The problem-oriented record system provides members of the health care team, whether gerontological nurse, social worker, psychologist, or physician, with a means to communicate and work together in the alleviation of each elderly client's health problems. But in order for it to be functionally efficient, each member must be instructed on its proper utilization. This chapter briefly explains the format for the problem-oriented recording system introduced by Lawrence Weed in 1960. The system has four components: data base, problem list, initial plan, and progress notes.

DATA BASE

The first component, or *data base,* consists of a client's complete health history, including the chief complaint, history of present illness, past history, psychosocial history, family history, and review of systems (see chapter 5). The mental health as-

sessment, described in chapter 7, is another integral element of the data base. The data base also includes the objective findings obtained from a complete physical examination and any diagnostic tests performed (see chapter 6).

For elderly clients the data base is often very lengthy because of their rich historical past and the numerous interrelated health complaints that they frequently identify. All of the information must be recorded comprehensively so that the gerontological nurse as well as other health care providers will be able not only to view these clients holistically but to perceive each as an individual. The data base must be structured to provide a firm foundation for the evaluation of each elderly client's physical, emotional, and social health status.

PROBLEM LIST

The second component of the problem-oriented record is the *problem list.* This portion includes all problems requiring evaluation or management by members of the health care team. Changes in lifestyle that affect the health of elderly clients, as well as emotional, financial, and social problems, should be included in the problem list. All members of the health care team are encouraged to make appropriate additions to the problem list. As illustrated in figure 8.1, each problem should be numbered and dated on a problem list sheet, which is placed at the front of the client's chart. Here the list serves as an index to the record and, when accurately maintained, is an overview of the client's holistic health picture.

When a problem on the list is no longer perceived as a problem, it becomes inactive or resolved. This status is documented by drawing a horizontal arrow to the inactive column and recording the date the problem was resolved in the designated column. Example 1 in figure 8.1 demonstrates the resolution of problem #2.

Significant problems that were resolved prior to accumulation of the data base should also be listed in the inactive column. Previous illnesses, hospitalization, and injuries, as well as serious emotional

FIGURE 8.1 Examples of the Problem List Portion of the Problem-Oriented Record System.

Example 1

Problem No.	Date	Problem	Date Resolved	Inactive Problems
#1	3/20/78	rheumatoid arthritis		
#2	3/20/78	pneumonia	4/1/79 →	
#3	4/1/78	financial problems		
#4	4/25/78	depression		

Example 2

Problem No.	Date	Problem	Date Resolved	Inactive Problems
#1	1/15/78	joint pain	→	#3
#2	1/15/78	facial rash	→	#3
#3	2/1/78	systemic lupus erythematosis		

Example 3

Problem No.	Date	Problem	Date Resolved	Inactive Problems
#1	3/5/78	loss of spouse	4/2/78 →	#4
#2	3/15/78	loss of appetite	4/2/78 →	#4
#3	3/5/78	insomnia	4/2/78 →	#4
#4	4/2/78	depression secondary to loss of spouse.		

problems, may be numerous in the elderly and should be included here. Minor, self-limiting problems that can be resolved without health care intervention and that do not require evaluation are usually not recorded in the problem list.

When a client presents with multiple complaints that appear unrelated, each is listed as a separate problem. If the diagnostic assessment demonstrates a relationship between these problems, this newly established assessment becomes the next problem on the list. The original problems are no longer considered separately but are referred to the newer diagnostic assessment as shown in the second example in figure 8.1. In this example joint pain and facial rash were no longer considered active problems after a diagnosis of systemic lupus erythematosus was made. In the third example in figure 8.1 the nurse carefully ruled out any physical problems and, after working collaborately with a psychologist, determined that the elderly client was suffering from a depression caused by her husband's death.

Because the problem list is the chart index and an overview of the health profile, the importance of thoroughness and accuracy is apparent. Gerontological nurses should thus be aware of an error commonly made in the compilation of a problem list. When dealing with an elderly client with more than one problem, some that are less prominent are often overlooked. Such oversight can be detrimental to the client's future health; it interferes with holistic care because health care team members are unable to observe interrelationships between all the client's health problems. The gerontological nurse should remember, then, that while younger clients often have single problems, problems do multiply with age

and interrelationships become more complex. Thus, a complete problem list is necessary to avoid overlooking problems that may be highly significant in the provision of effective health care.

INITIAL PLAN

The third component of the problem-oriented record system is the *initial plan.* Numbered according to the sequence identified in the problem list, the initial plan includes general plans of action for each problem listed. Each plan should be divided into three crucial parts.

The first part consists of the tentative nursing assessment and the means for evaluation of the assessment. This section includes the nursing diagnosis and the data that need to be gathered; it also lists specific diagnostic tests that need to be done to determine the accuracy of the initial nursing diagnosis. This portion of the plan is necessary before a specific plan of nursing management can be implemented. The diagnostic portion in figure 8.2 illustrates the diagnostic tests that were ordered for a patient complaining of joint pain.

The second part of the initial plan outlines the nursing interventions. The gerontological nurse may need to determine plans of therapy in collaboration with a physician or other health professional. The therapy indicated for each problem should be stated very clearly so that on subsequent encounters client compliance and effectiveness of therapy can be evaluated. Medications, dosages, and frequency of administration, as well as specific treatments, should be documented. The therapeutic portion in figure 8.2 documents the use of ASA and warm, moist soaks in the treat-

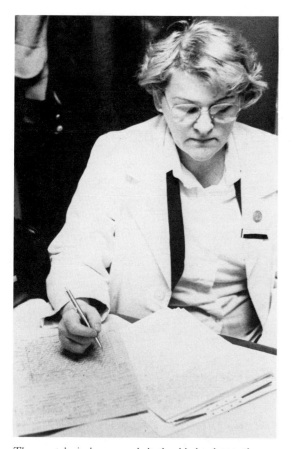

The gerontological nurse can help the elderly adapt to the aging process by utilizing the problem-oriented record system as a means to comprehensively identify their needs, to assess the quality of their care, and to help avoid fragmented care; elderly clients need a holistic approach that includes health care as well as concern for their social, emotional, and financial problems.

plans for client education. Plans should include provision for instructing the elderly client about normal aging, disease process, therapy, and the significance of these on lifestyle. The client should also be taught about basic health and how to promote health through exercise and good nutrition. In figure 8.2 a plan for teaching the client about joint pain is illustrated.

This portion of the plan demands clear documentation to facilitate client teaching and to avoid the possibility of confusion and repetition. An important point nurses should remember is that elderly clients must be educated in terms they can understand. To explain their health to them in unclear terms can create anxieties since they will become frustrated at being unable to understand what is being taught.

Overall the initial plan provides guidelines for the ongoing management of clients' problems and contributes to continuity of care by being available to all members of the health care team for consultation. Frequently, the plans are revised during subsequent evaluations that are documented in the next portion of the record.

PROGRESS NOTES

The fourth and final component of the problem-oriented record system is the *progress notes* section or continuation sheet. This section, which documents the client's progress at subsequent evaluations, is based on the initial plan. The notes provide an orderly format for recording additional data, as each note is numbered and titled to correspond with the items on the problem list.

The progress notes, or SOAP notes as they are called, are divided into four parts:

ment of joint pains. A precise statement of goals, projected termination of therapy, plans for follow-up, as well as alternative plans in case of treatment failure, should be included in this portion. Methods of emotional support for each elderly client should also be clearly documented.

The third part of the initial plan—the *teaching* portion in figure 8.2—includes

Problem: #1 joint pain, R/O rheumatoid arthritis, R/O osteoarthritis, R/O gout, R/O systemic lupus erythematosis.

Diagnostic (D$_x$): 1. sedimentation rate, rheumatoid factor, uric acid, antinuclear antibody.
2. Knee X-rays.

Therapeutic (R$_x$): 1. ASA 650 mg. q 4°.
2. Warm moist soaks to aching joints PRN.

Teaching: 1. Explain effects of ASA and the importance of taking it regularly.
2. Explain purposes of tests and what they may indicate.
3. Explain necessity of avoiding unnecessary stress to joints until assessment is completed.
4. Explain to client and family together the disease and how to best maintain and promote health. Discuss client's and family's anxieties about chronic disease and implications for client's lifestyle.

FIGURE 8.2 Problem-Oriented Record System: Initial Plan.

Subjective data, Objective data, Assessment, and Plan. Under *subjective,* the gerontological nurse includes what the elderly client states about the problem, as well as all unverifiable information. As illustrated by the example in figure 8.3, this portion should be as concise as possible, but should contain all relevant subjective information.

The *objective* part includes the observations made by the nurse in relation to the

FIGURE 8.3 Problem-Oriented Record System: SOAP Progress Notes. ▶

Name: Mary Brown   Date: 10/14/78

Problem: #3 Diabetes Mellitus

Subjective: Taking 45 units NPH insulin every a.m. Following 1800 cal. ADA diet carefully. Urine sugar testing +2 and +3 regularly. Acetone neg. Denies dizziness, thirst, or polyuria. States is feeling "well" and that daughter is visiting daily to draw up her insulin and give foot care. Client also states she is feeling less lonely.

Objective: Client is smiling and talkative. Wt. —160 lbs. Fasting blood sugar (FBS) — 274. (See flow sheet.)
        Eyes: Ophthalmic Exam. — no narrowing, exudates, microaneurysms, or hemorrhage.
        Heart: Rate 82 and regular. No murmurs.
        Lungs: Clear to auscultation and percussion. Respirations—18.
        Extremities: Pedal pulses strong and equal. Vibratory and position sense present bilaterally.

Assessment: Blood sugar still elevated despite insulin increase. Weight loss of 2 lbs. in one week. Increased family support causing better emotional status and decreased loneliness.

Plan:
  Dx: FBS on 10/21/78.
  Rx: Increase NPH insulin to 50 units every a.m.
Teaching: 1. Continue 1800 cal. ADA diet faithfully.
  2. Continue testing urine four times a day and record.
  3. Contact daughter about results of visit & instruct on increase in insulin. Determine emotional response of daughter to her daily visits to mother. Give support & enthusiasm on mother's improved emotional state.
  4. Ask to return to clinic on 10/21/78 for FBS & reevaluation of diabetes. Continue assessment of client's social support system.

specific problem. As can be seen in figure 8.3, it should also include physical findings and diagnostic test results.

The *assessment* may be the most difficult portion for the nurse, for the information obtained in the subjective and objective portions must be synthesized to determine the client's progress, be it satisfactory or poor. The assessment, the criteria used, as well as the client's response should all be clearly documented.

The *plan* for nursing intervention is formulated based on the assessment portion of the notes. In preparing a plan for one problem all the client's problems should be considered to avoid initiating interventions contraindicated by other problems. Each plan should consist of the same format as the initial plan and include any additions or revisions that will improve the management of the given problem. As shown in figure 8.3, the plan for Mary Brown includes an FBS, an increase in the client's daily insulin, and dietary instruction.

Flow Sheets

Flow sheets may also be utilized as part of the progress notes. Their use should be limited to repetitive data that can be used to assess progress in resolving each elderly client's health problems. Information provided in flow sheets may be referred to in the objective portion of the progress notes. Flow sheets should be individualized for clients and contain parameters for monitoring their care. For example, figure 8.4 illustrates parameters for monitoring a client with diabetes mellitus. On weekly visits the

FIGURE 8.4 Problem-Oriented Record System: Progress Notes Flow Sheet.

Problem: #6 Diabetes Mellitus

Date	5/1/77	5/8/77	5/15/77	5/22/77	6/5/77
Blood Pressure	150/94	146/90	136/90	136/88	140/88
Pulse	86	84	86	86	84
Respiration	24	24	22	22	20
Weight	193	192	189	185	188
Fasting Blood Sugar	235	230	200	144	168
Urine Sugar & Acetone	+3/neg	+2/neg	+2/neg	+1/neg	+1/neg
Insulin	NPH 30 units 7 a.m.	NPH 32 units 7 a.m.	NPH 40 units 7 a.m.	NPH 40 units 7 a.m.	NPH 40 units 7 a.m.
Diet	1800 ADA	1800 ADA	1800 ADA	1800 ADA	1800 ADA
Emotional Status	Fair	Poor	Fair	Good	Good

nurse recorded findings according to the parameters previously established on the flow sheet.

SUMMARY

The implications for the gerontological nurse's use of the problem-oriented record system in health care settings are many. This system not only contributes to quality care, but furthers the education of gerontological nurses by permitting an ongoing audit. Each practitioner is able to analyze the critical thinking and decision making used in the management of clients' problems through the systematic format of the progress notes. Thus, they are able to evaluate the quality of care they are rendering.

The problem-oriented record also facilitates communication between members of a multidisciplinary health team. Because all members utilize the same type of progress notes, they are more readily aware of what plans other health care providers have formulated for the management of problems. This awareness contributes to more comprehensive modes of health care delivery and allows for discussion of client problems on a sophisticated level between all members of the team.

The major advantage of the problem-oriented record is that it is a permanent and easily understood documentation of the client's health problems. The record system, ideally, should be begun early in life for each client and then maintained throughout the life span. This record should be in a readily retrievable, accessible form that accompanies the client. It would then provide the gerontological nurse with an accurate, lifetime, health profile of each elderly client regardless of the health care setting. Such a comprehensive record would contribute not only to the continuity and comprehensiveness of care, but might also serve to improve the quality of life of the elderly client maintained through the health care system.

REFERENCES

ANSLEY, B. 1975. "Patient-Oriented Recording: A Better System for Ambulatory Settings." *Nursing '75* 5(8):52–53.

ATWOOD, J., P. H. MITCHELL, and S. R. YARNALL. 1974. "The POR: A System for Communication." *Nursing Clinics of North America* 9(2):229–34.

BLOOM, J. T., et al. 1971. "Problem-Oriented Charting." *American Journal of Nursing* 71(11):2144–48.

CORBUS, H. F., et al. 1977. "The Problem-Oriented Medical Record in Long-Term Facilities: A Teaching Method." *Journal of Gerontological Nursing* 3(4):24–31.

HURST, J. W., and H. K. WALKER. 1972. *The Problem-Oriented System.* New York: Medcom Press.

LEITCH, C. J., and R. V. TINKER. 1978. *Primary Care.* Philadelphia: F. A. Davis.

MITCHELL, P. H. 1973. "A Systematic Nursing Progress Record." *Nursing Forum* 12(2):187–209.

ROBINSON, A. M. 1975. "Problem-Oriented Record: Uniting the Team for Total Care." *R.N.* 38(6):23–28.

SCHELL, P., and A. CAMPBELL. 1972. "POMR—Not Just Another Way to Chart." *Nursing Outlook* 20(8):510–14.

WEED, L. L. 1971. *Medical Records, Medical Education, and Patient Care.* Ohio: Case Western Reserve.

WOODY, M., and M. MALLISON. 1973. "The Problem-Oriented System for Patient-Centered Care." *American Journal of Nursing* 73(7):1168–75.

YARNALL, S., and J. ATWOOD. 1974. "Problem-Oriented Practice for Nurses and Physicians." *Nursing Clinics of North America* 9(2):215–28.

ZIMMER, M. J. 1974. "Quality Assurance for Outcomes of Patient Care." *Nursing Clinics of North America* 9(2):305–15.

III

GERONTOLOGICAL NURSING MANAGEMENT

Overview

NURSING MANAGEMENT OF HEALTH PROBLEMS IN THE OLDER ADULT

Throughout life, humans change not only with respect to the kinds of illness they suffer, but also in their response to the illness. Progressive mortality appears to be related to a gradual decline of the functional reserve capacity of the various organs responsible for the maintenance of homeostasis. Management of health problems in the older adult requires a balancing of senescence against the severity of the stress. If the organism is allowed to stray too far or too long out of balance, homeostasis will be irretrievably lost and death results.

CELLULAR AGING

Cell aging and death occur at all stages of development. In fetal life, cells form and die in an orderly, timed sequence. Limb buds form hands, renal development passes through several stages, and solid structures form hollow organs by means of the death of specifically located cells occurring at the proper moment. In childhood the thymus develops and then involutes. In the mature adult this process of involution leads to diminishing organ-reserve capacity in the kidney (Rowe et al. 1976), depressed bone marrow (Yasukazu and Toksu 1976), as well as decreased temperature regulation capacity (Watts 1971) and diminished cardiac reserve (Dock 1956).

In addition to these changes, other striking clinical alterations are well known. Central nervous system cell loss leads to an altered response under stress known as an acute brain syndrome. Arteriosclerosis reduces blood flow, thus rendering tissues more susceptible to anoxia when metabolic demand is increased. Additionally, a delay in pancreatic response to a glucose load poses difficulty in diagnosing diabetes in the older client.

267

Whatever the cellular mechanisms involved may be—genetic loss, mutation, or suppression; protoplasmic sludging; or a limited energy reserve—the inexorable result for all complex organisms is death.

Acquired changes add their burden to these processes. Health problems intervening over the lifetime destroy cells and leave nonfunctional scars that hasten the end. In addition, genetic mutation causes hyperlipidemia, hypertension, coronary artery disease, diabetes, intestinal polyposis, gout, and medullocystic renal disease, all of which further reduce the target organ's stress reserves and add to the health problems.

Thus the combined attack of heredity and environment determine the true biological age of the client. Future research may permit a slowing or reversal of cellular aging; however, until that time nursing care of the older adult requires assessment of reserve capacity and its maintenance for as long as possible by acting to diminish the effects of stress upon the organism. Diminishing the effects of stress requires an understanding of how aging affects both the cellular response to pathology and the early diagnostic findings of health problems in the older adult.

NURSING MANAGEMENT

The gerontological clinical specialist/nurse practitioner caring for elderly individuals in a primary care site utilizes the nursing process (assessment, planning, intervention, evaluation). Health management depends on each preceding step, not on any particular step. Part III is concerned with the examination of age-related pathological conditions and their subsequent effect on health in older adults. Each chapter will cover the pathophysiology of age and illness related to the health problem, followed by nursing assessment, diagnostics, and management. Assessment is described in terms of nursing subjective and objective findings; management examines care in terms of treatment, evaluation of care, and client counseling and health education.

As nursing expanded its scope of practice, nursing intervention naturally expanded into the realm of health problem management. The lines of health management provide overlapping areas between what was traditionally the nurse's domain and what was traditionally the physician's domain.

Practitioners of nursing find a high degree of variability in the types of services and practice they provide. These services are highly dependent upon the needs of the consumer group being serviced, the judgment and knowledge base of the nurse, the practice arrangement, reimbursement arrangements, acceptance of other health professionals, and state practice laws. Regardless of these conditions that influence practice, the nurse needs to have a knowledge base concerning health management. In addition to counseling and health teaching, management may include drug therapy and collaboration on specific health problems with other members of the health team, and referral when indicated.

PRESCRIBING DRUGS TO THE ELDERLY

While nurses in a number of states are already prescribing drugs under protocols or provider numbers, all nurses need to know drug ranges regardless of whether the nurse or the physician prescribes the drug. When prescribing drugs to any individual, reactions must be carefully documented. Recording such data is especially important in treating the elderly, who frequently take many drugs and who often present with iatrogenically drug-induced health problems. These facts are discussed by J. W. Long (1977) in relation to drugs and the elderly:

Advancing age brings changes in body structure and function that may alter significantly the action of drugs. An impaired digestive system may interfere with drug absorption. Reduced capacity of the liver and kidneys to metabolize and eliminate drugs may result in the accumulation of drugs in the body to toxic levels. By impairing the body's ability to maintain a "steady state" (homeostasis), the aging process may increase the sensitivity of many tissues to the actions of drugs, thereby altering greatly the responsiveness of the nervous and circulatory systems to standard drug doses. If aging should cause deterioration of understanding, memory, or vision or physical coordination, people with such impairments may not always use drugs safely and effectively.

Adverse reactions to drugs occur three times more frequently in the older population. Unwanted drug response can render a functioning and independent older person—whose health and reserves are at marginal levels—confused, incompetent, or helpless. For these reasons, drug treatment in the elderly must always be accompanied by the most careful consideration of the individual's health and tolerances, the selection of drugs and dosage schedules, and the possible need for assistance in treatment routines. [From the book *Essential Guide to Prescription Drugs: What You Need to Know for Safe Drug Use,* Copyright © 1977 by James W. Long, MD. Reprinted by permission of Harper & Row, Publishers, Inc.]

Table III.1 lists the hazards of commonly used drugs when they are given to the elderly.

TABLE III.1
Drug Hazards in the Elderly

	Increased Possibility of Adverse Reactions	Possible Confusion and Behavioral Disturbances	Possible Orthostatic Hypotension	Possible Constipation and Urinary Retention	Possible Urinary Incontinence
Amantadine	X	X			
Antacids (high sodium)					
Antianxiety Agents		X			
Anticoagulants (oral)*					
Antidiabetic Drugs*		X			
Antihistamines*		X			
Antihypertensives*			X		
Antiparkinsonism Drugs				X	
Atropine and Atropinelike Drugs		X			
Barbiturates*	X	X			
Belladonna Preparations		X			
Cortisonelike Drugs*					

TABLE III.1 (continued)

	Increased Possibility of Adverse Reactions	Possible Confusion and Behavioral Disturbances	Possible Orthostatic Hypotension	Possible Constipation and Urinary Retention	Possible Urinary Incontinence
Digitalis Preparations*	X				
Dihydroergotoxine		X		X	
Diuretics*		X	X		X
Ephedrine*					
Haloperidol*					
Hypnotics*		X			X
Indomethacin	X				
Levodopa		X			
Meprobamate		X			
Methyldopa		X			
Nalidixic Acid*					
Neproxen					
Narcotics*		X			
Oxphenbutazone	X				
Pentazocine		X			
Phenacetin	X				
Phenylbutazone	X				
Phenytoin		X			
Primidone		X			
Pseudoephedrine*					
Quinidine*					
Resperine		X			
Sedatives		X	X		X
Tetracyclines	X				
Thiothixene		X			
Thyroid Preparations*					
Tranquilizers (all types)			X		X
Tricyclic Antidepressants*		X	X	X	
Trihexphenidyl		X			
Vasodilators			X		

* Reduced dosage necessary until full effect seen.

Source: Table 12 (pp. 735–736) from The Essential Guide to Prescription Drugs by James W. Long, M.D. Copyright © by James W. Long, M.D. Reprinted by permission of Harper & Row, Publishers, Inc.

REFERENCES

DOCK, W. 1956. "Aging of the Myocardium." *Bulletin, New York Academy of Medicine* 32:175–78.

LONG, JAMES. 1977. *The Essential Guide to Prescription Drugs.* New York: Harper and Row.

ROWE, J. W. et al. 1976. "The Effect of Age on Creatinine Clearance in Men: A Cross-Sectional and Longitudinal Study." *Journal of Gerontology* 31:155–63.

WATTS, A. J. 1971. "Hypothermia in the Aged: A Study of the Rise of Cold Sensitivity." *Environmental Research* 5:119–26.

YASUKAZU, T., and I. TOKSU. 1976. "Fatty Marrow in the Vertebrae: A Parameter for Hematopoietic Activity in the Aged." *Journal of Gerontology* 31:527–32.

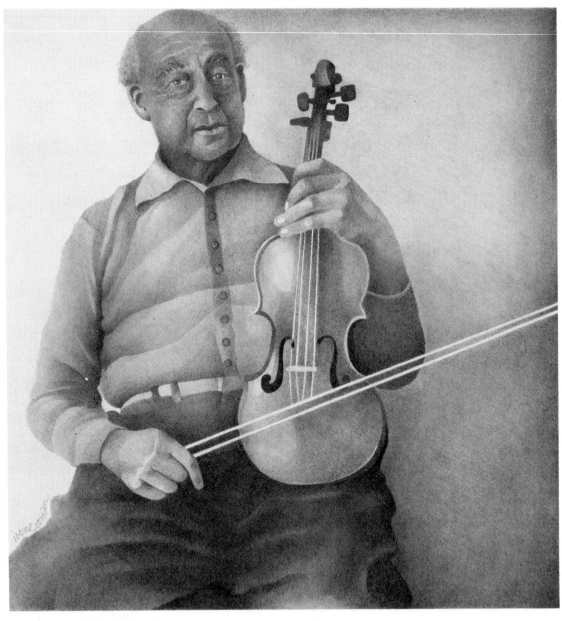

Chapter 9

GERONTOLOGICAL NURSING MANAGEMENT
THE ELDERLY CLIENT WITH A NEURO/EMOTIONAL HEALTH PROBLEM

Elderly people do not necessarily suffer mental decline, and many are extremely alert. Intellectual function often remains stable until shortly before death; in fact, a decline need not occur even in that period. For the cognitively impaired elderly, organic and functional disorders often overlap with labile or deteriorating behavioral manifestations. Many older clients show markedly advanced arteriosclerosis on autopsy, yet during life they either had good social support systems or were able to adapt to cognitive impairment in such a manner that organic changes only minimally affected their behavioral functioning. These findings have led to further studies that link socioeconomic factors, psychodynamic aspects, and premorbid personality to adaptation of cognitive impairment in the aged (Verwoerdt 1976).

In this chapter we discuss nursing management of problems that interfere with elderly clients' interpersonal relationships or independent living. Common emotional problems related to aging were discussed in chapter 7.

MENTAL HEALTH IN THE ELDERLY

The two major divisions of mental health problems in old age are *functional problems* and *organic brain problems*. Organic brain problems relate to the physical changes of brain tissue; functional problems describe changes of mood and thought content. Butler and Lewis (1977, p. 52) suggest that the true proportion of psychiatric problems among older people has not been fully documented; they estimate that 15 percent of the older population is in need of some mental health services.

The older population with mental health problems can be divided into two categories based on time of onset. The first includes people confined to mental institutions at a young age. Formerly the mentally ill grew old in institutions; now, however, they are being transferred to community settings or nursing homes. The second category is made up of persons who develop mental illnesses for the first time in late life. This group may have organic brain syndromes, a functional illness, or a combination of the two.

Too frequently, aberrant behavior has been thought to be part of the aging process. In addition mental illness in the aged has long been thought to be related to irreversible brain damage. Research and clinical work with the elderly have disproved these views. Kahn, Goldfarb, and others (1960) helped to clarify the differences between organic damage and affective behavioral changes. They tested orientation and memory with a "Mental Status Questionnaire" (described in chapter 7). Their findings show that some disorders are reversible and that organic tissue and personality changes are not necessarily a corollary to old age.

ORGANIC BRAIN SYNDROMES

Pathophysiology

The tissue of the brain is completely dependent upon a continuous blood supply in order to obtain the glucose and oxygen essential to its metabolism and function. Brain tissue stores virtually no energy; when deprived of its oxygen supply for more than three to four minutes, the tissue undergoes ischemic necrosis. Compounding the problem of the brain's critical need for a constant supply of blood is the fact that the brain is supplied by arteries and arterioles that are much thinner walled than systemic arteries and arterioles. The difference between cerebral and systemic vessels is due to the fact that the media in cerebral vessels contain very little muscle and are therefore less resistant to blood pressure elevations.

Since organic brain syndromes are most frequently related to cerebral arteriosclerosis, understanding the vascular changes that characterize this syndrome is important. Atherosclerosis is the chief form of sclerosis in the arteries of the brain. The most commonly accepted theory of atherogenesis is the filtration theory (Timiras 1972). This theory states that plasma lipids continually filter through arterial walls and that some of the lipid becomes trapped within the vessel wall. Consequently, the lipid acts as a foreign body. Mucopolysaccharides are then released by cells in the wall, and scar tissue is formed, causing a fibrous plaque to appear on the vessel wall. This plaque narrows the lumen and interferes with the critically needed blood supply. The plaques generally tend to form at arterial branches and bifurcations.

Organic brain syndromes are divided into two categories: an *acute* syndrome, which is reversible, and a *chronic* syndrome with irreversible organicity. Organic brain syndromes are often associated with various types of neurotic and psychiatric disorders. Chronic organic brain syndrome with generalized loss of functional brain cells may begin as early as the middle years. The mean age of onset for Alzheimer's disease is 53 years (Reichel 1978, p. 131).

Nursing Assessment

Chronic Organic Brain Syndrome (Dementia): Subjective and Objective Findings. In the very early stages of chronic organic brain syndrome, few symptoms may appear; but as cell loss becomes more marked, the client begins to have difficulties in everyday functions, manifested in personal, family, and community problems. Memory changes are among the most overt symptoms of chronic OBS; an initial effect is loss for recent events. Nocturnal confusion is prevalent in the early stages. The client may be oriented during the day but confused and frightened when awakening at night. The client may suffer from sleeplessness and restlessness. The family may complain that the client cannot manage the checkbook; a previously neat person may become slovenly; and a client with severe brain deterioration may wander or get lost.

As chronic OBS progresses, the client becomes disoriented to time, place, and person. Memory loss for both remote and recent events occurs, along with inability to provide general information of the simplest kind, such as "The grass is green" or "The sky is blue"; inability to do ordinary addition and subtraction; and loss of judgment. Delusions and hallucinations may occur in the advanced stages of chronic OBS.

Acute Organic Brain Syndrome (Delirium): Subjective and Objective Findings. Acute organic brain syndrome is abrupt, transient, and reversible. The client may have a fluctuating level of awareness. Hallucinations, when present, are of the visual type. Remote as well as recent memory loss occurs. Acute OBS must be differentiated from a transient acute OBS superimposed on a chronic OBS. Acute OBS and acute OBS superimposed on a chronic OBS are related to general health problems, such as septicemia secondary to infection, pain, fractures, malnutrition, heart failure or coronary thrombosis, malignancy, drug intoxication, or cerebrovascular accident. Attention span is shortened and recent memory and immediate recall are diminished.

A sudden deterioration in the subjective or objective findings of the client with chronic OBS may be induced by the development of the acute syndrome in the client. Thus increased agitation and confusion may be the sign of pneumonia, a metabolic disturbance, or an untoward effect of drug therapy instituted to control the client's behavioral problems.

For clients presenting with symptoms of a brain syndrome, the nurse should assess functioning through the use of a "Mental Status Questionnaire" and/or the face-hand test. Activities of daily living should also be assessed. Assessment may require a home visit, especially when a family member is not present or is unable to assist in providing data.

Diagnostics

Hamilton and Cowdry (1976, p. 337) suggest that an initial thorough diagnostic workup be obtained for the data base. Blood studies include a CBC, postprandial glucose, SGOT, SGPT, BUN, serum creatinine, electrolytes, blood bromide level, carbon dioxide tension, and serum thyroxine level. Additionally indicated are an EKG and urinalysis. Chest and skull x-ray films should be ordered. A brain scan and electroencephalography will rule out brain

275

tumor or hydrocephalus. Other specific blood tests will determine whether the client has diabetes, syphilis, or thyroid or renal disease.

Nursing Management

Treatment. The management goal in both acute and chronic organic brain syndromes is to reduce the symptoms manifested by the client. To reduce disorientation to reality in the home or institution, the following guidelines are suggested: (1) diminish stress by avoiding frequent change and by creating a calm and unhurried environment, (2) maintain privacy by clearly designating the client's territory, (3) allow the individual to maintain as normal a lifestyle as possible within existing condition, (4) call the client by name, (5) maintain reality by repeating factual data, (6) maintain a warm, supportive relationship with the client, (7) facilitate sensory awareness at night by using night lights.

A client with impaired cognitive functions has an increased need for cognitive stimulation. This stimulation, however, is frequently diminished as a result of the client's sensory deficits, loss of family and friends, and narrowing social sphere. Mentioning current events and seeking the client's opinion on a variety of topics are simple ways to provide ongoing cognitive stimulation.

The nurse can also provide sensory and cognitive stimulation through the use of group work. This technique is more effective than individual psychotherapy for the elderly. The nurse can function as a group leader or facilitator in a variety of settings, including day care programs, senior citizen centers, and long-term care institutions.

Both small- and large-group sessions can help to increase self-esteem and social integration while giving support and reassurance to the individual. Burnside's (1978) book on group processes and techniques is an excellent resource for nurses practicing in institutional settings. Many of the techniques can be adapted to community settings.

A number of groups in community settings initially begin in response to social needs. Others are organized to spread health information and then serve to socially integrate the cognitively impaired elderly residing in the community. For example, a "soft-therapy"-group program in assertiveness training is currently being conducted by the Douglas Gardens Community Mental Health Services in Miami for the elderly of the community. The Northside Neighborhood Family Center, Inc., composed of an inner-city group of elderly, uses the concept of the "surrogate family" (Glasscote, Gudeman, and Miles 1977, p. 59). Other group approaches focus on religion, current events, or common concerns.

Evaluation of Care. The starting point in nursing care management must be focused on identifying the personal assets of the client. Measures to amplify personal assets should be identified and initiated. A trial period is often necessary when the nurse is selecting among various techniques; even a successful technique must be reassessed constantly and changed when it is no longer effective.

The nurse must know and use community resources when attempting to help the client set up social support systems. The advocate role of the nurse is time consuming, as seeking and obtaining a community resource often takes many hours. Efforts should be directed toward establishing a support system that will determine the need for institutional placement. A nurse-staffed clinic for senior citizens can provide these services as well as act as a central referral agency for needy elderly (Stanley, Brovender, and Anderson 1979).

Improving or maintaining the highest level of functional capacity is a major responsibility for the nurse. Existing metabolic stress should be alleviated in an attempt to eliminate any reversible component. Infection should be treated, pain controlled, and sedatives reduced.

The client may have a tendency to overextend energy levels. The management plan must consist of a balance between rest and activity. Treatment of anemia, dehydration, electrolyte imbalance, and vitamin deficiencies will guide nutritional requirements and dietary supplements as well as help determine how much energy can be expended (Hirschfield 1976). In the event that death is imminent, the nursing focus should be shifted from rehabilitative management to helping the person attain a peaceful and comfortable death.

CEREBROVASCULAR ISCHEMIC PROBLEMS

Pathophysiology

Two conditions can arise from atherosclerosis: the formation of a thrombus and the progressive narrowing of cerebral arteries.

Thrombus Formation. A thrombus is most likely to form at a plaque site; since plaques frequently form at arterial bifurcations, thrombus formation is not uncommon at the origin of the internal carotid and at junctions of the middle cerebral, vertebral, and basilar arteries. Plaques are composed of a mixture of disintegrated platelets and fibrin. Such plaques have proved to be the source of embolic showers that cause transient ischemic attacks (TIAs). Further, clinicians agree that if the source of the embolic showers is in one of the internal carotids, the resultant TIAs are harbingers of a completed stroke (Dalessio 1978).

Thrombi also form frequently at bifurcations of the circle of Willis vessels. If emboli or thrombi occlude a vessel, ischemic necrosis will result. Necrosis occurs because brain tissue has been deprived of blood; it is reflected peripherally by impaired motor functions, such as hemiplegia, or by altered central functions, such as a speech disturbance. The clinical picture is variable and depends on the location of the focal necrosis that results from cerebral vessel occlusion by the thrombus.

Progressive Narrowing of Arteries. If progressive narrowing of cerebral arteries and arterioles is severe enough to reduce blood flow to a trickle or to occlude the vessel entirely, the brain tissue upstream is deprived of essential oxygen and glucose. The tissue becomes necrotic, and, just as in the case of cerebral thrombosis, the clinical picture is variable. Peripheral manifestations of the neurological deficit again will depend on the focal necrosis.

While the pathological events of both cerebral thrombosis and progressive narrowing of cerebral vasculature occur over a period of time and may or may not be pre-

277

ceded by transient ischemic attacks, a *cerebral embolism* causes a stroke to develop very rapidly. The source of the embolic fragment is usually a thrombus within the heart, and if the embolus is large enough, it will generally lodge in a proximal cerebral bifurcation or at a point of vascular narrowing. Again the clinical picture depends on the location of the ischemic necrotic brain tissue.

Two other causes of stroke with an abrupt onset are hypertensive intracerebral hemorrhage and saccular aneurysm. *Hypertensive intracerebral hemorrhage* occurs within the brain tissue; damage to the tissue is due to compression by the hematoma and to interruption of blood flow. The neurological signs and symptoms again depend on the extent and location of the hemorrhage.

In stroke caused by ruptured *saccular aneurysm,* the cerebral vessel rupture occurs at the site of a developmental defect or thin-walled blister in the vascular wall. Ruptures occur most frequently in persons age 40 to 65. The most common sites of the rupture are in the anterior portions of the circle of Willis. Because these vessels lie in the subarachnoid space, blood is discharged there. Thus spinal fluid taken in a tap will be very bloody. The severity of the clinical signs and symptoms can range from a temporary loss of consciousness to death. Again the extent and locations of the hemorrhage will determine the clinical findings and outcome.

Pathology of vasculature in the brain can lead to both mild and severe cerebrovascular diseases. The same can be said of pathological changes in vasculature in any organ of the body. Vascular pathology will be discussed in greater detail in chapter 10, on cardiovascular disorders.

Nursing Assessment

Cerebrovascular ischemic disease may present as a transient ischemic attack (TIA) or as a true stroke with prolonged motor and sensory impairment.

Transient Ischemic Attacks: Subjective and Objective Findings. Transient ischemic attacks are temporary impairments of motor and/or sensory function. They may last from several minutes to 24 hours (Hardin 1976). Frequently the client will note temporary visual loss (amaurosis fugax) and muscle weakness on the affected side. Transient slurring of speech may be found in dominant side problems. During the attack a variety of neurological changes with or without loss of consciousness may be present, with evidence of loss of central control over peripheral function. Hoffman's or Babinski's signs with hyperactive reflexes may be found. After the attack neurological changes may be absent. Auscultation of the carotid or vertebral artery will often reveal a systolic bruit on the side opposite the peripheral signs. The episodes are caused by embolization from the extracranial vascular stenosis; without further therapy the risk of a major stroke is 80 percent.

Intracerebral Vascular Occlusion (True Stroke): Subjective and Objective Findings. The client with more prolonged impairment has suffered intracerebral vascular occlusion, which is associated with cerebral infarction and irreparable loss of functional tissue. At the time of assessment, a stroke may be either in progress or completed. Since this condition is determined by observation and a stroke in progress may be life threatening, the client should be hospitalized for evaluation and treatment during the acute phase.

In the *acute phase* the client may be alert or unconscious. If alert, the client usually complains of functional loss of some portion of the body. Examination reveals peripheral evidence of long tract, central nervous system impairment, motor impairment being the most common. Paralysis is often flaccid, with decreased or absent reflexes. Upper extremities are more frequently and more severely involved than lower. When speech is impaired, right-sided peripheral signs are usually present.

Sensory impairment is less frequent and usually involves the spinothalamic functions of pain, touch, and thermal sensation. The impairment is contralateral to the motor loss. Hoffman's and Babinski's signs indicate the central origin of the motor dysfunction. Kernig's sign, indicating meningeal irritation, is found with hemorrhage. Fever may be present and rise dramatically, signaling a terminal condition.

Spasticity and reflex hyperactivity appear later. Clients may complain of severe cramping of the extremities. The affected upper limb is held in flexion, the lower in extension. A scissors gait is often seen. Speech impairment may consist of receptive aphasia (inability to understand) or motor aphasia (inability to speak). The latter may produce a partial paralysis of the speech muscles of the tongue or palate and cause slurring.

A *home visit* can be invaluable in the nursing assessment of the stroke victim. Physical aspects of the home are evaluated in terms of the client's needs. Doors must be wide enough to accommodate a wheelchair if necessary. Steps of access to rooms must be taken into account, as well as potential dangers, such as scatter rugs or highly polished floors. The bed should be at a height to facilitate transfer and ease of care. The home is the best place to assess family dynamics. Is the family or significant other able to be firm when necessary? Is the attitude one of caring or of resentment and deep-seated anger? What are the coping strategies of the family or significant other? (Wilcoxson 1966, p. 67).

Nursing Management

Treatment. Medical management of a client who is having TIAs should be carried out under the direction of a physician. Treatment is focused on either surgical intervention or some form of long-term anticoagulation. For the client with the completed stroke, treatment is aimed at controlling any etiologic factors that might be present, such as smoking, hypertension, gout, or diabetes mellitus, and at rehabilitation of the existing motor deficits.

Health Education and Counseling. The client most often has problems in maintaining personality organization. Both client and family will require support and counseling from the nurse. The principles of short-term goals should be employed to prevent overstressing the client and to improve chances of success (Matheney 1966). Frequently family members will be so distressed by the changes in the client that they will do too much for the client, thereby deterring rehabilitative aims. Family members should be taught how to satisfy the client's need for proper exercise and nutrition and how to cope with changes in the client's mental status. When long-term therapy is indicated, the client should receive home health nursing services. The nurse clinical specialist or practitioner should keep informed of the client's progress through the home health nurse.

Evaluation of Care. The nurse employs a multidisciplinary approach, including the use of orthopedic, speech, and physiotherapy consultants, and also gives ongoing support and encouragement to the client and family.

The convalescent period may be prolonged. A simple, nondominant, unilateral stroke may require up to 90 days for amelioration, while a dominant side stroke with aphasia may require 6 months.

FUNCTIONAL DISORDERS

Depression is the most common functional disorder seen in the aged. According to Butler and Lewis (1977), "depression reactions increase in degree and frequency with old age as a corollary to the increased loss of much that is emotionally valued by the elderly person." Reassessment of one's life can bring depression, acceptance, or satisfaction. Unresolved grief, guilt, or anger are expressions of both mild and severe depression. All too frequently, depressed elderly people are incorrectly labeled as having an organic brain syndrome or being apathetic.

Busse and Pfeiffer (1973) found that the elderly tolerate loss of significant others better than loss of physical health. Many elderly try to cope with loss by using the mechanism of denial. This response can cause maladaptation if the client denies such things as a decrease in vision.

Nursing Assessment

Subjective Findings. Depression in the elderly client is frequently overlooked be-

cause the client does not always present with the classic signs of a younger depressed person. The affective manifestations, such as sad feelings or despair, self-depreciatory thoughts or loss of initiative, and crying spells, may not be present or prominent. The prominent complaints are of a somatic origin: insomnia, anorexia, fatigue, loss of energy, and constipation. Psychomotor retardation is evident, as the depressed older individual moves and thinks more slowly than the normal aged person (Verwoerdt 1976, p. 46). Frequent visits to the nurse because of varying somatic concerns should be a clue to a possible depression.

Objective Findings. In contrast to individuals with chronic brain syndromes, depressed persons remain oriented to time, place, and person. The MMPI ("Minnesota Multiphasic Personality Inventory") and the absence of evidence of OBS may provide objective data.

Nursing Management

Treatment. Management of depression in the elderly can follow several patterns. One pattern is to *acknowledge the depression and help the individual realize that someone cares.* Caring can be shown by phone calls, the use of touch, and other forms of communication. Another pattern is to *help the individual regain feelings of self-worth* by encouraging improvement of physical appearance and expansion of relationships with others. The nurse must be aware of community facilities available to the elderly. Most areas have senior clubs and senior citizen centers. Additionally many high schools and community colleges are offering course work that is specifically geared to leisure time.

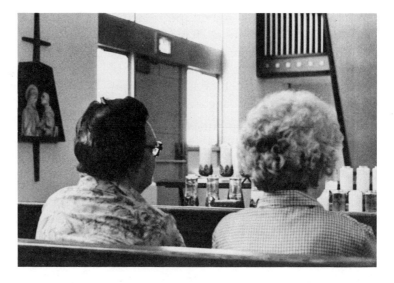

The gerontological nurse can help the elderly adapt to the aging process by encouraging religious and social activities; elderly clients need to have a source of spiritual strength and a sense of belonging.

Still another pattern of management is to *use group dynamics and processes* or group memberships where individuals can socialize and share feelings. The use of groups for the cognitively impaired elderly was previously discussed. Groups can also be very beneficial for the psychologically impaired. Traditional group therapy for the elderly should be led or assisted by a trained psychologist, psychiatrist, or nurse mental-health therapist.

Untreated depression may lead to self-destructive behavior. The suicide rate is higher for older individuals than for younger persons and higher for older males than for older females. Suicide attempts in nursing homes may be indirect or subtle (examples of subtle suicide attempts are refusing medication, striking windows or walls, climbing out of wheelchairs and falling, and not eating). Since depression-based suicide is thought to be preventable (Butler and Lewis 1977), health providers need to be alert to warning signs. Nurses should sensitively explore with the depressed client any covertly or overtly ex-pressed suicidal tendencies. Clients with expressed suicidal thoughts should be immediately referred for psychiatric evaluation.

In the severely depressed or suicidal client not rapidly responding to group therapy, *medication* can be a useful adjunct. The most commonly used medications are derivatives of tricyclicamines, either alone or in combination with a phenothiazine. The initial dose for the elderly should be one-third that for the younger patient and should be carefully increased every 5 to 7 days until either the therapeutic response is attained or the side effects become too bothersome to the client. The tricyclics may take 10 days to 2 weeks to produce therapeutic results. If, after an adequate trial of antidepressant drugs, life-threatening depression is not alleviated, hospitalization should be considered and the client referred to a psychiatrist.

Impramine hydrochloride (Tofranil) 10 mg three times daily to 150 mg a day in divided doses; amitriptyline hydrochloride (Elavil) 10 mg three times daily to 150 mg a day in divided doses; and desipramine hydrochloride (Norpramine) 25 mg daily four times a day are the most commonly used tricyclicamines. Dosage changes should be made slowly to allow observation for a potential reaction to the drug as well as for the therapeutic response of the client. These medications can cause hypotension and cardiac arrhythmias and exacerbate anxiety-related complaints.

PARKINSONISM

Pathophysiology

Parkinsonism is a common health problem in the elderly and is due to multiple pathology. It is caused by a dysfunction of the dopaminergic-nigro-neostriatal system of the brain. Parkinsonism is characterized by extrapyramidal neurological and autonomic systemic manifestations. The inhibitory extrapyramidal system controls posture and movement. Briefly, this motor system consists of several areas of the cerebral cortex; multiple pathways leading from the cerebral areas; several "ganglia" of the cerebral hemisphere, midbrain, pons, and medulla oblongata (including the basal ganglia); and the numerous pathways leading from these ganglia (Duvoisin 1976, p. 3).

Parkinsonism is usually divided into primary and secondary types. However, the nurse must also distinguish forms of pseudoparkinsonism, which have a superficial resemblance to the disease but a different evolution and do not respond to the same modes of treatment (see table 9.1).

In Parkinson's disease the extrapyramidal structures, which are thought to be diseased, are the substantia nigra and the globus pallidus of the corpus striatum. The extrapyramidal system is now thought to innovate, control, activate, and inhibit the same musculature controlled by the pyramidal system. "It is now known that in primates there are numerous connections between the precentral cortex and the basal ganglia, but many of the details of these connections, both as regards structure and function, are still unknown" (Vick 1976, p. 327). More recent findings show that the intact normal substantia nigra and corpus striatum have significant amounts of the catecholamine dopamine, an inhibitory neurotransmitter. Further, in clients with Parkinson's disease the level of dopamine is depleted, as it is in animals with experimental lesions of the substantia nigra (Duvoisin 1976, p. 4).

Other important discoveries include the recent identification of pathways in the basal ganglia. Some pathways are mediated by acetylcholine; others by gamma-aminobutyric acid (GABA). Acetylcholine is an excitatory transmitter in the basal ganglia; GABA is an inhibitory synaptic transmitter. The most recently proposed pathophysiological explanation for parkinsonism states that "when the basal ganglia is diseased . . . neural mechanisms (are) 'released' from the control or inhibition of the structures (substantia nigra) which have been destroyed" (Vick 1976, p. 329). Recall that the substantia nigra contains significant amounts of the inhibitory neurotransmitter dopamine.

Among the manifestations of the "release" phenomenon are rigidity and tremors. Both of these clinical findings may be present in clients with parkinsonism, but they may be manifested in varying degrees.

282

TABLE 9.1
Classification of Parkinsonism by Etiology

Clinical Form	Etiology or Associated Illness

Primary Parkinsonism
  Parkinson's disease, idiopathic
  Parkinson's disease, paralysis agitans,
  shaking palsy
	Degenerative disease of unknown etiology

Secondary Parkinsonism
  Postencephalitic
	Encephalitis lethargica (Von Economos's
	  disease), suspected viral illness,
	  virus never isolated

Iatrogenic	Phenothiazine medication

Parkinsonism-plus	Progressive supranuclear palsy,
	  familial olivopontocerebellar atrophy,
	  Shy-Dager syndrome with dementia

Juvenile form	Hepatolenticular degeneration (Wilson's disease)
Symptomatic form	Trauma, ischemia, hemorrhage, tumor, neurosyphilis, neurotuberculosis

Pseudoparkinsonism	Arteriosclerotic or senile tremor;
	  familial, essential tremor; hypo- or
	  hyperthyroidism; hyperparathyroidism;
	  depression with psychomotor retardation;
	  normal-pressure hydrocephalus

" 'Tremor-at-rest' is most commonly associated with lesions of the substantia nigra or the globus pallidus [of the corpus striatum] or both" (Vick 1976, p. 331).

Examination of diseased substantia nigra and the corpus striatum reveal "cell loss with a broad range of regressive alteration in the remaining neurons. [There is also] prominent depigmentation, and the presence of intracytoplasmic hyaline inclusions" (Vick 1976, p. 335).

Nursing Assessment

Primary parkinsonism is an insidiously progressive and disabling illness of un-known etiology, rarely encountered in persons under age 40. It affects 1 percent of persons over age 50, causing 1 million cases in the United States and 50,000 new cases annually. The course of the disease is variable. Some cases are rapidly progressive, with total invalidism within five to ten years after onset. Others may linger in the early stages over a course of twenty years. Whatever the evolution, the ultimate result is a severe invalidism and an associated susceptibility to infections and other complications, leading to a diminished life expectancy. Primary parkinsonism is characterized by a triad of *tremor, loss of postural reflexes,* and *rigidity.* Secondary forms often

283

have other distinguishing findings, such as oculogyric crises, dystonic spasms, dementia, or liver disease, grafted onto the classic triad.

The severity of the findings varies according to the stage of illness. In early cases these changes may be quite subtle; in the more advanced ones, findings are pronounced, and the nurse should have little difficulty in recognizing the illness.

Subjective Findings in the Early Stage. The early stage is characterized by unilateral involvement. Subjective complaints include periarthritis of the shoulder; cramps; figiting; a one-sided tremor, often localized to the upper limb; and difficulty in performing simple acts, such as buttoning a shirt. Frequently clients seek help at the insistence of their families, who have noted handwriting changes, slowness of movement (bradykinesis), or diminished facial expression (hypomimia). On direct questioning, the nurse may often elicit a history of vague aches and pains or of cold and burning sensations (thermal paresthesias), which precede the onset of the tremor (Duvoisin 1976).

Objective Findings in the Early Stage. Objective findings are limited to the affected side and include a tremor at rest, which improves with movement and sleep and is worsened by suspension or anxiety. The body often tilts slightly away from the affected side. The affected arm is carried in slight abduction at the shoulder and is flexed at the elbow. Speech may be low pitched, slow, and measured. Hypomimia gives the face a blank expression. The affected limb is somewhat rigid. The nurse feels this decreased mobility as a plastic resistance or *cogwheel* phenomenon through-

out passive flexion and extension. Rapid alternating movements (dysdiadochokinesis), such as tapping the thigh with the palm and back of the hand alternately, become progressively slower. Finger dexterity is diminished and handwriting changes are characteristic in dominant side disease. These changes include micrographia (small writing), shakiness, and poorly formed loops in letters such as *e* and *l*.

Subjective Findings in the More Advanced Stages. In the more advanced stages, the findings become bilateral and more obvious. Subjective complaints now include weakness, tiredness, and lethargy, with increasing difficulty in the performance of simple tasks.

Objective Findings in the More Advanced Stages. Objective examination reveals a mild, generalized slowness. The postural tilt changes to a stooped forward position of the trunk and neck when the client is standing or walking. In addition to shoulder abduction and elbow flexion, the hand is in ulnar deviation and is flexed at rest. The gait is shuffling and the body held rigidly, so that all movement becomes deliberate. Akinesia occurs and the client appears to be frozen and unable to complete an action. Eye blinking is diminished, but blepharospasm (recurrent spasmodic blink) is induced by tapping the glabella with a hammer or fingers (Myerson's sign). All of these findings will progress to cause increasing disability, often forcing early retirement from work, reducing social participation, and leading to the abandonment of hobbies and interests. Depression is a frequent complication.

Retropulsion and propulsion are particularly disturbing. The client takes a step backward and is unable to stop, or the client walks forward and the steps become shorter and faster while the body leans forward. These episodes are extremely frightening and often terminate in a fall, which may cause injury. Loss of postural reflexes is also revealed by the fact that if the client is pushed, a fall ensues without any effort to block it by arm or leg movements.

Further progression is associated with increasing stiffness and bradykinesis. The gait slows and becomes even more hesitant. Rising from a chair or changing position becomes difficult. Cutting and eating food become a problem. Seborrheic dermatitis and constipation become increasingly severe. The client may note increased perspiration.

Objective Findings in the Final Stage. In the final stage invalidism is total. The client is confined to the bed or a chair. The tremor lessens or is absent, but voluntary motor activity is minimal. The face is expressionless; the hands are clenched; the feet are in flexion, with the big toe in extension; the eyelids are retracted in an unblinking stare; and a continuous drool issues from the open mouth. Chewing and swallowing are extremely slow, leading to malnutrition and dehydration. The cough reflex and respiratory excursions are diminished, predisposing the client to pneumonia. Diminished bladder emptying frequently results in a urinary infection, while the immobility causes decubitus ulcers. Thus death often results from infection or other complications.

Nursing Management

Although much information is available about the pathological evolution of parkinsonism, the etiology is still unknown or unidentified, except in a few cases of iatrogenic or symptomatic disease. For the present no way of preventing, arresting, or reversing the illness is known.

Treatment. Iatrogenic disease is treated by withholding or reducing the dose of the offending medication. Symptomatic Parkinson's disease responds to the treatment of the primary illness if such treatment is possible. For the largest number of cases, treatment remains palliative, supportive, and symptomatic.

Levodopa is the drug of choice, given in doses of 3 to 10 g daily in three or four doses. Although this medication does not prevent progression, it can give long periods of symptomatic relief. Levodopa passes the blood-brain barrier and enters the nigrostriatal system, where it increases the intracellular levels of the neurotransmitter dopamine (Duvoisin 1976). To minimize side effects, levodopa is begun in small doses of 250 to 500 mg three or four times daily, and then is raised by increments of 250 or 500 mg every 48 hours or more. In some clients the dose should not be raised until after intervals of a week. These increases are continued until maximum relief with minimal side effects is attained (Yahr et al. 1969). Recently combinations of levodopa 100 mg with methyldopa 10 mg have been effective at small dosages. The advantage is that the dose of levodopa is decreased and the side effects are reduced. The usual dose is 1 tablet four times daily.

Low-dosage side effects are anorexia, nausea, and vomiting. These effects usually subside spontaneously. They may be minimized by giving the medication after meals. The high-dosage side effects are cardiac arrhythmias, orthostatic hypotension, insomnia, mental disturbance, agitation, and choreiform movements of the face and arms. These effects require lowering the dosage. Over time the maximally tolerated dose gradually decreases, forcing adjustment downward and diminishing the effectiveness of the medication. This reduced tolerance is most likely an expression of disease progression.

Centrally acting synthetic anticholinergics can give effective, symptomatic relief in large numbers of clients. The medications may be used in combination with each other; if the client is taking one, it should not be withdrawn prior to instituting treatment with levodopa.

Trihexyphenidyl hydrochloride (Artane) is given orally. The initial dose is 2 mg three times daily before meals. It may be increased in 2-mg increments every 48 hours to the maximum tolerated dose, which may be as high as 20 mg per day. Rarely does a higher dose have any significant effect. Congeners of this medication exist and may be useful for clients who have not responded to Artane.

Benztropine methanesulfonate (Cogentin) is a similar, long-acting medication. The initial oral dose is 2 mg daily. Increments of 2 mg every 48 hours are added to tolerance. Going beyond the maximal dose of 6 to 8 mg daily is rarely useful.

When short- and long-acting medications are used in combination, the dose of each should be lowered. The side effects of these medications include dry mouth and constipation, which are treated directly by giving the client sour balls to suck and increasing dietary bulk with raw bran, using laxatives only when necessary; blurred vision, confusion, and hallucinations, which require dose reduction; urinary retention with prostatic hypertrophy; and glaucoma.

The last two side effects must both be appropriately treated.

Evaluation of Care. Response to medication will vary from client to client and in the same client over time. Thus constant supervision is required, with frequent assessments for evidence of toxicity. In particular, drug reactions should be evaluated in any client who, while on the drug, presents with psychotic behavior. The nurse should decrease the dosage of the medication and observe the client's behavior. Once an appropriate drug is found, it should never be totally withdrawn without first obtaining good control from another medication. Otherwise a complete recurrence of the physical manifestations of this disorder will result.

Some clients do better on a dose lower than the one maximally tolerated (Yahr 1972). In such cases small doses of an antihistamine may achieve additional results. *Diphenhydramine* (Benadryl) 25 to 50 mg three or four times daily, *orphenadrine hydrochloride* (Disipal) 50 mg three times daily, or *orphenadrine citrate* (Norflex) 1 mg orally twice daily may give good results if they are administered in small doses and slowly increased to tolerance or the desired effect.

Side effects for antihistamines are similar to those described for the anticholinergics. An additional one is drowsiness, which may be quite disconcerting for the client with parkinsonism. Fortunately this effect often disappears after a time or may be eliminated by trying another drug.

Counseling. Supportive counseling for both client and family is a very important aspect of management. The family may be embarrassed or overly anxious by the client's appearance. They usually tend to assist the client in stressful situations, thereby hastening the disabling effects of Parkinson's disease. The family needs to know when to help and when to encourage the client to be self-sufficient. This behavior promotes a healthy interdependence. Adaptation to the progressive nature of this chronic disabling neurological problem is most important for emotional adjustment. The client experiences a grieving process for the losses of self-esteem, independence, social interactions, and work capacity and for other effects of the disabling process. Often the nurse will have to assist in grief work. The nurse should identify how the client coped with problems in the past in order to capitalize on coping mechanisms. The primary goal of counseling and therapy is to assist the client in maintaining a degree of independence as long as possible (Jones, Dunbar, and Jirovec 1978, p. 29).

Sociocultural adjustments to the effects of the disorder must also be achieved. The client often withdraws from all social interaction. The nurse should encourage both client and family to seek meaningful social interchange in a supportive environment. The adjustment of sexual patterns to satisfy sexual needs must also be explored. Often family roles change as a result of parkinsonism. The nurse should assist both client and family to work through feelings and adapt to changes if role conflict occurs.

Anxiety exacerbates disabilities. Explaining the nature of new complaints or findings helps to allay anxiety and provides the client with the strength to surmount handicaps. Indeed, clients can be reassured that progression of the disease is usually slow and that many productive years lie ahead. However, the nurse must also be realistic and help the client adjust employment patterns in order to remain active as long as possible (Jones, Dunbar, and Jirovec 1978).

Many of the behavioral changes, such as aggressive behavior, delirium, delusions, and paranoid behavior, are often due to medication side effects from both anticholinergics and levodopa. Reduction of dosages should always be tried in these cases (Matheney 1966).

Severe depression can be treated with both supportive therapy and with a tricyclicamine, such as amitryptiline 80 to 100 mg at bedtime. The action of the tricyclic antidepressants is potentiated by levodopa (Duvoisin 1976).

Health Education. Adequate nutrition is difficult to maintain as mastication and swallowing become increasingly difficult. The client often turns to a soft, bland diet and decreases fluid intake. When getting food to the mouth is a problem, the nurse should advise the client to use a spoon. Increasing roughage and fluids will mitigate the constipatory effects of increasingly poor muscle tone and lowered physical activity. A flexible drinking straw will help when the client has difficulty handling fluids. The client should eat in an unhurried atmosphere, and finger foods, especially of high-residue quality, should be provided when possible. Rinsing the mouth before eating may help alleviate the metallic taste caused by medications. After eating, oral hygiene rids the oral cavity of food particles. These particles lead to odor formation and can be an aspiration hazard. The use of a bib to help the drooling client depends on the individual, as some will consider this measure demoralizing.

A regularly maintained physical activity schedule is of utmost importance in providing independence. When corrective physi-

287

cal therapy is needed, the nurse should recommend a physiotherapist. Activity is enhanced when it is goal oriented. Thus the client should be encouraged to take walks. Local heat applications diminish muscle rigidity and associated pain. Gait training and exercise serve to prevent muscle contractures. Clients should be taught to walk by lifting the leg high, taking large steps, and placing the heel first to the floor. Turning can be assisted by taking a series of small steps or by raising the toes while turning, thereby placing the weight on the heels. To deal with the problem of "freezing" in social situations, clients should be advised to arrive before the crowd comes and to leave after the crowd clears. Sometimes a hand to lead the way may be all that is necessary to initiate movement; but the hand may unbalance the client who must begin forward movement by taking an initial step backward. Care and health instruction must be individualized by trying different methods to discover what can best assist the client (Langan 1976).

Special teaching involving the performance of mimicry in front of a mirror is indicated for eye and facial exercises. The nurse should observe how the client gets in and out of a chair and should offer instruction if necessary. Speaking may become increasingly difficult. Clients should be encouraged to speak often and to coordinate articulation with expiration. When difficulty in speaking becomes more pronounced, the client may require the guidance of a speech therapist.

Safety factors must be considered to prevent falls in walking and in the bathroom area. A bar next to the toilet can assist the client in getting up and down. A firmly placed stool or chair may be necessary when the client takes a shower. Some clients feel more secure when walking with a cane; others consider the cane an obstacle.

Clothing should be loose fitting and easy to put on; for ease in dressing, front-fastening zippers and other aids should be considered (Fischbach 1978). Good hygiene is essential. To control the problem of seborrheic dermatitis, the client should use one of the commercial preparations available for this purpose. Greasy eyelash scale can be removed with a moistened cotton swab. Corneal inflammation may occur as a result of reduced blinking; the use of artificial tears will provide corneal lubrication and prevent inflammation.

The pooling of saliva results from decreased automatic swallowing. In early stages the chewing of gum will strengthen jaw muscles and assist in swallowing saliva. For the client in a more advanced stage, a bulb syringe can be used to remove pooled saliva (Langan 1976).

The client and family should receive instruction on the necessity of taking medications and should be warned about the untoward effects of the medications. As the illness progresses and disabilities increase, nursing care will become directed toward the prevention of complications such as decubiti and pulmonary stasis. Measures to prevent dehydration and malnutrition will become essential to prevent the development of infections and other complications that lead to early death.

SUMMARY

Neuro/emotional health problems in the elderly are multicausal. Differentiation must be made between organic brain syndromes and functional problems. The most important factor to remember is that elderly individuals with these conditions can be treated when a proper assessment is made. An aggressive management plan will improve the quality of life for these persons.

REFERENCES

BURNSIDE, I. M. 1976. "Overview of Group Work with the Aged." *Journal of Gerontological Nursing* 2(6):14–17.

———, ed. 1976. *Nursing and the Aged.* N.Y.: McGraw-Hill.

———. 1978. *Working with the Elderly: Group Processes and Techniques.* North Scituate, Mass.: Duxbury Press.

BUSSE, E., and E. PFEIFFER. 1973. *Mental Illness in Later Life.* Washington, D.C.: American Psychiatric Association.

BUTLER, R., and M. LEWIS. 1977. *Aging and Mental Health: Positive Psychosocial Approaches.* St. Louis: C. V. Mosby.

DALESSIO, D. J. 1978. *Journal of the American Medical Association.* Vol. 239, January 16. Editorial.

DUVOISIN, R. 1976. "Parkinsonism." *Clinical Symposia* (Ciba Pharmaceutical Corp.) 28(1):1–26.

FISCHBACH, F. T. 1978. "Easing Adjustment of Parkinson's Disease." *American Journal of Nursing* 78(1):66–69.

GLASSCOTE, R., J. E. GUDEMAN, and D. MILES. 1977. *Creative Mental Health Services for the Elderly.* Washington, D.C.: The Joint Information Service of the American Psychiatric Association.

GOLDFARB, A. I. 1964. "The Evaluation of Geriatric Patients Following Treatment." In P. H. Hock and J. Zubin, eds., *Evaluation of Psychiatric Treatment.* New York: Grune and Stratton.

HABER, M. E. 1969. "Parkinson's Disease Challenge to the Health Professions." *Nursing Clinics of North America.* 4(2):263–73.

HAMILTON, J., and E. V. COWDRY. 1976. "Psychiatric Aspects." In F. U. Steinberg, ed., *Cowdry's The Care of the Geriatric Patient.* St. Louis: C. V. Mosby.

HARDIN, W. B. 1976. "Neurological Aspects." In F. U. Steinberg, ed., *Cowdry's The Care of the Geriatric Patient.* St. Louis: C. V. Mosby.

HIRSCHFIELD, M. J. 1976. "The Cognitively Impaired Older Adult." *American Journal of Nursing* 76(12):1981–84.

JONES, D. A., C. F. DUNBAR, and M. M. JIROVEC. 1978. *Medical Surgical Nursing: A Conceptual Approach.* New York: McGraw-Hill.

KAHN, R. L., et al. 1960. "Brief Objective Measure for the Determination of Mental Status in the Aged," *American Journal of Psychiatry* 117:326–32.

LANGAN, R. J. 1976. "Parkinson's Disease: Assessment Procedures and Guidelines for Counseling." *The Nurse Practitioner* 2(2):13–16.

———, and G. C. COTZIAS. 1976. "Do's and Don'ts for the Patient on Levodopa Therapy." *American Journal of Nursing* 76(6):917–18.

MATHENEY, R. V. 1966. "Cerebrovascular Accident and Personality Organization." *Nursing Clinics of North America* 1(3):443–49.

REICHEL, W. 1978. "The Evaluation of the Confused, Disoriented, or Demented Elderly Patient." In W. Reichel, ed., *Clinical Aspects of Aging.* Baltimore: Williams and Wilkins.

STANLEY, L., S. BROVENDER, and D. ANDERSON. 1979. "The Senior Citizen's Primary Care Clinic: An Experiment in Collaborating Service and Education." *Journal of Gerontological Nursing,* 5(3):49–55.

TIMIRAS, P. S. 1972. *Developmental Physiology and Aging.* New York: Macmillan.

VERWOERDT, A. 1976. *Clinical Geropsychiatry.* Baltimore: Williams and Wilkins.

VICK, N. 1976. *Grinker's Neurology.* Springfield, Ill.: Charles C. Thomas.

WILCOXSON, H. 1966. "Cerebrovascular Accident: The Role of the Public Health Nurse." *Nursing Clinics of North America* 1(March):63–72.

YAHR, M. D. 1972. "The Parkinsonian Syndrome." In P. B. Beeson and W. McDermott, eds., *Cecil-Loeb Textbook of Medicine.* Philadelphia: W. B. Saunders.

———, et al. 1969. "Treatment of Parkinsonism with Levodopa." *Archives of Neurology* 21:243–46.

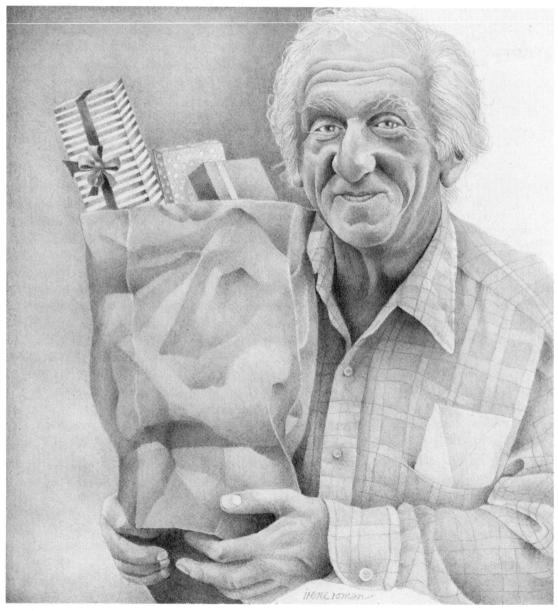

Chapter 10

THE ELDERLY CLIENT WITH A CARDIOVASCULAR PROBLEM

Distinguishing between changes in organ morphology and function caused by biological aging and organic changes that are secondary to disease is often difficult. Nevertheless, age-related changes have been identified in hearts having no clinically evident disease. Cardiac problems and their associated changes are described in this chapter.

CONGESTIVE HEART FAILURE

Heart failure in elderly clients is most often due to multiple factors, but it may also be associated with other disorders. The clients present with a difficult assessment and management picture. An older person with a diminished cardiac reserve is more susceptible than a younger person to overtaxation by physical or emotional stress (Resnick and Harrison 1962; Hershey 1974; Dock 1956). Therefore, diagnosing failure is not sufficient; the underlying pathology must also be clarified. Heart failure complicated by pneumonia may be resolved by curing the latter. Examples of other high-output failures that are completely reversible are those induced by anemia, A-V fistula, hyperthyroidism, and fever. Pulmonary emboli from peripheral veins can cause congestive failure, as can endocarditis, which causes valvular insufficiency. Valvular lesions are amenable to surgical repair. In many cases recognition of the underlying pathology and appropriate therapy can dramatically improve longevity and the quality of life.

But the vast majority of elderly clients with congestive heart failure do not have reversible disorders. They have either hypertensive disease, electrocardiographic findings of ischemic heart disease, or evidence of a previous myocardial infarction.

291

The frequent association of heart failure with irreversible disorders is supported by at least one autopsy study that demonstrated ischemic heart disease in 48 percent of clients with congestive failure (Pomeranz 1968). A history of elevated blood pressure is always found in clients with hypertensive heart disease. Myocardial amyloidosis also must be considered, as its incidence tends to increase with advancing age. Febrile clients with elevated sedimentation rate, anemia, and heart murmur should be evaluated for bacterial endocarditis. The nurse should check for Ossler's nodes or pea-size, cutaneous, tender lesions on the tips of fingers and toes or on the palms of hands and feet, as well as for subungual splinter hemorrhages. Acute myocardial infarction is frequently associated with congestive failure because it diminishes left ventricular output (Ebsani et al. 1975; Rahimtoola et al. 1972).

Pathophysiology

With aging the cavity of the left ventricle frequently becomes smaller because of muscle-wall atrophy, and both the left atrium and aorta become enlarged as a result of a loss of elasticity. These changes, in addition to an increased rigidity and thickening of the heart valves, reduce the effectiveness of the pumping action of the heart.

Gross changes in the endocardium include diffuse, thickened, whitish patches in atria, ventricles, and papillary muscles. More patches are present in the left than in the right chambers. Further changes include a decrease in the number of myocardial fibers and a fibrotic thickening of the sinoauricular node, the pacemaker of the heart. The effect of the above changes on heart function will be described later, after a brief review of the anatomy and physiology of the normal heart.

Anatomy and Physiology of the Heart. The four-chambered heart and blood vessels of the body constitute a closed circuit that conducts blood to and from all of the tissues of the body. Although the heart is frequently referred to as the pump in the closed circuit, the organ is probably more accurately described as two separate pumps, each separated from the other by muscular walls.

The thin walled atrium of one pump, the right heart, accepts deoxygenated blood from both the coronary and systemic circulation; the blood then enters the ventricle below. This slightly muscular right ventricle pumps this blood into and through the lungs. The thin walled atrium of the left heart receives this oxygenated blood from the lungs and delivers it to the thick walled, muscular left ventricle. This chamber subsequently pumps the blood out into the coronary and systemic circulatory systems.

Muscle tissue of the heart, or myocardium, must be structurally and physiologically sound in order for the heart to function as an efficient pump. Structural changes such as fat infiltration and atrophy of myocardium can weaken the pumping function. Physiological changes such as decreased force and velocity of contraction of myocardial cells also contribute to this decreased efficiency.

Over time the hemodynamic stress to which all four valves are subjected during each cardiac cycle causes them to thicken and become increasingly rigid with advancing age.

For the young, healthy male adult at rest, cardiac output is approximately 5.6 liters a minute; in the healthy aged client under similar conditions, cardiac output is approximately 5 liters a minute. After age 25 cardiac output drops 1 percent each year because of a decrease in both the amount of blood pumped out of the left ventricle during each cardiac cycle (stroke volume) and the heart rate (Harris 1970). Stroke-volume drop is due in part to the decrease in ventricular compliance, which results in a reduction in diastolic filling, and in part to an increase in age-related resistance offered by peripheral blood vessels.

Signs and Causes of Congestive Heart Failure. Based on the fact that the function of the heart is to pump sufficient blood to meet the body's metabolic needs, heart failure occurs when an abnormality of myocardial function interferes with the ability of the ventricles to deliver adequate quantities of blood to the metabolizing tissues at rest or during normal activity. Although heart failure can be acute, occurring suddenly and dramatically, this discussion focuses on heart failure that develops slowly.

The signs and symptoms of congestive heart failure (CHF) are related to whether the ventricle of the left or right heart has become deficient. We must emphasize, however, that because the circulatory system is a closed system, failure of one side of the heart will eventually affect the other side. This reaction is especially true in advanced congestive heart failure.

Right-sided heart failure very rarely develops independently of left-sided heart failure. The right ventricle, or right heart, is said to have failed when it can no longer effectively pump venous blood returning by way of the superior and inferior vena cava and coronary sinus into the lungs. In this event end-diastolic volume is increased, as are the pressures and volumes in the right atrium and systemic veins and capillaries. This disorder is sometimes referred to as *backward failure*. Because of the elevated pressure and volume in the venous system and capillaries, fluid escapes into tissue spaces. In renal veins the elevated pressure causes increased renal tubular reabsorption of sodium. The signs of right-sided failure, then, are systemic edema, usually dependent venous congestion within organs such as the liver, and an elevated central venous pressure, or pressure measured in the right atrium.

Pulmonary embolism and chronic pulmonary diseases such as emphysema can cause pulmonary hypertension and subsequent right-sided heart failure. The right heart fails because of the excessive workload placed on the right ventricular myocardium as it is forced to pump against additional resistance of damaged pulmonary vasculature. Other disorders such as valvular pulmonic stenosis and pulmonary hypertension also increase the workload of the right ventricle. Mitral stenosis also affects the right heart and is characterized by an increase in pulmonary vascular resistance. The adherent mitral valve causes a narrowed mitral orifice, thereby limiting left atrial emptying into the left ventricle. This resistance creates a cycle of congested pulmonary circulation, which again increases the workload of the right ventricle.

Although congestive heart failure can be classified as right or left sided, it most often begins in the left ventricle. One of the primary causes of *left-sided failure* is myocardial weakness resulting from coronary artery

293

disease, which diminishes or occludes the blood supply to the various segments of the myocardium.

A second cause of left-ventricular failure is an excessive workload on this chamber. As with right-sided failure, workload increases when resistance to ejection is increased. This increased resistance occurs in hypertension and in aortic valvular disease. In hypertension degenerative changes cause narrowing of arterial walls. In turn, the workload of the left ventricle is increased in order to overcome the resistance caused by the narrowing. Contractile force is increased by three compensatory mechanisms: (1) hypertrophy of the myocardial fibers with increased fiber length, (2) chamber enlargement, and (3) sympathetic nervous system stimulation. In aortic stenosis the added workload placed on the left ventricle is due to the narrowed aortic orifice through which blood must be pumped. In such cases the increasing work needed to maintain cardiac output eventually surpasses the ability of the heart to compensate; venous return cannot be ejected, and cardiac failure results.

In left-sided heart failure, the end-diastolic volume of the left ventricle increases, and pressure and volume in pulmonary vasculature rise. When the hydrostatic pressure in the pulmonary vasculature rises above the osmotic pressure of plasma, fluid transudes into the interstitial spaces of the lungs. The lungs become congested and edematous, and the patient exhibits dyspnea on exertion.

The loss of pumping effectiveness of the left heart results in an inadequate discharge of blood into the arterial system. The resultant diminished renal blood flow lowers the glomerular filtration rate and also causes an increase in sodium reabsorption by renal tubular cells, leading to water retention, expanded blood volume, and edema.

Nursing Assessment

Left-Sided Failure: Subjective Findings. A careful evaluation of subjective complaints and their effects on activities of daily living is essential. In the initial phases the subjective complaints usually precede the objective signs (Levine 1958). Fatigability and dyspnea are by far the most prominent complaints. The dyspnea is progressive, initially occurring only in the performance of an activity requiring moderate effort; eventually it will be present even at rest.

Left-Sided Failure: Objective Findings. The development of orthopnea and paroxysmal nocturnal dyspnea point to increasing failure. Acute pulmonary edema, which can dramatically awaken and cause marked distress to a sleeping client, also indicates acute left-ventricular failure. This medical emergency should be immediately referred to a physician.

Dyspnea must be differentiated from breathlessness due to obesity, pulmonary disease, or poor physical conditioning. Orthopnea may manifest itself as insomnia (Rodstein 1971), and the associated hypoxia may induce nocturnal confusion. Coughing and wheezing due to failure must be differentiated from bronchitis and other lung problems (Harris 1978).

Fatigue, or "loss of pep," may persist in spite of adequate treatment. Anorexia and nausea leading to malnutrition may be due to the failure itself or it may be induced by digitalis therapy. The dietary intake should be scrutinized for excessive sodium intake.

Right-Sided Failure: Subjective Findings. Subjective complaints include digestive problems, nausea, vomiting, abdominal distension, right upper quadrant pain, and edema of the lower extremities (Harris 1978). Clients may complain that their shoes are too tight at the end of the day. Initially disappearing overnight, this swelling becomes persistent and increases as the condition progresses. However, the client with advancing age poses diagnostic problems of ankle swelling due to venous obstruction in an extremity or in the pelvis, varicose veins, intraabdominal disease, or prolonged immobility with dependent lower limbs.

Right-Sided Failure: Objective Findings. Auscultation of the lungs in an aged, confused client with underlying pulmonary fibrosis or senile kyphosis and diminished tidal volume is particularly difficult. Basal rales are the traditional clue to both diagnosis and the evaluation of treatment. The elderly pose the problem of differentiating the origin of respiratory signs, which may also be due to atelectasis, prolonged bed rest, or inactivity.

Oliguria with low sodium concentration and high specific gravity is common and reversed by diuretic therapy. Prerenal azotemia and mild proteinuria are frequently found and may be aggravated by an overzealous diuresis.

Several objective findings appear with the advance of congestive failure. Cheyne-Stokes respirations and gallop rhythm may be found. Pulsus alternans—a variation in the strength of alternate radial artery pulsations—may also occur. Cheyne-Stokes respirations are characterized by alternate periods of apnea and hyperpnea. Cheyne-Stokes respirations also may be found in stroke clients; when present in failure, they usually indicate concomitant cerebrovascular disease (Fishneau 1971). An S3 ventricular gallop sound early in diastole is a reliable sign of failure. The S4 atrial gallop sound occurring in presystole is more likely related to the decreased ventricular compliance that often occurs in the normal elderly (Beard 1976; Harris 1975).

Premature ventricular contractions also may be found both in the client with congestive failure and in the client who has digitalis toxicity or ischemic heart disease without failure.

Cardiac enlargement is often difficult to evaluate. Age-related changes cause ventricular atrophy as well as chest wall expansion and emphysema. Therefore, diagnosis may necessitate serial chest x-rays to demonstrate progressive dilation. Echocardiography can demonstrate dilation and has the additional advantage of identifying existent intracardiac pathology (DeMaria et al. 1976; Abassi 1976). The objective findings of venous congestion are manifested by peripheral edema, tender hepatomegaly, jugular vein distension, and the development of pleural effusion. Ascites, scrotal edema, and sacroiliac edema may be found in extreme cases of congestive failure.

Careful assessment of signs of electrolyte imbalance must be performed at all times. Potassium depletion may occur from a number of causes other than diuretics. Vomiting, diarrhea, stress, low-sodium diets, and starvation can cause electrolyte imbalances. Although early signs of hypokalemia are not readily detected, anemia, mental confusion, irregular pulse, and muscular weakness occur as depletion progresses (Ritchie 1968, p. 670).

Diagnostics

Typically an EKG and chest x-ray are ordered. The EKG demonstrates the presence of arrhythmias or myocardial changes. Chest films provide information on pulmonary congestion due to left-sided heart failure, pulmonary infection and infiltrates as well as information on pulmonary infarction, emphysema, or bronchitis, which simulate heart failure. Blood studies include electrolytes, blood urea nitrogen, and glucose levels. On occasion diagnosis may require pulmonary function studies, arterial blood gas determinations, radioactive lung scanning, and/or echocardiogram. Usually blood gas determinations in pulmonary edema show hypoxia with PO_2 less than 60 mmHg and hypocapnea secondary to hyperventilation due to hypoxia. Complete evaluation of potentially curable heart lesions may require referral for chest fluoroscopy and cardiac catheterization. Thyroid function studies may be necessary, as thyroid disease is often masked in the elderly.

Nursing Management

Health Education. The nurse must inform clients with congestive failure of the underlying and precipitating causes of heart failure in order to help them accept modifications of activity and diet. Many booklets are available from the American Heart Association, such as *Heart of the Home*, which simplifies housework.

Waxler (1976) describes how nurses can provide health education to clients with congestive problems. Her teaching plan is based on a model that is divided into five areas: (1) understanding the disease process, (2) recognizing signs of failure, (3) medications, (4) diet, and (5) activity, rest, and the avoidance of other illnesses.

1. *Understanding the Disease Process:* To attain compliance with therapy requires some understanding of the disease process by the client and family. Even the terminology may be frightening, since the heart symbolizes life to most people. Waxler suggests two helpful analogies: the loss of contractility of the heart can be compared to an overstretched elastic band that has lost its snap or power; and the congestive aspect can be compared to a river that overflows its banks into surrounding lands (tissues) and results in flooding (swelling, congestion, edema).

2. *Recognizing Signs of Failure:* Next the nurse helps the client to recognize impending or worsening failure. Asking the client to memorize a long list of signs and symptoms is rarely useful. A more effective technique is to review symptoms experienced at the onset of illness in order to encourage the client to report such symptoms and to seek help early. Clients should be taught to recognize weight gain by ankle swelling or increasing tightness of shoes and clothes as well as by coughing episodes, tiredness, and a general slowing of ability to perform chores. The person who has a bathroom scale and can read it should report seemingly insignificant gains of 2 to 3 pounds within one or two days (Waxler 1976).

3. *Medications:* Clients taking digitalis should know that it is for heart failure. So

many medications for heart conditions are available that the client might mistakenly take digitalis for chest pain and dangerously alter the dosage without obtaining relief. If capable of taking a pulse, the client should be instructed to do so at rest and report a rate below 60 or above 100 as well as changes in regularity. Even if the client cannot take a pulse, other signs of digitalis toxicity, such as loss of appetite, nausea and vomiting, visual problems, and palpitations or skipped beats can still be recognized.

The person on diuretics should know that such drugs will increase voiding and consequently should be taken at times when they will not interfere too greatly with daily activities. The nurse must avoid giving the impression that this discretion is license to omit a dose. Explaining the function of potassium supplements is easier if the client is told that the "fluid pill" causes loss not only of fluid but also of a substance essential for normal body functioning. Thus the special substance must be replaced either with foods high in potassium (like tea, orange juice, etc.) or with supplements in medication form. All potassium supplements cause gastric irritation, so the elixirs should be diluted or taken after meals. For the diabetic client the diluent should be sugar free; but basically whatever makes the supplement palatable to the client should be used. Also the client should be told that weakness, faintness, and leg or abdominal cramps are indicators of insufficient potassium. Elimination of excess fluid is accomplished through diet and medication.

4. *Diet:* Adherence to low-sodium diets is influenced by cultural factors, by the person doing the cooking, and by the degree of the client's motivation and self-discipline. To place the problem into perspective, estimates are that the average per capita sodium intake in the United States is between 5 and 10 g daily. One teaspoon of salt contains 2,300 mg of sodium (Ziesche and Joseph 1977). Thus, a reduction to 2 or 3 g daily requires a drastic change in eating habits. The best technique is to provide the client with a list of foods to avoid and definite instructions on how much salt, if any, can be added to cooking foods. Many people are not aware of the less obvious sources of sodium used in processing and preserving foods and as leavening agents. The water supply in certain areas is extremely high in sodium, and certain medications also contain sodium and can cause fluid retention. Such medications include antacids (Maalox, Gelusil, baking soda), corticosteroids (Cortisone, Prednisone), and antiarthritics (Indomethacin). In mild failure a limitation of 4 g of sodium daily is sufficient. Severe restriction to 0.5 g is necessary only in advanced disease. The debilitated elderly client with diminished taste may find salt restriction intolerable. Thus noncompliance and treatment failure or anorexia and malnutrition may result from overzealous therapy. If the client can tolerate mild restriction, a 1 g sodium diet may be used with an additional allowance of one teaspoon of salt sprinkled on food during the day. Pepper, paprika, and other spices may be used liberally, and, in the absence of renal disease, a commercial salt substitute may be used for more flavor. Such spices added to food just before ingestion give a much better flavor than if they are added to cooking food.

5. *Activity, Rest, and Avoidance of Other Illnesses:* In the final segment of the teaching

297

plan, the nurse explains the necessity of avoiding physical exertion or stressful situations that cause the heart to work harder. The client will probably experience fatigue and dyspnea if limits are exceeded. Mild heart failure usually can be managed by a decrease in motor activity and by naps and more rest at night. This regimen may require a leave of absence from work, fewer work hours each day, or a reorganization of household tasks. The client should sleep in a warm room and avoid activities that increase cardiac output, such as walking against the wind or uphill. The best position is sitting or reclining, which permits drainage of fluid away from the lung apices and decreases breathlessness. The obese client can reduce cardiac workload by losing weight. The nurse should suggest that the client eat several small meals rather than two or three larger ones each day. Constipation can be avoided by including ample roughage in the diet. Mild exercise and eating two tablespoons of raw bran a day will reduce laxative use.

Tranquilizers and sedatives for the anxious older client must be used with caution to avoid oversedation, which may manifest itself as confusion or dementia. The danger of sedatives in clients with chronic hypercapnea is well known, and great care should be exercised in such cases.

Clients should also be reminded that other illnesses will probably further burden the heart and exacerbate congestive failure. Consequently they should seek help early and avoid people with respiratory infections and influenza.

Treatment. In congestive heart failure due to a curable disorder, the client will benefit most from treatment directed toward the primary condition. When such conditions are properly diagnosed and treated, their clinical course and the associated heart failure will improve markedly. Transfusion of the symptomatic anemia, treatment of the thyroid disorder, or closure of an arteriovenous fistula can cure the associated myocardial insufficiency. Likewise the treatment and resolution of a pulmonary infection can reverse the associated failure. To be sure, supportive therapy is necessary during the period of illness.

Unfortunately, however, curable disorders are the least common causes of heart failure. In a client who has a noncurable heart problem due to the prolonged stress of a high peripheral load, as in malignant hypertension, failure will require sustained symptomatic treatment aimed at improving cardiac output and mobilizing excess fluid from the body.

Because they do best in their own environment, most older clients should be treated at home. But if the nurse finds evidence of hypoxemia, renal impairment, bradycardia, or ventricular arrhythmia, the client should be referred to a physician and probably hospitalized.

Mild congestive failure may be treated by reduction of physical activity, moderate salt restriction, and diuretics without digitalis. Diuretic medications, like all drugs, can cause problems. These medications work by depression of renal tubular function, thereby causing decreased resorption of water and electrolytes. This effect leads to a decrease in blood volume and a subsequently reduced load. The contracted fluid volume also causes a decrease in the glomerular filtration rate (Lohmuller et al. 1975).

The existence of potent *diuretics* has permitted some liberalization of diet and has generally improved therapy. However, because of the side effects only as much medication as necessary should be prescribed. Electrolyte loss can lead to hypokalemia and digitalis intoxication in clients taking both diuretic and digitalis preparations. Decreased glomerular function can cause hyperuricemia and, rarely, gout. When used with severe sodium restriction, diuretics can lead to weakness, oliguria, and azotemia. The chloruretic sulfonamide diuretic may cause diabetes mellitus, but this effect is rare in the elderly. If the diuretic ethacrynic acid is used, it can produce vertigo, tinnitus, and acute hearing loss. In the elderly male with an enlarged prostate, use of any diuretic may precipitate acute urinary retention.

In prescribing diuretics, one differentiates between first-line, potent drugs and second-line, less potent ones usually used as additives. The potent group consists of chloruretic sulfonamides (Chlorthiazide, Hydrochlorthiazide, etc.), mercurial diuretics (Mercuhydrin), and the most potent, furosemide (Lasix) and ethacrynic acid (Edecrin). The mercurials generally are effective only by injection and are rarely used. Current treatment usually consists of an oral sulfonamide given intermittently for a few days, followed by a few days of rest. Chlorthiazide 0.5 to 2 g or Hydrochlorthiazide 50 to 200 mg are most commonly used. In the presence of advancing failure and the increased need for a daily diuretic, hypokalemia may develop. Instead of unpalatable potassium chloride solutions, triamterene (Dyrenium) 25 to 100 mg or spironolactone (Aldactone) 25 to 100 mg may be added to prevent this complication.

The most powerful medications are usually kept in reserve and should be used in collaboration with a physician. Furose-mide (Lasix) 20 to 200 mg or ethacrynic acid (Edecrin) 40 to 300 mg, used orally or parenterally, have replaced the mercurials. Lasix or Edecrin may be used intermittently to supplement a basic regimen or they may be substituted for the oral sulfonamide. They are given intravenously in the treatment of acute pulmonary edema.

One of the important rationales underlying treatment of heart failure is to improve cardiac output. Improvement may be directly attained through the use of *digitalis*. Digitalis has a direct action on the myocardial fiber, where it improves the force of contraction. The stronger contraction increases cardiac output and renal perfusion while it decreases venous congestion, regardless of the etiology of the failure. Digitalis is indicated in congestive failure because it improves myocardial exercise tolerance. In cases of reversible failure, digitalis may be discontinued when the offending stress has been removed. It is given after breakfast, provided that pulse rate and appetite are normal.

Since an effect of digitalis on the myocardium is to block the cellular sodium pump, the intracellular concentration of sodium increases while potassium decreases. The resultant intracellular potassium depletion can lead to ventricular arrhythmias in clients taking digitalis. This effect is a real danger in the older client who may have a poor nutritional status, particularly if diuretics are used. Because digitalis increases ventricular irritability, it must be used with caution or avoided in acute myocardial infarction.

Further action of digitalis occurs at the junctional tissue, where it slows conduction through the atrioventricular node. This block is particularly useful when failure is accompanied by atrial fibrillation. In these cases the ventricular response to the atrial impulse is slowed by digitalis, thus decreasing the tachycardia and improving cardiac output. In atrial fibrillation the blocking effect of digitalis permits use of the ventricular rate as a guide to dosage. When a rate of 80 to 100 beats a minute is obtained, maintenance therapy is begun. Toxic levels can lead to a high degree of atrioventricular block.

Digitalis exists in a variety of forms derived from Digitalis plant extracts. All digitalis pharmaceuticals are pure glycosides and are usually classified according to their speed of onset and duration of action. However, their activity, side effects, and contraindications are identical. The most commonly used short-acting oral preparation is Lanoxin; the long-lasting preparation is Digitoxin (Fishneau 1971).

Treatment is based on the principle of an initial loading dose and a lower maintenance dose. If a single dose of Lanoxin is given and the rate of urine excretion is followed, the dose will be gradually excreted at a rate dependent upon the plasma concentration and the creatinine clearance (Smith 1973). Thus if a dose of Lanoxin is given daily, it will gradually accumulate in the body at a rate inversely proportional to the body's urinary excretion rate. When any given dose is greater than the daily excreted dose, it will accumulate to the point of toxicity.

Digitalis toxicity is manifested first by complaints of increasing anorexia, nausea, vomiting, and diarrhea, which may be accompanied by abdominal discomfort and pain. Occasionally clients may complain of disturbances in color vision. The heart is also affected by digitalis poisoning. The changes of rate and rhythm can mimic every known clinical condition. Increasing

congestive failure may be the only manifestation. Ventricular extrasystoles are very common, as is A-V block, particularly with a ventricular rate below 60 beats per minute. Other changes include atrial tachycardia with block and, rarely, atrial fibrillation. If serious digitalis arrhythmia is suspected, the nurse must withhold medication and immediately refer the client to a physician.

Although the usual daily maintenance dose of Lanoxin is 0.25 to 0.5 mg, the creatinine clearance tends to fall progressively with age and the decline accelerates with advancing age (Rowe et al. 1976). This tendency explains the higher incidence of digitalis toxicity occurring in the older client. A maintenance dosage of 0.125 mg daily, 5 days or less a week, may be enough to maintain the therapeutic effects of Lanoxin in an older client. A similar situation applies for Digitoxin, where maintenance dosages may be decreased with age (see table 10.1).

Digitalis loading may be accomplished rapidly in the absence of any digitalis use in the previous 2 to 4 weeks. Thus a full loading dose may be given rapidly (table 10.1) or slowly over a week through the use of 0.25 to 0.5 mg of Lanoxin daily or 0.1 to 0.2 mg of Digitoxin daily. EKG monitoring should show a digitalis effect of a lengthened P-R wave with S-T depression. The appearance of toxic symptoms or signs requires a temporary cessation of medication. An appropriate maintenance dose may be instituted once these symptoms are controlled. The blood level of the specific glycoside may also be obtained for monitoring.

Occasionally congestive heart failure is encountered in elderly clients with a marked bradycardia. In such clients car-

TABLE 10.1
Digitalis Preparations

Preparation	Absorption by Oral Route	Time of Onset of Action	Time for Maximum Effect	Average Oral Digitalizing Dose	Usual Oral Daily Maintenance Dose
Deslanoside C (Cedilanid)	Poor	10–30 min.	1–2 hrs.	I.V.—use only 1.6 mg	—
Digoxin (Lanoxin)	60–85%	15–30 min.	1½–5 hrs.	1.25–1.5 mg	0.25–0.5 mg 0.125 in elderly
Digitoxin	90–100%	25–120 min.	4–12 hrs.	0.7–1.2 mg	0.1 mg*

* *Older clients may require less (see text).*

Source: *T. W. Smith, "Digitalis Glycosides,"* New England Journal of Medicine *288 (1973):791–822. Reprinted by permission of the publisher and the author.*

diac output may be improved by direct acceleration of heart rate, accomplished by the use of a pacemaker. This treatment is particularly effective in clients with heart block and a ventricular rate below 40 beats per minute (Furman 1976). Such clients should be referred to a physician for evaluation.

Once failure is controlled, the client will often have improved exercise tolerance. However, the nurse must recognize that in most cases the condition is progressive and control becomes increasingly difficult over the remaining years. Recognition and correction of certain etiologic factors prior to the onset of failure is more successful and is discussed in the next section.

HYPERTENSION

Pathophysiology

Factors Regulating Blood Pressure. Although blood pressure is regulated by many factors, such as cardiac output and blood volume, one factor of great importance in the aged is *peripheral resistance.* This resistance is either increased or decreased according to the needs and demands of the body by neural mechanisms acting on muscular arterioles. Arteriolar constriction increases resistance to blood flow and elevates blood pressure. Arteriolar relaxation, or dilation, reduces resistance to blood flow and lowers blood pressure.

A modest increase in arterial pressures is seen with age. Decreased aortic elasticity causes a rise in systolic pressure and an expanded pulse pressure. Vasomotor lability increases the diastolic pressure as the medium-size muscular arteries become more resistant to blood flow at a rate of 1 percent a year (Harris 1975). This increased resistance slows the peripheral runoff from the aorta and raises the diastolic pressure, since the rise in pressure is associated with a known fall in cardiac output (Harris 1970).

Malignant hypertension is rare in persons over age 70 (Kincaid-Smith et al. 1958). More common is benign essential hypertension (Caird and Dall 1973). The probable mechanisms involved in the development of hypertension are discussed below.

Mechanisms of Hypertension. Arterial pressure is usually defined as the product of

301

cardiac output and peripheral resistance. These two factors are actually controlled by the blood volume. An increase in blood volume augments the venous return and causes an increase in cardiac output. The rise in output increases the peripheral blood flow and provokes constriction of the precapillary arterioles, thus raising the peripheral resistance.

The observations of Douglas and others (1964) reveal that expanded extracellular fluid volume is the primary factor causing hypertension in anephric animals maintained by renal dialysis. An increase in blood pressure and extracellular volume also occurs in renal patients when salt and water are ingested beyond the level that the kidneys can handle.

Augmented fluid volume is the common factor in the various forms of secondary hypertension. This increase in fluid may be due to excessive circulating corticosteroid in Cushing's syndrome and hyperaldosteronism; to renal hypoperfusion and diminished glomerular filtration in aortic coarctation, Goldblatt kidney, and sympathetic vasoconstriction due to anxiety, frustration, and pain; or to diminished glomerular filtration in glomerulonephritis and glomerulosclerosis. In each of these disorders, sodium and water retention cause increased blood volume and hypertension. In essential hypertension the kidneys appear to function normally. However, a fall in arterial pressure to normal levels always results in an accumulation of urinary waste products (Guyton et al. 1972). This diminished urinary excretion at normal pressure levels leads to salt and water retention, expanded blood volume, and an increase in cardiac output.

Fulkow and others (1973) suggest that increased arteriolar resistance in sustained hypertension is due to hypertrophy of the vascular wall in response to a sustained circulatory load. Thus, irrespective of the precipitating event, the resulting vascular resistance is secondary to the increase in cardiac output. Some form of renal or renovascular lesion is likely to be present in essential hypertension. This lesion causes fluid retention and an expanded blood volume and provokes an increase in cardiac output. Vasoconstriction due to the high output raises the peripheral resistance. This resistance restores the output to normal, but with a resultant increase in the systemic pressure.

Essential Hypertension. The terms *essential* or *idiopathic hypertension* are used to designate conditions in which the pathology causing the elevated pressure is unknown. The incidence of essential hypertension increases with age; more than 90 percent of all cases of identified hypertension are placed in this category (Engelman and Brunwald 1974).

Increases in pressure variants should not be viewed as age-intrinsic phenomena, since clients who exhibit higher pressures at any age are in a higher risk category than cohorts with lower pressures (Kannel 1976). The systolic pressure variant is more uniformly linked to cardiovascular sequelae than is diastolic pressure. This finding is contradictory to past emphasis on closer monitoring of diastolic pressure (Kannel 1976). Generally in benign essential hypertension, elevated pressure develops slowly with little untoward effort. Clients who not only exhibit an accelerated course but also have a diastolic pressure of 110 mmHg and a systolic pressure of 200 mmHg are said to have malignant essential hypertension (Robbins 1974). In either event the elevated pressures frequently lead to cardiovascular, renal, and cerebral disorders because of secondary organ damage. Complications usually occur after a long, latent period of asymptomatic arterial hypertension. Taken together, these complications account for over 50 percent of deaths in the United States.

Nursing Assessment

Even episodic pressure elevations or single-casual pressure elevations have a high correlation to subsequent morbidity and mortality. However, a conclusive diagnosis of hypertension should be determined only after multiple observations and recordings (Kannel 1976).

Support for the diagnosis of systemic hypertension requires that one of two criteria be met: (1) the presence of sustained, elevated systolic or diastolic pressures or (2) the presence of elevated arterial pressure and evidence of end-organ disease—cardiac, vascular, or renal. In middle-aged adults, levels exceeding 145 mmHg systolic and 94 diastolic are accepted as elevated, representing an increased risk. Effective treatment will increase the life expectancy of such individuals. Although the statistical benefit of treatment is less evident for older clients, Babu and Luisada (Babu et al. 1977) diagnose as hypertensive any client with levels above the middle-aged norms. The validity of this thesis appears confirmed by one large national study (National Health Survey 1975). Others recommend that systolic levels rise above 170 (Harris 1970) or 200 mmHg (Rodstein 1971) before treatment is instituted in the older client. In the absence of more precise studies, given the general tendency to overtreat the elderly and in view of their poor

tolerance for hypotension, the authors' tendency has been to diagnose as hypertensive clients with systolic pressures exceeding 180 mmHg or diastolic surpassing 99 mmHg.

Subjective Findings. Hypertension is asymptomatic unless severe, and as a general rule the older client will not have any hypertension-related complaints. Clients with accelerated hypertension may complain of occipital headache, which is present on arising and relieved by vomiting. Vague feelings of tension and anxiety are described by the clients. Commonly these symptoms disappear as the pressure is brought to normal levels.

A past history of hypertension, stroke, renal disease, or coronary artery disease is helpful. Also useful is a history of rejection from military service or for life insurance because of elevated pressures. Toxemia or eclampsia in pregnancy or a history of labile hypertension may be significant. A positive familial history aids in the diagnosis, since essential hypertension has a strong familial tendency. Hypertension, stroke, and coronary artery disease in parents, siblings, or children of the client are highly suggestive.

Objective Findings. The physical examination includes a search for diagnostic, etiologic, and complicating factors. Pressures should be measured consistently in both the recumbent and sitting positions, and the cuff must be wide enough for the size of the limb, or false high readings will be obtained. Pressures should be taken in both arms. Pulses are obtained in all extremities. These measurements will demonstrate vascular occlusion and coarctation

303

of the aorta. An atheromatous plaque in the lumen of a subclavian artery can cause false low pressure readings on the affected side. Elevated pressures should be rechecked after 10 to 20 minutes. If the findings are questionable in any way, the client should be brought back for further measurements. If any of these readings combines abnormal with normal systolic and diastolic levels, the pressures are termed *labile* and are of lesser but still significant import compared with sustained hypertension. Such clients should be followed. All clients should be weighed. The correlation between obesity and hypertension is high.

All hypertensive clients should have a *funduscopic examination* performed by the nurse at the initial visit and at each subsequent one. The state of the optic disc and vessels as well as the presence of any degenerative changes should be determined. Hypertensive changes are classified by the Keith-Wagner grading of progressive severity:

Grade I: Loss of parallelism and arteriolar narrowing,
Grade II: Segmental spasm and arteriovenous nicking,
Grade III: Hemorrhages and exudates,
Grade IV: Papilloedema.

Grade IV indicates malignant, accelerated hypertension and should be immediately referred to a physician for rapid induction of treatment. The nurse must differentiate these hypertensive changes from atherosclerotic changes, characterized by a widened light reflex and a copper- or silver-wire appearance of the retinal arteries, and from the microaneurysms and hemorrhages of the diabetic retina.

In hypertensive clients, *the lungs* must be examined for congestive failure. In such clients basal rales will be heard. To avoid incorrect diagnoses, care must be taken when examining clients with chronic bronchitis and pulmonary fibrosis or in elderly bedridden clients whose rales may not indicate failure at all.

Examination of *the heart* includes searching for ventricular hypertrophy and other evidence of failure. Palpation of the apical thrust helps to gauge not only the size of the heart but also its force of contraction. In left ventricular hypertrophy the heart tends to move outward toward the midclavicular line and downward into the sixth intercostal space. At auscultation the aortic second sound is accentuated and may be clacking. The fourth heart sound, heard frequently in hypertensive clients, also may be present in the elderly because of diminished ventricular compliance. In such clients this sound is of lesser diagnostic value. An S3, or middiastolic gallop, suggests decompensation. The electrocardiogram may demonstrate left ventricular hypertrophy by a heightening of the QRS complex. S-T depression and T wave inversion are indicative of hypertrophy plus "strain." The chest x-ray may show left ventricular enlargement and early heart failure.

The neck is examined for thyroid enlargement and the skin of *the abdomen* for the purple stria of Cushing's syndrome. The abdomen should be palpated for abdominal masses, the kidneys checked for enlargement, and a careful search made for an aortic aneurysm. Auscultation of the abdomen also includes searching for vascular bruits. The systolic bruit of renal artery stenosis is usually heard in the epigastrium, lateral to the midline or in the flank.

Diagnostics

Laboratory studies help to diagnose the presence of secondary forms of hypertension and to evaluate the effects of the high pressures on other organs. Since 90 to 95 percent of hypertension cases are idiopathic and since the incidence of hypertension rises with advancing age, performing an elaborate workup in a client over age 40 is rarely necessary. A complete blood count should be done. Serum electrolytes measured prior to treatment may disclose the hypokalemia of Cushing's syndrome or hyperaldosteronism. A serum creatinine or BUN is useful in assessing renal function. An elevated serum creatinine is evidence that renal tissue has been damaged, and the prognosis regarding the hypertension is grave (Perry 1969). The nurse must refer clients with high serum creatinine to a physician for evaluation and treatment.

Urinalysis should be performed. Proteinuria and an abnormal sediment are found in glomerulonephritis: pus cells and bacteria should suggest pyelonephritis (Wollan and Gifford 1976). Because of the frequency of high blood pressure in clients with urinary obstructive disease, intravenous pyelogram x-rays should be obtained. In the client whose hypertension is of sudden onset or who has a history of abdominal trauma, the films should be of the rapid sequence type (1, 2, 3, IVP). A post-void film should also be obtained.

Nursing Management

The use of nurse specialists and nurse practitioners as the primary care providers for clients who suffer from elevated pressures has been demonstrated to be highly efficacious by a large number of lay high-blood-pressure clinics as well as by Veterans Administration clinics (Alderman and Schoenbaum 1975; Runyan 1975; Brovender and Anderson 1978). The nurse's consistent methods of empathetic counseling and of health teaching have greatly enhanced client compliance (Foster and Kousch 1978).

Health Education and Counseling. Health instruction should center on the nature of the problem, with emphasis on its lifelong character. Clients must also be told about the potential side effects of medication. Consider the male client who, on awakening in the morning, urinates a thick, mucousy stream of whitish yellow urine. Imagine how anxious he would be if he had never been told about the possibility of retrograde ejaculation.

The greatest problem in hypertensive clients is their tendency to discontinue medication when they feel well. In the elderly "resistive hypertension" is most often caused by their neglecting to take medication. Clients must be told that they have a chronic illness that will require monitoring and treatment for the rest of their lives.

Mild hypertension may be controlled by weight loss coupled with a well-balanced, moderate exercise regimen (Stamler et al. 1978). All too often health practitioners forget to instruct clients about the importance of healthful living habits as a preventive measure; they consider therapy only in terms of control through medication. Varying results have been obtained through teaching relaxation measures. Among the techniques in use are autogenic suggestion, yoga, transcendental meditation, and biofeedback training. A well-known book describing the biofeedback

305

technique is Herbert Benson's *The Relaxation Response* (Hassett 1978). However, too great an emphasis on changing the lifestyle augments noncompliance and the rate of dropout from treatment (Mushlin and Appel 1977).

For the client with truly elevated pressure, evidence has repeatedly shown that consistent lowering of blood pressure to normal levels not only prolongs life but also prevents the serious complications of stroke, congestive failure, and renal insufficiency. Treatment efficacy has been demonstrated in large population studies (Veterans Administration 1970) by the diminution of heart size on x-ray and by improvement in renal function. Therefore, the diagnosis must be made during the latent period and the elevated arterial pressures effectively lowered to normal levels and maintained at these levels for the rest of the client's life.

Evaluation of Care. Drug therapy should be instituted as soon as the diagnosis of hypertension is made and should be followed up to check for effectiveness on blood pressure levels, improved health parameters, compliance with treatment, and the existence of any medication side effects.

The nurse must consider that sexual performance may be important in the elderly client's lifestyle and must be particularly adept in eliciting information about the effects of drug therapy. Questions regarding changes in libido, in frequency, and in obtaining or maintaining an erection are appropriate irrespective of the client's age. Presumably the nurse possesses enough sensitivity to consider a client's reluctance to discuss these intimate details. However, the nurse should not assume that the aged lose sexual desire or cease to have encounters. If medication disturbs sexual patterns, other drugs should be tried.

After institution of drug treatment and during changes of medication, clients should be seen at a time when maximum therapeutic effectiveness can be expected from the medication, bimonthly or monthly, until the desired pressures are obtained. Stable clients with normal levels should be seen every four to six months to insure continued optimal results and compliance.

Treatment. The cornerstone of an effective program is a diuretic. The most commonly used are the thiazide diuretics—chlorthiazide (Diuril) 500 mg to 1 g once or twice daily or hydrochlorthiazide (Hydrodiuril) 50 to 100 mg once or twice daily. The second dose should be taken between 4:00 and 5:00 P.M. to minimize nocturia. After the medication is started, the client should be seen again in one month, at which time a serum potassium level is obtained and blood pressures are taken. If hypokalemia develops or if the client complains of weakness, muscle cramping, or other symptoms of hypokalemia, triameterene 25 mg and hydrochlorthiazide 25 mg (Dyazide) or spironolactone 25 mg and hydrochlorthiazide 25 mg (Aldatazide) may be substituted. These aldosterone antagonists minimize potassium loss and prevent secondary hyperaldosteronism; thus many of the side effects of the thiazide diuretic are avoided. If the blood pressure levels are still elevated, either the dosage of diuretic is increased or a second medication is added to reduce cardiac output.

Clients should be instructed not to add excessive salt to food and especially to avoid such heavily salted foods as brine

306

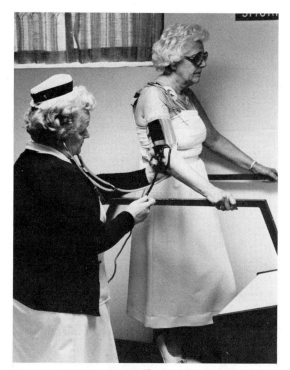

The gerontological nurse can help the elderly adapt to the aging process by recommending physical activities and exercise regimens suitable to their needs and capabilities; elderly clients should be encouraged to exercise after undergoing careful assessment procedures, such as cardiac stress testing.

pickles, potato chips, salted peanuts, smoked foods, meat tenderizer, soy sauce, bacon, and ham, as well as baking soda and Alka-Seltzer. With effective medication further sodium restriction is probably unnecessary.

Given the concept of increased cardiac output as the etiologic agent in hypertension (Keele and Neil 1971), the second most appropriate medication to use is propranalol hydrochloride 40 to 160 mg twice daily. This adrenergic blocking agent decreases heart rate and cardiac output. Propranalol also has a beneficial effect in angina pec-

toris; however, it may precipitate congestive heart failure. The drug is contraindicated in clients with asthma. Clients begun on this medication should be rechecked within one to two weeks. If withdrawn, propranalol must be tapered, as abrupt cessation may cause myocardial infarction.

If blood pressure levels remain elevated, a third medication should be added to the regimen. The third drug, usually a vasodilator, acts to lower peripheral resistance. Hydralazine hydrochloride (Apresoline) 25 or 50 mg four times daily to 200 mg is effective and has a minimum of side effects. However, in doses above 250 mg it may cause lupus erythematosis.

Medications other than adrenergic blocking agents are also useful in the treatment of hypertension either as second- or third-level treatment or as fourth and fifth drugs in severe cases. Alphamethyl-dopa (Aldomet) 250 mg to 1 g in divided doses is given two or three times daily. This drug operates by interfering with norepinephrine formation and may cause drowsiness in the first few days of treatment. The effect of Aldomet is of short duration and is gone within 48 hours after cessation of treatment. Rare cases of jaundice and Coombs positive hemolytic anemias as well as secondary-treatment failure have been reported with the use of this drug. Aldomet usually is well tolerated and attains peak effect one week after commencement of therapy.

Reserpine 0.25 mg given every other day to 0.5 mg daily must be taken up to one month to become effective; its effects may still be noted for an equal period after it has been withdrawn. Reserpine acts by depleting peripheral norepinephrine and decreasing the vasoconstrictive activity of

307

catecholamines. Because it also blocks central nervous system catecholamine uptake, it may cause severe depression and suicidal tendencies. It also can aggravate peptic ulcer disease and cause gastrointestinal bleeding. The drug should be used cautiously in the older client.

Another drug used to treat hypertension is guanethidine sulfate (Ismelin), a peripheral norepinephrine depleter. As it causes orthostatic hypotension, it is best avoided in the elderly client. It is given initially in 10 mg doses daily and may be increased to 25 mg daily and then further increased in increments of 25 mg up to 50 mg three times daily. The effects of Ismelin are blocked by tricyclic antidepressants, such as imipramine (Tofranil) and amitryptaline (Elavil), as well as by amphetamines and ephedrine, a common ingredient of commercial cold decongestants (Woosley and Nies 1976). Since Ismelin lowers blood pressure in the upright position, pressures should be measured in this position before changing dosage. The drug may cause considerable orthostatic hypotension, which may result in unsteadiness and falls. In the older client the risk of falling increases the possibility of fractures; therefore, Ismelin should be avoided in the elderly.

Drug therapy for hypertensive clients begins with a diuretic. When the diuretic is insufficient to bring the pressures to desired levels, a second drug is added. The second medication is gradually increased until either the desired pressure levels are attained or undesirable side effects are encountered. If maximal dosage has not sufficiently lowered the pressure, a third drug is begun. Treatment here follows the same rules outlined above. Clients can almost always be controlled by this stepwise approach. Secondary failure usually indicates that the client either is not taking the medication, is using a vasoconstrictor (e.g., ephedrine), or has resumed the use of large amounts of salt. The nurse must inquire about these possibilities prior to increasing or changing medication. Any client whose blood pressure unexplainably rises after institution of treatment—as well as any client with malignant hypertension, papilloedema, or evidence of renal impairment—must be quickly referred to a physician.

The treatment of hypertension is a long-term, joint effort shared by the nurse, the physician, the client, and the family. Complex medication regimens require that several persons have complete understanding of what is involved. Any evidence of memory lapse is sufficient reason to involve the family. Clients and family should be taught how to take blood pressures accurately. Again, weight loss, decreased alcohol use, moderate exercise, and a regular, relaxed life will help. The nurse must stress the outcome of untreated hypertension and the fact that symptoms may not be readily felt. However, the effects of iatrogenically induced hypotension may be equally dangerous in the elderly, leading to an acute brain syndrome, a fall, and a hip fracture. Any of these effects may lead to prolonged hospitalization, debilitation, or even death. The nurse is well advised to proceed cautiously and to see the client often when starting new medication or when changing dosage.

ISCHEMIC DISEASE

Pathophysiology

Arteriosclerotic changes in arteries and arterioles interfere with the ability of these vessels to increase or decrease their caliber in response to the needs of the tissues. These changes cause a loss in the elasticity of the vessels due to a structural change in the intima and medial layers. The morphology varies and has led to the adoption of descriptive terms such as atherosclerosis, Mönckeberg's medial calcific sclerosis, and hyaline arteriosclerosis.

In *atherosclerosis* fatty streaks appear in the intima. These streaks may disappear or continue to develop and be replaced by fibrous and calcified plaques, which diminish the lumen and weaken the wall of the vessel. The atheromatous lesion may be covered over by endothelium. Under this layer the fatty deposit may liquify, forming an atheromatous abscess. If the weakened intimal cover tears off, this roughened undersurface will permit the formation of a clot. This intraluminal thrombus may occlude the lumen or tear off to form an embolis.

The changes of *Mönckeberg's medial calcific sclerosis* occur in the media of medium and small muscular arteries. Here cartilaginous rings are formed. This distinct and unique disorder may be seen, along with atherosclerosis, in the same individual and even in the same vessel. Clinically this arteriosclerotic change is not significant.

In *hyaline arteriosclerosis* the vascular change is seen as hyaline thickening beneath the basement membrane. The hyaline also entraps the vascular smooth muscle. This form of arteriosclerosis is frequently seen in the kidneys, where the narrowing of the arteriolar lumina interferes with renal blood flow and causes a diffuse renal ischemia.

Ischemic diseases of the cardiovascular system involve the heart and the central and peripheral vascular systems. The major ischemic disorders of the heart include angina pectoris and myocardial infarction. Those of the central and peripheral vascular systems include aneurysmal and occlusive diseases as well as those that involve progressive arterial narrowing.

ISCHEMIC HEART DISEASE

Pathophysiology

The nature of cardiac energy production is strictly aerobic, and the myocardium normally extracts about 65 percent of the total oxygen present. The caliber of coronary vessels, their patency, aortic pressure, and the effective pressure gradient between the aorta (pressure head) and the right atria are of profound significance in coronary blood flow. A diminution in any of these factors can result in myocardial ischemia. The ischemia, in turn, causes changes in metabolic biochemistry and in the electrophysiology and myocardial contractility of the heart.

The caliber of coronary arteries and arterioles can be narrowed by atherosclerosis and by arteriospasm. When a segment of myocardium becomes ischemic under these conditions, the clinical syndrome called *angina pectoris* ensues. The pain is thought to be due to an accumulation of metabolites in the area temporarily deprived of blood flow. The pain is transient, and myocardial necrosis, such as that accompanying coronary occlusion, does not occur.

When a blood clot occludes a coronary artery, myocardial infarction results. The thrombotic occlusion usually involves one or more of the major coronary arterial trunks. The myocardium downstream of the occlusion becomes ischemic, and necrosis follows.

309

Coronary flow is also reduced when the effective pressure gradient between the aorta, often referred to as the *pressure head,* and the venous blood returning to the right atria from heart muscle is reduced. This situation is caused by pressure elevations in both the right atria and ventricle and is frequently seen in congestive heart failure.

Some less well-known causes of coronary insufficiency are increased blood viscosity, as in dehydration, shock, or polycythemia. Abnormal cardiac rhythms, such as premature contractions, which decrease cardiac output, also cause diminution of coronary flow. Whatever the cause, the resulting myocardial ischemia causes pain and usually interferes with the efficiency of the pump.

Nursing Assessment

Angina Pectoris: Subjective and Objective Findings. Identification of the angina pectoris syndrome will usually lead to a diagnosis of arteriosclerotic heart disease. However, the examiner must be alert to the possibilities of anemia, hyperthyroidism, subaortic or aortic stenosis, and aortic insufficiency, in addition to the other etiologic factors mentioned previously.

The classic syndrome is one of exertional pain. The client complains of distress, usually a pressure, squeezing, or burning in the region of the midsternum or to the left of the sternum. The pain may be referred to the shoulders and down the arms, to the epigastrium, or to the root of the neck. Rarely is it described in the face, teeth, jaw, or back. Breathlessness and fear of death often accompany the attack. In the elderly the pain may be blunted; more of a dull, burning character or breathlessness may be the prominent complaint. Often associated with belching, the pain may be confused with indigestion. Always sudden in onset, beginning during an effort (usually walking out of doors), angina is particularly aggravated if the effort is performed in cold weather or after a meal. Walking up a slight hill is difficult. Heated arguments or emotions such as anger may provoke an anginal attack. Clients quickly learn that the pain subsides in a few minutes with cessation of the activity and that performance at a slower pace prevents or delays the onset of pain. The elderly usually diminish their activity to a level below that pace (Rodstein 1971).

During an anginal attack, examination may reveal pallor and diaphoresis. Diaphoretic episodes, particularly on the face and neck, may be the first warning of decompensation. On cardiac auscultation, tachycardia or premature beats are often heard. Pressure exerted on the carotid sinus, if it slows the heart, may terminate the attack. This test is diagnostic if positive; however, carotid sinus pressure may be dangerous in the older client. The pressure may cause asystole or may decrease cerebral perfusion and cause a stroke. To avoid suggestion, the clients should be asked if the pressure on the neck makes the pain worse (Levine 1958; Feruglio 1975). Additionally the nurse must be aware that an electrocardiogram may reveal S-T depression, T wave inversion, or, rarely, transient infarction patterns, all reverting to normal with termination of the episode.

Between anginal attacks physical findings of significance are few. Evidence of peripheral atherosclerotic disease of the retinal, brachial, or pedal arteries is helpful but not diagnostic. Hypertension and cardiomegaly are findings with high diagnostic value, as these are often associated with angina.

Myocardial Infarction: Subjective and Objective Findings. Infarct in the aged, both initially and throughout its course, is markedly different than in younger clients. When it follows long periods of ischemia, it may be silent or it may present with subtle symptoms, such as fever or increased shortness of breath and fatigue. Myocardial pain differs in that it may be mild and of brief duration, agonizing and persisting for several hours to one to two days, or intermittent and prolonged for several days. Symptoms associated with infarction include nausea and vomiting, faintness, sweating, palpitation, and weakness (Patty 1976).

Diagnostics

A chest x-ray may demonstrate cardiomegaly or congestive failure. Fluoroscopy can detect specific heart chamber enlargement, coronary artery calcifications, or the presence of calcifications in the aortic valve. The electrocardiogram may reveal arrhythmias, fixed ischemic patterns, or evidence of old infarction, confirming the presence of arteriosclerotic heart disease.

Laboratory studies include a 2-hour postprandial blood sugar test to screen for diabetes, thyroid function tests (T3 and T4), and a luetic serology (Hinton, VDRL, etc.). Hemoglobin and hematocrit tests are helpful in screening for anemia. Enzyme studies of SGOT and SGPT are indicated to differentiate the cardiac pain origin, since hiatal hernia can present with similar bouts of pain (Feruglio 1975). Other isoen-

zyme tests in current use for myocardial infarction include CPK and LDH.

In the elderly even leukocyte elevations, serum enzyme changes, and EKG data may be masked, thereby placing diagnosis on the clinical findings. EKG changes in S-T interval and T wave inversion may not be as marked (Feruglio 1975, pp. 127 and 130).

In clients with the classic history of effort-induced pain, suggestively abnormal electrocardiograms showing ischemia, and a typical response to nitroglycerine, one may consider that the diagnosis has been made. In clients with equivocal histories, with or without the other findings, stress testing should be performed by a cardiologist.

Nursing Management

Treatment for *angina* in the elderly differs from that for angina in a younger client, for whom emphasis may be placed on a change of lifestyle. For the elderly client emphasis is placed on health instruction, counseling, and the appropriate use of medication.

Health Education and Counseling. Since physical activity is of cardinal importance in maintaining health, the client with angina should be advised that activity is helpful and may even reduce the severity and frequency of the attacks. After assessment by stress testing, clients with stable angina should be started on a sustained program of regular daily walking for at least 20 minutes, weather permitting. If the pain occurs, they should stop, take nitroglycerine, then continue to walk after relief is obtained. The aim is to achieve a sustained, tolerated pace. In most cases exercise will decrease the frequency and severity of attacks. This approach, however, may be difficult in older arthritic clients who are limited by musculoskeletal problems, but it should nonetheless be encouraged since it will greatly benefit these clients also.

Examination of the activity that consistently produces pain may permit changes that can reduce the frequency and severity of angina attacks. Anxiety may be lessened by teaching the client relaxation and anxiety-reducing techniques. Many paperback books such as *The Relaxation Response* by Herbert Benson are available and may be suggested for clients capable of reading. Clients must be reassured that angina attacks are not heart attacks and do not cause damage to the heart; but they should also be told that the attacks can be precursors of a myocardial infarction. Instructions should include explaining the character of myocardial infarction pain and, in particular, the necessity of reporting an increase or change in pain patterns.

The overweight elderly client should be counseled on the necessity of weight reduction and the role of cholesterol and triglycerides. Smoking and the excessive use of alcohol must be discouraged. Clients with unstable angina at rest or with angina of increasing frequency should be managed by a physician.

For the client who is suspected of, or diagnosed as, having a *myocardial infarction,* medical supervision is necessary. The nurse's role is primarily to teach prophylactic measures for cardiac rehabilitation. Sexual counseling may be indicated, as clients may have sexual dysfunction due to post–myocardial infarction (MI) fear.

Many elderly clients have a "silent MI" and may note only a change in pain character. They and their family need instructions to be alert for signs and symptoms such as dyspnea, fatigue, or a slight increase in temperature.

Treatment. For the anginal client the mainstay of drug therapy is nitroglycerine 0.15 mg to 0.4 mg sublingually. This drug works by relaxing smooth muscle, which permits coronary artery dilation and increased coronary artery blood flow. Nitroglycerine should be taken promptly at the onset of pain. Relief occurs in less than five minutes; this rapid response is almost diagnostic of angina pectoris. The prescribed dosage should be sufficient to relieve pain with minimal headache. Clients must be reassured that the medication is neither dangerous nor addictive, that it is actually helpful, and that tolerance is not a problem. They should be advised to renew the tablets about every 6 months and to keep the stock bottle in the refrigerator. They should carry a dozen or so tablets in a small box at all times. The unused tablets should be discarded and replaced from the stock every 2 weeks. When angina is produced by a particular activity that cannot be avoided, the client should take a tablet just prior to performing this activity. The attack will often be lessened or even aborted. Side effects of nitroglycerine include transient headache and, rarely, hypotension and fainting. These effects are relieved by decreasing the strength of the tablet. When attacks occur one or several times each day, further medication may be tried.

Propranalol 10 to 40 mg four times daily may be used. This medication induces bradycardia, decreases cardiac output, and often lessens the frequency of angina. The drug should not be stopped abruptly, as cessation may precipitate myocardial infarction. Propranalol is contraindicated in clients with asthma, heart block, or congestive heart failure. Experience with this medication in the elderly is still somewhat limited (Caird and Dall 1973). However, studies show that it decreases the frequency of resting and exercise arrhythmia (Nixon et al. 1978), a frequent cause of sudden death in coronary artery disease (Lown and Wolf 1971).

Longer acting nitrates may also be helpful either taken orally or applied to the skin as nitroglycerine paste: sustained-action nitroglycerine 2.5 to 6.5 mg taken every 12 hours; erythrityl tetranitrate 10 to 30 mg, pentaerythrital tetranitrate 10 to 20 mg, or isorbide dinitrate 5 to 30 mg, all taken orally every 6 to 12 hours; or nitroglycerine paste applied to a 6-cm–by–6-cm square of skin every 12 hours. These medications may diminish the number of episodes suffered by the client.

CENTRAL AND PERIPHERAL ARTERIAL DISEASES

Central and peripheral arterial diseases may be brought on by a variety of conditions. In the older client arterioatherosclerosis is the most frequent cause, with overt clinical manifestations appearing from the fourth decade on. Congenital vascular malformations, syphilitic aortitis, diabetic angiopathy, periarterites nodosa, and rheumatic fever are rare causes. Central and peripheral arterial diseases usually manifest themselves as vascular aneurysms or occlusive diseases, either sudden or progressive.

Central Arterial Disease: Nursing Assessment

Aneurysmal Disease: Subjective and Objective Findings. Weakened vessel walls undergo dilatation or dissection (Braunstein 1963). Most often this aneurysm will be an asymptomatic finding on a chest x-ray, or a pulsating mass, or a widened aorta palpated during the abdominal examination. Rarely clients may complain of pain due to pressure of the aneurysm on adjacent organs or bones. Occasionally ischemic pain distal to the aneurysm may occur because of diminished flow in these vessels. Severe, prolonged pain along the distal path of the dilated vessel is often due to dissection. This condition is a true emergency indicating possible, imminent rupture (Hurst 1971). Treatment is surgical, and clients should be referred to a physician.

Occlusive Disease: Subjective and Objective Findings. The site and rapidity of the blockage determines the clinical presentation. Sudden closure in any area with few collateral vessels leads to tissue death, scar formation, and functional loss. Initially, severe pain occurs for prolonged periods of time, as in mesenteric infarction or femoral artery occlusion. Functional loss may predominate, as in a stroke. These situations have a high mortality rate and require physician evaluation.

Progressive Arterial Narrowing: Subjective and Objective Findings. The findings in cases of progressive arterial narrowing are less dramatic. Blood flow may be normal at rest. Any increase in tissue oxygen needs—as a result of activity or fever, for example—will cause ischemic pain and diminished functional capacity. Progressive occlusion of the mesenteric arteries causes postprandial abdominal anginal pain that can mimic peptic ulcer. As evaluation and treatment require special radiographic studies and surgical intervention, these clients should be referred to a physician.

Peripheral Arterial Disease: Nursing Assessment

Intermittent claudication (painful, intermittent limp) is the syndrome of ischemic limb pain with effort. Peripheral arterial disease is commonly due to *arteriosclerosis obliterans* of the femoral artery. It occurs earlier and more frequently in the diabetic client (Coffman 1971) and has a significant association with a history of smoking. Peripheral arterial disease is rarely due to thromboangitis obliterans (Buerger's disease). Claudication may also be precipitated by chronic ergot ingestion, methysergiside medication, or emboli in clients with rheumatic heart disease or subacute bacterial endocarditis. Severe anemia also may present as claudication.

Arteriosclerosis Obliterans: Subjective Findings. Pain and a sensation of cold are the main complaints of arteriosclerosis obliterans. The pain is felt distal to the level of arterial occlusion or stenosis. The pain is described as a cramp or as a squeezing or fatigue in a muscle group, which begins during a sustained effort with the affected limb. Most commonly it occurs while walking. Slackening the pace or stopping relieves the pain in a few minutes. The necessary effort remains rather constant in a given client. The calf is usually affected; however, pain also can occur in the low back, buttock, thigh, or foot. Bilateral complaints may be associated with impotence and usually are due to aortoiliac disease (Leriche's syndrome). In a more advanced stage, the client may complain of pain at rest, which indicates insufficient blood flow to maintain skin integrity. Pain is relieved by dependency or by cooling the limb and, when expressed as night pain, by hanging the foot out of the bed and out of the covers. Other complaints include numbness, paresthesias, coldness, and color changes in the limb.

Arteriosclerosis Obliterans: Objective Findings. On physical examination distal pulses will be absent or markedly reduced. In unilateral disease the difference between the two limbs is sharp. Having the client exercise will often abolish the pulses; use of an oscillometer can confirm findings or disclose normal arteries covered by edema or in spasm. Color changes are either elevation pallor (decreased circulation), dependent rubor (anoxic injury), or cyanosis (diminished flow).

Skin changes may be present. The subcutaneous tissue becomes puffy and the skin atrophic, dry, shiny, pale, tightly drawn, and hairless. Ischemic ulcerations can develop. The nails become thickened, hard, brittle, ridged, and deformed. In later stages indolent, painful, sensitive fissures and ulcers of the toes and heels form and can progress to gangrene.

Auscultation of the abdomen and over the affected limb often reveals a systolic bruit, indicating obstruction or stenosis. A continuous bruit indicates deficient collateral circulation. Coolness of a limb is difficult to evaluate, but if it occurs in a warm room or is unilateral, it is definitely abnormal. Circulation can be evaluated from vascular flush and venous-filling time. With the client recumbent, the limb is elevated to 45°. Normally the plantar surface remains pink; pallor on elevation indicates circulatory compromise. The client is then moved rapidly to a seated position. A blush should appear instantly. Persistent pallor, beyond 20 seconds, is definitely abnormal. Venous filling should occur in 10 seconds; a venous-filling time greater than 30 seconds is abnormal. The presence of varicosities invalidates this portion of the test (Coffman and Maverick 1966). Any difference between the two limbs should also be noted.

Peripheral Arterial Disease: Nursing Management

Health Education and Counseling. The principal function for the nurse in the care of clients with a peripheral arterial problem again lies in health teaching and counseling. Warmth to the extremities is essential because of the vasodilatory effect. The client should be instructed to wear socks to bed. Special care should be taken to promote tissue perfusion and to prevent trauma to affected extremities. The client should be told that the affected limb is susceptible to infection. Mild soaps and attention to hygiene is necessary. For any client who uses tobacco, the vasoconstrictive effects of smoking must be explained in detail, and ongoing counseling to diminish smoking habits is indicated.

To avoid drying, cracking, and fissures of the skin, the client should apply skin emollients every night and morning and vigorously massage both legs. Each toe should be massaged individually. Clients who perspire should apply a mild medicated powder, such as Ammens or Diaperene, to their feet daily. Toenails should be cut regularly and straight across, with only a toenail clipper. The client should be advised against the use of other instruments such as files and emory boards because of decreased sensation due to peripheral ischemic neuropathy.

Shoes should be comfortable; if necessary special space shoes should be used. The client should sleep on a firm mattress, since a soft one will permit trunk flexion and impede circulation to the lower extremities. The nurse may advise the use of an electric blanket to avoid heavy bedding. The client can place a small board at the foot of the bed to elevate the bedding and diminish pressure on the feet.

The client should be instructed about the importance of frequently changing the position of the extremities. Either sitting with legs dependent or standing for too long exacerbates the condition. The client should avoid crossing the knees and should perform simple rotating leg-raising exercises if required to sit for a long time. The client should also be instructed to wear elastic support hose.

The nurse must be aware that the chronicity of the pain and condition will have a significant psychological effect on the client. These clients definitely need continual encouragement. This support is even more significant in the obese client who refuses to lose weight or the client who refuses surgical intervention or skin grafting for a chronic ulcer. The elderly client who has lived with a chronic ulcer for a lengthy period may consider the condition to be hopeless. Dressing changes as well as other pre-cautions may be neglected. A home visit seems to be most appropriate for further assessment of such a client. Dealing with the noncompliant client is difficult, but the nurse must maintain a caring, accepting attitude in order to help the client.

Treatment. Clients with peripheral vascular occlusive disease should be evaluated by a physician for bypass surgery. Conservative treatment of ulcers includes the application of an antibiotic ointment and a clean pressure dressing when necessary, alternating with attempts to heal the ulcer through solar or open-air drying. Diabetic and neurotrophic ulcers are best treated without wet compresses. Such compresses often extend the lesion, except when they are used as hydration prior to careful mechanical debridement (Tindall 1978).

The pressure dressing reduces interstitial fluid stasis. The effect of the dressing can be enhanced through movement. Therefore, the client should be instructed to walk as much as possible and to avoid sitting for any length of time.

Local treatment includes cleansing the ulcer and debridement for removal of necrotic tissue. When stasis dermatosis is present, corticoid ointment such as hydrocortisone 1% or triamcinolone 0.05% may be applied to the region surrounding the ulcer (Schmidtke and Schoop 1975, p. 177).

An ointment with neomycin and hydrocortisone provides an anti-inflammatory function while treating any secondary infection. A Gelocast boot, also known as an Unna boot, may be applied and changed once or twice a week by the nurse. A thin gold leaf applied directly to the ulcer has been found to stimulate tissue granulation (Brunner et al. 1970, p. 338).

Evaluation of Care. Some clients may benefit from endarterectomy, grafting, or amputation and therefore require physician evaluation. Arteriosclerosis obliterans can be treated conservatively in clients with normal-appearing limbs and minimal claudication. Weight loss, discontinuance of tobacco use, and reduction in the rate of exercise will lessen the attacks. An attempt to improve collateral circulation by graded, increasing exercises may be helpful. The client should be encouraged to walk until pain begins, to stop until the pain clears, and then to walk on. The goal is to exercise the limb for at least 20 minutes daily. Rest pain may require pain-relieving medication, such as aspirin 600 mg every 4 hours, propoxyphene 65 mg every 4 hours, or a mild narcotic (Codeine 3 mg every 4 hours). Gangrene is a complication of arteriosclerosis obliterans and may require amputation; a physician must be consulted.

When the peripheral arterial problem is due to causes other than arteriosclerosis, the elimination of ergot, either in medication or in moldy rye, or of methylsergiside medication specifically alters the disease induced by these agents. Clients with atrial fibrillation, evidence of rheumatic heart disease, or subacute bacterial endocarditis should be referred to a physician for specific evaluation and therapy.

SUMMARY

Cardiovascular disorders are a major source of disability for the older client. Recognition and proper management are essential for the maintenance of optimal health and activity as well as for the prevention of severely limiting and life-threatening conditions of stroke and congestive failure.

REFERENCES

ABASSI, A. S. 1976. "Echocardiography in the Differential Diagnosis of the Large Heart." *American Journal of Medicine* 60:677–86.

ADLERMAN, M., and E. SCHOENBAUM. 1975. "Detection and Treatment of Hypertension at the Worksite." *New England Journal of Medicine* 293:65–68.

BABU, T. N., et al. 1977. "What is Normal Blood Pressure in the Aged?" *Geriatrics* 32:73–76.

BEARD, O. W. 1976. "Congestive Heart Failure." Presented at a symposium on "Cardiovascular Problems of Aging" at the American Gerontological Society Meeting, New York, October 14.

BRAUNSTEIN, H. 1963. "Pathogenesis of Dissecting Aneurysm." *Circulation* 28:1071–75.

BROVENDER, S., and D. ANDERSON. 1978. "Quality Care Assessment in Hypertension: An Audit in a Joint Practice Clinic." Lecture presented at the 31st Annual Meeting of the Gerontological Society, Dallas, November 19.

BRUNNER, L. S., et al. 1970. *Textbook of Medical Surgical Nursing,* 2nd ed. New York: J. B. Lippincott.

BRUNWALD, E. 1974. "Heart Failure." In M. W. Wintrobe et al., *Harrison's Principles of Internal Medicine.* New York: McGraw-Hill.

CAIRD, F. I., and J. L. C. DALL. 1973. "The Cardiovascular System." In J. C. Brocklehurst, *Textbook of Geriatric Medicine and Gerontology.* Edinburgh: Churchill Livingstone.

COFFMAN, J. D., and J. A. MAVERICK. 1966. "An Objective Test to Demonstrate the Circulatory Abnormality in Intermittent Claudication." *Circulation* 33:177–79.

————. 1971. "Diseases of the Peripheral Vessels." In P. B. Beeson and W. McDermott, eds., *Cecil-Loeb Textbook of Medicine,* 13th ed. Philadelphia: W. B. Saunders.

DeMARIA, A. N., et al. 1976. "Echocardiography: Applications in Office Practice." *Cardiovascular Medicine* (October):105–18.

DOCK, W. 1956. "Aging of the Myocardium." *Bulletin of the New York Academy of Medicine* 32:175–78.

DOUGLAS, B. H., et al. 1964. "Hypertension Caused by Salt Loading. II: Fluid Volume and Tissue Pressure Changes." *American Journal of Physiology* 207:669–79.

DOVENMUHLE, R. H., E. W. BUSSE, and G. NEWMAN. 1970. "Physical Problems of Older People." In E. Palmore, ed., *Normal Aging.* Durham, N.C.: Duke University Press.

EBSANI, A., et al. 1975. "Left Ventricular Performance after Acute Myocardial Infarction." *Archives of Internal Medicine* 135:1539–47.

ENGLEMAN, K., and E. BRUNWALD. 1974. "Elevation of Arterial Pressure." In M. W. Wintrobe et al., eds., *Harrison's Principles of Internal Medicine.* New York: McGraw-Hill.

FERUGLIO, F. S. 1975. "Heart Diseases." In H. P. von Hohn, ed., *Practical Geriatrics: Guidelines for General Practice.* New York and Basel: S. Karger, A.G.

FISHNEAU, A. P. 1971. "Diseases of the Cardiovascular System." In P. B. Beeson and W. McDermott, eds., *Cecil-Loeb Textbook of Medicine.* Philadelphia: W. B. Saunders.

FORD, R. V. 1958. "The Vascular Status of a Heterogeneous Group of Patients with Hypertension with Particular Emphasis on Renal Function." *American Journal of Medicine* 24:164–76.

FOSTER, S., and D. KOUSCH. 1978. "Promoting Patient Adherence." *American Journal of Nursing* 78:829–32.

FRIEDBERG, C. K. 1950. *Diseases of the Heart.* Philadelphia: W. B. Saunders.

FULKOW, B., et al. 1973. "Importance of Adaptive Changes in Vascular Design for Establishment of Primary Hypertension, Studied in Man and in Spontaneously Hypertensive Rats." *Circulation Research* (Supplement 1) 32(2):2–15.

FURMAN, S. 1976. "Artificial Pacemakers." Presented at a symposium on "Cardiovascular Problems of Aging" presented at the 29th Annual Meeting of the Gerontological Society, New York, October 14.

GRAY, R., et al. 1975. "Hemocynamic and Metabolic Effects of Isorbide Dinitrate in Chronic Congestive Heart Failure." *American Heart Journal* 90:346–52.

GUBNER, R. S., and H. E. UNGERLIEDEN. 1959. "Life Expectancy and Insurability in Heart Disease." *Modern Concept of Cardiovascular Disease* 28:565–70.

GUYTON, A. C., et al. 1972. "Arterial Pressure Regulation: Overriding Dominance of the Kidneys in Long-term Regulation and in Hypertension." *American Journal of Medicine* 52:584–92.

HARRIS, R. 1970. *The Management of Geriatric Cardiovascular Disease.* Philadelphia: J. B. Lippincott.

_____. 1975. "Cardiac Changes with Age." In R. Goldman and M. Rockstein, eds., *The Physiology and Pathology of Human Aging.* New York: Academic Press.

_____. 1977. "Cardiopathy of Aging: All the Changes Related to Congestive Heart Failure." *Geriatrics* 32:142–46.

_____. 1978. "Special Problems with Heart Disease." In W. Reichel, ed., *Clinical Aspects of Aging.* Baltimore: Williams and Wilkins.

HASSETT, J. 1978. "Teaching Yourself to Relax." *Review* 2(11):17–24.

HERSHEY, D. 1974. *Life Span and Factors Affecting It.* Springfield, Ill.: Thomas Publishing.

HURST, J. W. 1971. "Disease of the Aorta." In P. B. Beeson and W. McDermott, eds., *Cecil-Loeb Textbook of Medicine,* 13th ed. Philadelphia: W. B. Saunders.

JOHNSON, R. H. 1976. "Blood Pressure and Its Regulation." In F. I. Caird, J.L.C. Dall, and R. D. Kennedy, eds., *Cardiology and Old Age.* New York: Plenium Press.

KANNEL, W. B. 1976. "Blood Pressure and Cardiovascular Disease in the Aged." In F. I. Caird, J. L. C. Dall, and R. D. Kennedy, eds., *Cardiology and Old Age.* New York: Plenium Press.

KEELE, C. A., and E. NEIL. 1971. *Samson Wright's Applied Physiology,* 12th ed. London: Oxford University Press.

KINCAID-SMITH, P., J. McMICHAEL, and E. A. MURPHY. 1958. "The Clinical Course and Pathology of Hypertension with Papilloedema (Malignant Hypertension)." *Quarterly Journal of Medicine* 27:117–53.

LEVINE, S. 1958. *Clinical Heart Disease,* 5th ed. Philadelphia: W. B. Saunders.

LOHMULLER, G., et al. 1975. "Mechanism of Immediate Hemodynamic Effects of Chlorthiazide." *American Heart Journal* 89:487–92.

LOWN, A., and G. WOLF. 1971. "Approaches to Sudden Death from Coronary Heart Disease." *Circulation* 44:130–42.

MOST, A. S., H. G. KEMP, and R. GORLIN. 1969. "Postexercise Electrocardiography in Patients with Arteriographically Documented Coronary Artery Disease." *Annals of Internal Medicine* 71:1043–50.

MOYER, J. H., et al. 1958. "The Vascular Status of a Heterogeneous Group of Patients with Hypertension with Particular Emphasis on Renal Function." *American Journal of Medicine* 24:164–66.

MUSHLIM, A. J., and F. A. APPEL. 1977. "Diagnosing Potential Non-Compliance: Physicians' Ability in Behavioral Dimension of Medical Care." *Archives of Internal Medicine* 137:318–21.

National Health Survey. 1975. *Blood Pressure of Persons 18–74 Years, United States 1971–1972, Rockville, Maryland.* National Center for Health Statistics, U.S. Department of Health, Education, and Welfare.

NIXON, J. V., et al. 1978. "Efficacy of Propranalol in the Control of Exercise Induced or Augmented Ventricular Ectopic Activity." *Circulation* 57:115–22.

PATTY, M. S. 1976. "Myocardial Infarction." In F. I. Caird, J. L. C. Dall, and R. D. Kennedy, eds., *Cardiology in Old Age.* New York: Plenium Press.

PERRY, M. 1969. "Survival of Treated Hypertensive Patients, Grand Rounds, No. 20," *Journal of the American Medical Association* 210:890–92.

POMERANZ, A. 1968. "Cardiac Pathology in the Aged." *Geriatrics* 23:101–08.

RAHIMTOOLA, S. H., M. M. DiGIKO, and A. EBSANI. 1972. "Changes in Left Ventricular Performance from Early after Acute Myocardial Infarction to the Convalescent Phase." *Circulation* 46:770–79.

RESNICK, W. H., and T. R. HARRISON. 1962. "Diseases of the Heart." In T. R. Harrison, ed., *Principles of Internal Medicine.* New York: McGraw-Hill.

RITCHIE, M. 1968. "Heart Failure—The Geriatric Patient." *Nursing Clinics of North America* 3:4.

ROBBINS, S. 1974. *Pathologic Basis of Disease.* Philadelphia: W. B. Saunders.

RODSTEIN, M. 1971. "Heart Disease in the Aged." In I. Rossman, ed., *Clinical Geriatrics.* Philadelphia: J. B. Lippincott.

ROWE, J. W., et al. 1976. "The Effect of Age on Creatinine Clearance in Men: A Cross-Sectional and Longitudinal Study." *Journal of Gerontology* 31:155–63.

RUNYAN, J. 1975. "The Memphis Chronic Disease Program: Comparison in Outcome and the Nurse's Extended Role." *Journal of American Medical Association* 231:264–67.

"Salt and Hypertension." 1975. *Lancet* 14:1325.

SCHMIDTKE, I., and W. SCHOOP. 1975. "Peripheral Vascular Disorders." In H. P. L. von Hahn, ed., *Practical Geriatrics.* New York and Basel: S. Karger, A.G.

SMITH, T. W. 1973. "Digitalis Glycosides." *New England Journal of Medicine* 288:719–22.

STAMLER, R., et al. 1978. "Weight and Blood Pressure. Findings in Hypertension Screening of 1 Million Americans." *Journal of American Medical Association* 240:1607–10.

TAYLOR, W., et al. 1975. "The Hemodynamic Effects of Nitroglycerine Ointment in Congestive Heart Failure." *Circulation* 51 and 52 (Supplement 2):135–38.

TIMARIS, P. S. 1972. *Developmental Physiology and Aging.* New York: Macmillian.

TINDALL, J. P. 1978. "Geriatric Dermatology." In W. Reichel, ed., *Clinical Aspects of Aging.* Baltimore: Williams and Wilkins.

Veterans Administration. 1970. "Cooperative Study Group on Antihypertensive Agents. Effects of Treatment of Morbidity in Hypertension II. Results in Patients with Diastolic Blood Pressure Averaging 90–114 mmHg." *Journal of the American Medical Association* 213:1143–52.

WAXLER, R. 1976. "The Patient with Congestive Heart Failure—Teaching Implications." *Nursing Clinics of North America* 11(2):297–308.

WEINBLATT, I. S., S. SHAPIRO, and F. R. CAUDSAGER. 1968. "Prognostic Factors in Angina Pectoris—A Prospective Study." *Journal of Chronological Diseases* 21:231–40.

WOLLAM, G. I., and R. W. GIFFORD. 1976. "The Kidney as a Target Organ in Hypertension." *Geriatrics* 31:71–79.

WOOSLEY, R. I., and A. S. NIES. 1976. "Guanethidine." *The New England Journal of Medicine* 295:1053–56.

ZIESCHE, S., and F. JOSEPH. 1977. "Clinical Application of Sodium Nitroprusside." *Heart and Lung* 6(1):3–5.

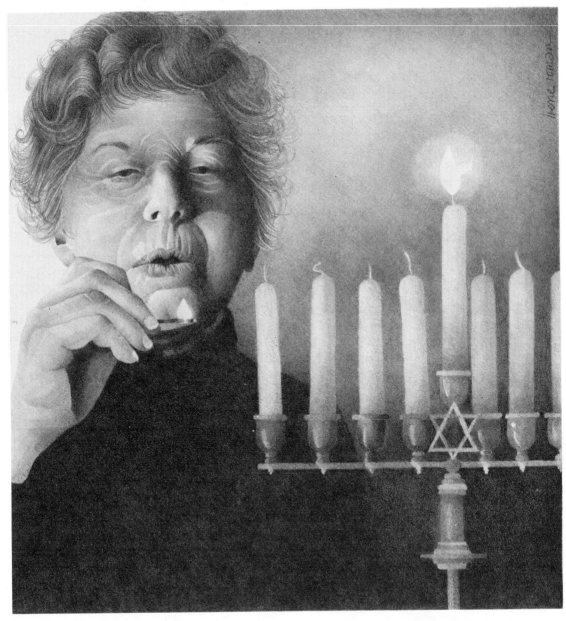

Chapter 11

GERONTOLOGICAL NURSING MANAGEMENT
THE ELDERLY CLIENT WITH A RESPIRATORY PROBLEM

Respiratory problems in the elderly can be either acute or chronic. Most frequently the client has had a long-standing problem of the lungs, such as emphysema or bronchitis. The major acute respiratory diseases seen in the aged client are pneumonia, pulmonary embolism, and lung cancer. This chapter discusses both acute and chronic conditions.

PULMONARY FUNCTION

Pathophysiology

Normal Pulmonary Function. The two pulmonary functions are *ventilation* and *respiratory gas exchange.* Ventilation involves the conduction of air down to and through the respiratory tree. The structures involved in conducting air are the nasal passages, larynx, trachea, bronchi, and terminal bronchioles; however, only the latter three structures are included in the term *respiratory tree.* Respiratory gas exchange occurs in the most distal segment, the respiratory membrane, which includes alveoli and pulmonary capillaries. The lungs of a 70 kg adult male have approximately 300 million alveoli (Guyton 1976).

The walls of the larynx, trachea, and large bronchi contain a high proportion of hyaline cartilage, which gives these passageways a degree of rigidity. The smaller bronchi contain progressively less cartilage and more smooth muscle. At the level of bronchioles, cartilage is absent and the walls are predominately smooth muscle arranged in a circle. All of these structures are lined with ciliated cells, which, through their constant motion, propel trapped airborne dust and other particulate matter away from the terminal bronchioles and respiratory membrane. The conducting passageway also is heavily endowed with mucus-secreting cells. Mucus not only traps foreign material so that it can be expelled, but it also moistens inspired air.

The structure of the respiratory membrane has been established by the electron microscope and is highly suitable for performing gaseous exchange. The respiratory membrane is comprised of several layers of membranes. Oxygen must first penetrate surfactant, the layer of fluid that lines each alveolus, and then cross the thin epithelial wall of these sacs. Once through the cell wall, oxygen penetrates the alveolar basement membrane, crosses an interstitial space, and then penetrates the basement membrane of the adjacent capillary. Oxygen then passes through the capillary endothelial wall and finally enters erythrocytes in the blood.

Note that throughout the lungs there are many elastic fibers. These fibers, along with the surface tension of the fluid lining the alveoli, give the lungs the ability to stretch and recoil. Volumetric capacity of the lungs is greatly influenced by both elasticity and surface tension, which, when altered by disease, affect the amount of air delivered to the respiratory membrane.

Ventilation is a function performed primarily through the respiratory muscles, such as the diaphragm and the intercostals. These muscles, plus the elastic properties of lung tissue, control the volumetric capacity of the lungs. Diseases of the lungs affect pulmonary capacities and volume. For this reason, the nurse must know the ventilatory function tests used to establish the values for the average normal adult.

Volumetric Capacities of the Lungs

Tidal Volume (TV): 500 ml—the amount of air breathed in or out during quiet breathing

Inspiratory Reserve Volume (IRV): 3,000 ml—the amount of air that can be inspired over and above that inspired in a normal tidal volume

Expiratory Reserve Volume (ERV): 1,000 ml—the extra amount of air expelled by forceful expiration following a normal tidal expiration

Residual Volume (RV): 1,200 ml—the amount of air remaining in the lungs after a maximum expiration

Functional Residual Capacity (FRC): 2,300 ml = RV and ERV—the amount of air remaining in the lungs at the end of a normal expiration

Inspiratory Capacity (IC): 3,500 ml—the amount of air achieved when the deepest possible breath is drawn, begilning at the end of a normal expiration

Vital Capacity (VC): 4,600 ml—the maximum amount of air that can be expelled after a maximal inspiration.

Total Lung Capacity (TLC): 5,800 ml—the maximum amount of air present in the lung when a maximum inspiratory effort is made following a maximum expiration

Maximum Breathing Capacity (MBC): 82–169 l/minute—the maximum amount of air that can be breathed voluntarily in one minute

Causes of Decline in Pulmonary Function. Although up to 4 liters of oxygen can be delivered each minute across the respiratory membrane of a 20-year-old man, this value is reduced 1.5 liters in a 75-year-old man. Some of this difference is attributed to a decline in cardiac output seen in the elderly. Other reasons for the decline in pulmonary function are the decrease in the elastic property of lung tissue and chest wall, the decline in the strength of muscles that assist respiration, and the diminished efficiency of the nervous system. The lung tissue changes are related to thickening of ground substance and increasing cross-linkage in collagen and elastin fibers, which reduce elasticity. The diminished chest wall compliance is related to changes in costal cartilage. Changes in lung tissues and the neuromuscular changes described above contribute to a reduction of pulmonary vital capacity, which involves expiratory reserve volume, tidal volume, and inspiratory reserve volume.

Some disorders found in the older population further affect pulmonary function. For example, the changes of chronic bronchitis and emphysema limit lung excursion; deformities of thoracic vertebrae, as in the gibbous of osteoporosis, diminish maximum breathing capacity.

Resistance and normal defense barriers to airborne infections diminish with age; therefore, bacteria and viruses more easily invade the lungs of the elderly, especially those with a history of chronic bronchitis. The body responds to bacterial pneumonia in four stages, described below (Robbins 1974).

Once the bacteria are able to establish themselves in the lungs, the number of bacteria rises rapidly and serous exudation increases. The body's response includes vascular engorgement and an increase in the numbers of intraalveolar neutrophils. This response is the *first stage* of congestion within the alveoli. Other elements are added during the *second stage*—namely, the precipitation of fibrin and the extravasation of red blood cells into alveoli already engorged with serous exudate, bacteria, and neutrophils; thus the normal pulmonary structure of discrete alveoli is altered.

The alveoli are distended with the material; together they form consolidation. The area of respiratory gas exchange becomes proportionately reduced. The *third stage* is characterized by further precipitation of fibrin and disintegration of both inflammatory neutrophils and erythrocytes. In most cases the *fourth,* and final, *stage* is one of resolution of the consolidated exudate by phagocytic digestive enzymes. Any debris from this digestion is either resorbed or coughed up. During the acute phase the diminished area of gas exchange results in anoxemia and, of course, dyspnea.

Pulmonary embolism is another acute respiratory problem frequently seen in the aged, especially those immobilized by bone fractures or otherwise confined to bed. In this disorder the emboli become lodged in a blood vessel, effectively blocking blood flow to respiratory tissue upstream of the obstruction. This blockage leads to a reduction in blood oxygenation and thus again results in anoxemia and dyspnea.

PNEUMONIA—ACUTE PULMONARY DISORDER

Although pneumococcal (diplococcus) pneumonia is the most common cause of bacterial pneumonia, other significant etiologic agents include *streptococcus, pneumonia viruses* and the *influenza virus.* Together these latter account for two-thirds of all fatalities due to pneumonia and are particularly harsh on the elderly (Freeman 1973). The diagnosis of etiologic agents—in particular mycoplasma, influenza, and legionnaires disease—is suggested by an epidemic situation (Reichel 1978; Lattimer and Rhodes 1978).

Nursing Assessment

Subjective Findings. Only rarely does the elderly client present with the classic pneumonia findings, which are an upper respiratory infection for 2 to 3 days, followed by chills, vomiting, stabbing chest pain, and a productive cough. More commonly seen are dyspnea, a mucopurulent cough, listlessness, lethargy, and nocturnal confusion.

Objective Findings. On examination the client appears to be ill; the older client, less so. Pulse and respiratory rate are increased (Capell and Case 1976). Temperature may be high, slightly elevated, or, in the very ill, subnormal. The latter is a grave prognostic sign. Cyanosis of the lips and nail beds and hypotension indicate severe infection.

Checking the gag reflex of all elderly clients who present with respiratory problems is imperative. Neurological impairment may lead to an ineffective gag reflex and to aspiration problems. The cough mechanism should be checked to determine the existence of bulbar involvement from a neurological problem. The client should be instructed to take a deep breath and cough deeply. On examining the chest, the nurse will find dullness in the area of involvement, increased tactile fremitus and voice transmission, and crepitant rales. In bronchopneumonia percussion signs are less obvious, and a variety of rhonchi and bullous rales are often audible. In atypical pneumonia objective findings are less evident.

Nursing assessment of the client's hydration status may be performed by comparing the relationship between intake and output. Equally important are observation of skin turgor and mucous membranes. Daily weighing and changes in daily monitored vital signs of the client provide a quick reference to fluid loss.

Diagnostics

The chest x-ray may be extremely helpful by indicating the area of involvement; it also may be diagnostic as to the type of infection that is present. The pneumococcal pneumonia is less likely to cause the typical homogeneous consolidation of lobar pneumonia in the older client. The radiological findings usually appear as a mottled, patchy bronchopneumonia. Chest films in the virally infected client usually show a diffuse, bilateral, perihilar infiltrate. Pneumonia in a client infected with the staphylococcal organism can quickly progress to multiple abscess and cavitation, which will be demonstrated on x-ray. Mycoplasma infection will be demonstrated on x-ray as the classic perihilar infiltrate, although lobar consolidation is not unusual (Wanderer 1978). In legionnaires disease the image is of a migratory atypical pneumonia out of proportion to the clinical findings (Lattimer and Rhodes 1978).

Sputum smears and cultures for bacteria, pleuropneumonialike organisms, and acid-fast bacteria should be obtained. Blood cultures are frequently positive in clients infected with the pneumococcal organism. Diagnosis of mycoplasma infections and legionnaires disease requires complement fixation tests or antibodies from serum specimens collected early in the disease and 2 to 3 weeks later (Stark

1975; "Follow-up on Legionnaires Disease" 1977).

Nursing Management

Nursing management is aimed at alleviating symptoms and treating the client with an appropriate antibiotic when the causative organism is identified. Clients with chronic disease, hypotension, cyanosis, jaundice, or confusion and those not responding to treatment within 72 hours require hospitalization.

Health Education and Counseling. Hydration should be maintained, particularly in the presence of fever. Fever itself is not a problem, provided that it is not tiring the client. The nurse should encourage the intake of clear fluids, which will assist in the liquification of secretions. Additionally a cold-mist humidifier can be used.

The client should be instructed, in the presence of diaphoresis, to keep dry and warm and to avoid drafts and chilling. Rest is essential to minimize cardiopulmonary strain. The nurse can teach the client to splint the chest when coughing. Analgesics such as acetomenophen (Tylenol) or aspirin may be used for pain. Caution must be exercised in administering any sedative or hypnotic, such as codeine, as the elderly are very sensitive to these. Futhermore, since cough and sputum production are considered therapeutic, cough suppression is necessary only if it is tiring the client.

The nurse should teach the client how to avoid spreading the infection to other family members, such as by covering the mouth when coughing and special handling and disposal of tissues for sputum.

Dishes should be sterilized in a dishwasher, if possible, or soaked and washed in boiling water. When the client has an elderly spouse, a temporary change in sleeping arrangements to avoid cross-infection is advisable.

The client needs to be informed that recovery from pneumonia often requires a long-term period of convalescence and that this period is accentuated because of reduced health resilience. The client will need to take frequent rest periods, eat a well-balanced diet, and avoid overexertion. Furthermore, avoiding contact with persons who have respiratory infections is most important (Jones et al. 1978, p. 1058).

Treatment. Antibiotic management is quite specific. After sputum and blood cultures are obtained, the client with lobar patchy pneumonia may be treated with penicillin "V" 1 to 29 g daily in divided doses. The response is dramatic, and treatment should be continued until the client has been afebrile for 72 hours. Any client who fails to respond to treatment within 48 hours must be referred to a physician. When a concomitant urinary infection is present or if a gram-negative infection is suspected, ampicillin 4 to 8 g daily in divided doses may be tried first. Staphylococcal pneumonia requires 3 to 8 weeks of intravenous antibiotic therapy in the hospital. Either erythromycin or tetracycline can be used in the presence of a mycoplasma infection. Legionnaires disease resembles mycoplasma but is best treated with erythromycin 1 to 2 g daily in divided doses ("Follow-up on Legionnaires Disease" 1977). Chest x-rays should be repeated in 10 days and in 3 to 6 weeks after

325

completion of therapy, not only to measure the course of treatment, but also to ascertain the presence of late complications, such as delayed resolution, fibrosis, bronchiectasis, and cavitation. These disorders are possible forerunners to the development of chronic pulmonary problems, such as chronic obstructive pulmonary disease.

CHRONIC OBSTRUCTIVE PULMONARY DISORDERS (COPD)

Pathophysiology

The term *chronic obstructive pulmonary disease* (COPD) can be considered a misnomer because it implies that the disorder is a single disease (Wintrobe 1974, p. 1275). COPD is more accurately a syndrome seen in diseases characterized by persistent slowing of outflow during forced expiration ("Pulmonary Terms and Symbols" 1975). COPD can be observed in clients with chronic bronchitis, bronchiectasis, emphysema, and asthma. Persons who have asthma rarely develop COPD unless they have a positive smoking history. COPD is characterized by a generalized narrowing of airway structures and is usually accompanied by destruction of lung tissue. Although chronic bronchitis, emphysema, and bronchial asthma exhibit these common pathological features, each of these disease conditions has certain additional characteristic pathological features.

Chronic Bronchitis. The airway structures that are narrowed in chronic bronchitis are the large bronchi and smaller bronchioli; the trachea can also be involved. The pathological changes include an increase in the number and size of mucus-secreting cells and an excessive amount of mucus secreted. The mucus becomes thickened and may even become mucopurulent in exacerbated conditions. The thickened mucus interferes with ciliary activity in the airway and with the cough mechanism required to clear the airway. A classic symptom of chronic bronchitis, therefore, is the persistent productive cough. Other pathological changes in mucous tissue that result in airway narrowing and interfere with the cough mechanism are vasodilatation, congestion, and edema. In these disorders mucosa are infiltrated by lymphocytes and polymorphonuclear cells. Needless to say, areas of pulmonary membrane beyond the affected airways are underventilated; hypercapnia, hypoxemia, and cyanosis develop.

Emphysema. Smaller bronchioli become narrowed in chronic obstructive pulmonary emphysema. In addition, destruction of lung parenchyma occurs beyond the narrowed bronchioli. At the alveoli level, walls rupture and alveoli coalesce, thereby reducing the area for oxygen and carbon dioxide diffusion and exchange.

Some etiologic factors of emphysema include chronic bronchitis and bronchial asthma as well as serious pulmonary infections. The chief etiologic factor linked to the development of emphysema is a positive history of smoking. When bronchiolar mucosal walls become edematous or thickened because of an increase in the number and size of mucus-secreting, or goblet, cells, as seen in chronic bronchitis, the end result is a narrowing of the terminal airway. This narrowing also occurs when the muscular layer of bronchioli becomes hypertrophied, as in bronchial asthma. A consequence of this narrowing is the trapping of air in alveoli and an increase in the pressure exerted on the walls of these delicate structures. The excessive pressure causes disruption of the alveolar walls, and the normal air space is enlarged as alveoli coalesce. Blood capillaries in septa between alveoli are destroyed, thereby diminishing the area of effective respiratory membrane.

Since expiration consists of a passive recoil of lung tissue and relaxation of respiratory muscles, the outward flow of expired air in clients who have severe emphysema is slowed because of airway resistance. Residual volume is consequently increased. Typically such clients are dyspneic and are obliged to make every effort to exhale forcibly to get rid of trapped air. Respiratory acidosis can develop in severe emphysema.

Bronchial Asthma. The bronchi are involved in the pathological airway narrowing seen in bronchial asthma. Changes involve hypertrophy of the smooth muscle layers, engorgement of mucosa, and hyperactivity of goblet cells. Bronchial obstruction is generally diffuse and usually reversible because it is almost always allergenic in nature. However, with repeated attacks the airway narrowing can become permanent and lung parenchyma can become thickened and ultimately destroyed.

The incriminating agent causing smooth-muscle constriction has not been conclusively identified; however, the reaction is known to be caused by exposure to substances to which the individual is hypersensitive. These substances include inhalants, drugs, and food, including fluid. The autoimmune response also includes respiratory mucosal edema. Blood vessels become engorged and dilate, causing exudation of plasma and diapedesis of leukocytes. Hyperactivity of mucus-secreting cells results in the excessive production of mucus, frequently tenacious in consistency.

Nursing Assessment

As previously stated, COPD is a diffuse, nonspecific pulmonary disorder due to a variety of etiologic factors. It is characterized by cough and sputum, with or without an uncomfortable dyspnea; findings may be either intermittent or continuous. COPD has become one of the most frequently encountered pulmonary syndromes. It increases in incidence with aging and accounts for considerable morbidity, mortality, and economic loss.

Nursing assessment of a chronic obstructive pulmonary disorder requires the exclusion of a localized pulmonary disease or certain other generalized diseases due to granuloma, fibrosis, collagen disease, pneumoconiosis, primary cardiovascular disease, chest wall diseases, and functional disease (Knowles 1962). The breathing and coughing mechanisms of the COPD client must be carefully assessed. Often the client has an ineffective cough mechanism and therefore a defective cleansing mechanism.

Although respiratory obstruction occurs characteristically in primary pulmonary disorders, such as asthma, chronic bronchitis, and bronchiectasis, in most instances bronchitis and emphysema coexist in the same client. Causative factors include cigarette smoking, environmental pollution, recurrent infection, and bronchial irritation (Reichel 1978). Clinical presentation is due primarily to two abnormalities: generalized narrowing of bronchi

327

and destruction of lung tissue. These changes lead to a spectrum of subjective and objective findings irrespective of the etiology.

Subjective Findings. The initial subjective complaint is shortness of breath with exertion, often associated with wheezing. Frequently the client has morning dyspnea with a sensation of chest tightness relieved by expectoration of sputum. Asthmatics may have episodes of chest tightness and dyspnea occurring during the day or awakening them between 2:00 and 4:00 A.M. As the disease progresses, dyspnea becomes more prominent and is provoked by less exertion and by contact with bronchial "irritants," such as dust, smoke, perfume, or cold air. It is usually then associated with orthopnea and shortness of breath on stooping. At this point dyspnea begins to interfere with daily activities and may be provoked by emotional upset or arguments.

Commonly the client has a long history of cigarette smoking and a morning cough (usually ignored). The nurse should ascertain the number of packs normally smoked and the number of years the client has smoked. Additionally the nurse often finds a history of chronic bronchitis or an annual "winter bronchitis." Cough may be precipitated by lying down at night or by changing position in bed. Sputum production may vary from small amounts of thick, mucoid material to copious amounts of mucopurulent material or even frank pus. Sputum is usually most abundant in the morning on arising. Older clients with increasing hypercapnea and anoxia may develop mental confusion at night or even during the day, which is often sufficient reason for hospitalization. A history of asthma or of frequent or recurrent pulmonary infections is important to note.

Objective Findings. The nurse should be watchful for episodes of airway obstruction and ventilatory failure. The client will present with hypoxia, hypercapnea, and respiratory acidosis. This diagnosis can be made only by the measurement of arterial blood gases. If the client's $PaCO_2$ (partial pressure of CO_2) is above 50, or if PaO_2 (partial pressure of O_2) is below 50, or if these findings coexist, the client must be assumed to be in acute respiratory failure. Immediate hospitalization is indicated for this condition (Reichel 1978).

On physical examination the COPD client may present a large variety of findings that have been clinically and pathologically classified in recent years. The client is usually over 50 years of age. The extreme ends of the spectrum are the emphysematous type, or "pink puffer," and the bronchitic type, or "blue bloater." Between these two lie a large number of intermediate types of mixed clinical presentations (Howell 1971).

The type A, or emphysematous, client ("pink puffer") is usually underweight and presents with severe exertional dyspnea. The mucus membranes and nail beds are pink. No clubbing is seen. The chest is fixed and expanded, and the secondary respiratory muscles of the neck are prominent. The chest percussion notes are hyperresonant. Respiratory auscultation sounds are reduced and have a prolonged expiratory phase. Sibilant rhonchi are audible on forced expiration. Heart sounds as well as cardiac pulsations are most prominent in the epigastrium. Many older clients with emphysema have a persistent mild pulmonary infection, and when an acute episode occurs, it may only manifest itself as a slight change in the client's usual symptoms, such as increased shortness of breath, changes in sputum character, or increased cough. Such clients have a normal CO_2 sensitivity and do not suffer CO_2 narcosis when treated with oxygen therapy.

The type B, or bronchitic, client ("blue bloater") presents with a long history of chronic bronchitis and recurrent episodes of purulent sputum production. Exercise tolerance, initially good, gradually deteriorates or may deteriorate precipitously after an acute bout of infection. Along with the diminishing exercise tolerance, mild ankle edema appears. This condition is initially present at the end of the day and then becomes present constantly and more extensively. The "blue bloater" is plethoric, appearing with cyanosis at rest, and the extremities are warm. Slight chest expansion is present, and the expiratory phase is prolonged. Rhonchi and basal crepitant rales are present on auscultation. Cardiac enlargement, distended jugular veins, hepatomegaly, and edema of the lower extremities are often evident. These symptoms increase during acute exacerbations, which may precipitate cor pulmonale. Such clients have a diminished CO_2 sensitivity and are at risk of CO_2 narcosis if given oxygen therapy.

The nurse must distinguish between acute exacerbations of chronic bronchitis and emphysema on the one hand and asthmatic episodes on the other. A prior history of allergies or asthma with recurrent episodes of chest tightness or dyspnea during the day or episodes that awaken the client at night is suggestive of asthma. Asthma of itself rarely causes COPD unless the client has a positive smoking history. When asthma first begins in older adulthood, it is usually of the intrinsic type and may be resistive to desensitization.

Diagnostic

Laboratory studies of the emphysematous client reveal an increased total lung capacity and residual volume. Vital capacity and FEV_1 (forced expiratory volume) are decreased; $PaCO_2$ is normal; and PaO_2 is normal or slightly decreased. The chest x-ray shows hyperinflated lungs and a long, narrow heart.

Laboratory studies of the bronchitic client demonstrate a normal lung capacity with an increased residual volume. The FEV_1 is moderately diminished. $PaCO_2$ is increased and PaO_2 slightly decreased. Hematocrit and hemoglobin levels may be increased due to secondary polycythemia. The chest x-ray may show increased bronchial markings, right ventricular prominence, and, during exacerbations, evidence of congestive heart failure. In clients with a cough and morning chest tightness, one must suspect chronic obstructive pulmonary disease. Although prolonged expiration and a decreased FEV_1 are diagnostic of COPD, these findings appear late in the progression of the disease.

Eosinophilia in blood and sputum is a confirmatory sign of asthma with an allergic etiology. If any doubt is present, the client should be referred to a physician for ventilatory studies with appropriate bronchodilators (Howell 1971).

Nursing Management

Clients suffering from COPD require an aggressive management plan to alleviate symptoms and promote optimal functioning. Management is designed to permit normal daily activities with a minimum of

329

symptoms and to reduce the frequency and severity of the exacerbations. These effects are accomplished by decreasing bronchial irritation, controlling infection, increasing exercise tolerance, and minimizing bronchoconstriction and secretions. If etiologic factors can be eliminated early in the disease, evidence suggests that clinical improvement can be expected (Speir 1976).

Sputum studies of the client who has COPD usually reveal only normal oropharyngeal bacteria that have invaded the lower air passages because of the decreased ability of these passages to defend themselves. Viral infections of the passages increase secretions, permit secondary bacterial overgrowth, and, in clients with chronic bronchitis, are a cause of occasionally fatal exacerbation.

Treatment. Many studies have shown that antibiotics such as the penicillins and tetracyclines are useful in clearing these infections (Speir 1976). Penicillin "V," ampicillin, or tetracycline, all in dosages of 250 mg daily in four divided doses, should be used whenever cough and sputum increase or when sputum becomes purulent.

Occasionally clients with recurrent infection will require more frequent treatment. They may be given a prescription for tetracycline and advised to use this drug at the onset of a cold or if the sputum changes color. The drug should be continued for at least 5 days. Some clients will require prophylactic antibiotic treatment during the winter months.

Health Education and Counseling. The gerontological nurse should be involved in the primary prevention of infection. Clients should be instructed to avoid crowds or exposure to individuals with respiratory infections. Maintenance of good nutrition and adequate hydration, balanced with an exercise program, will help to ward off infection.

1. *Restorative Nursing Measures:* In order to obtain clinical improvement, a change in the client's lifestyle often is required.

> Medical management is usually centered on relief of symptoms, but a new way of living may have to be found if the symptoms are to be kept under control. This new life-style is not followed in response to a prescription—it must be taught to the patient in such a way that he will become actively involved in his own restoration. [Coulter 1974, p. 397]

Among the things that are important in altering the client's lifestyle are conservation of energy and avoidance of fatigue. Clients should be instructed to take frequent rests. They should seek out resting sites when shopping or walking. The progressive physical changes that may eventually incapacitate the client can be slowed by a program of regular exercises to increase muscular strength and retrain breathing patterns. In addition to relieving physical symptoms, the exercise program will help the client combat apathy and helplessness by demonstrating that something can be done to control the symptoms.

Exercise and good physical conditioning are important, but they take on increasing relevance for clients with chronic respiratory problems. Perhaps one of the most important benefits the nurse can accomplish for such clients is to instill in them the confidence necessary to learn to help themselves through breathing retraining and general exercise. Since the course of chronic respiratory ailments leads the clients to become more and more sedentary, a graded exercise program to build muscle strength is essential. The client's condition may preclude any exercise other than the practice of new breathing techniques. Seriously ill clients may experience shortness of breath even while sitting in a chair. The technique of blowing out a candle at increasing distances may be a starting point for an exercise regimen.

In the emphysematous client the chest cage is enlarged on both expiration and inspiration. The usefulness of the diaphragm muscle is decreased because of its flattened shape, caused by the chronic increase in lung volume, and consequent inability to rise on expiration. In an effort to compensate, intercostal muscles and accessory muscles, such as the sternocleidomastoids, the scalenus group, the trapezius, and the latissimus, become involved in the work of breathing. Such breathing requires a tremendous expenditure of energy. Therefore, the aims of therapy are directed toward minimizing the energy requirements of respiration by reducing noncontributory associated movements of respiration (Dirschel 1973, pp. 618–619).

To restore the mechanical advantages of the normal diaphragm, the client must learn to use the abdominal muscles to assist in pushing the diaphragm upward. Prior to initiation of the exercise, the nurse should instruct the client to practice pushing the abdomen out and pulling it back in. The client is instructed to lie on the back with bent knees supported by pillows and with hands on the lower ribs. Attention is drawn to suppressing chest movements and distending the abdominal muscles on inspira-

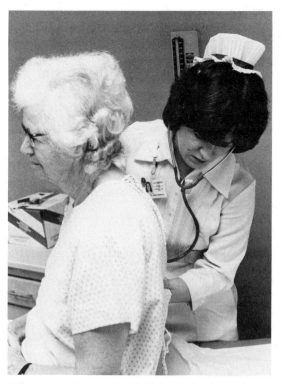

The gerontological nurse can help the elderly adapt to the aging process by emphasizing the importance of regular physical examinations and selective checkups; elderly clients need individualized instruction in the specific measures that will help them promote health and prevent illness.

tion and contracting the abdominal muscles on expiration.

Pursed-lip expiration establishes resistance by forming a mechanical obstruction with the lips. This resistance presumably increases pressure, which is reflected backward in the tracheobronchial tree. By holding the "pursed" breath for a count of 2 or 3, the airflow can be controlled in a slow stream.

Another measure that can assist breathing effort is aimed at using the abdominal viscera as a pressure lift for the diaphragm.

331

To accomplish this feat, the client must wear an abdominal belt daily. Daily abdominal exercises will also increase abdominal breathing ability. Weights can be applied to increase the workload of the abdominal muscles and eventually strengthen them. The weights are added in graded amounts, beginning with 1 pound the first week and adding a pound each week until a maximum of 10 pounds is reached. The maximum amount is used from that point daily in the exercise regimen (Dirschel 1973). When the nurse teaches these new breathing methods, an important principle to remember is to extend the excitement intervals. Maintaining a calm atmosphere and reducing emotional stress will decrease the client's need for oxygen. Emotional-stress factors may be observed in family relationships or in the lifestyle the COPD client is forced to lead. Both the client and family need ongoing encouragement and empathetic support. If the problems require long-term therapy or counseling beyond the nurse's ability, the client should be referred to an appropriate community mental health center or therapist.

2. *Reduction of Bronchial Irritation:* Clients must be encouraged to stop smoking or at least to diminish the number of cigarettes smoked. Cigarette smoke is by far the most common bronchial irritant. Although the chances of breaking the habit are small, the client must be convinced that cigarette smoke plays a vital part in the continued progression of the disorder.

The nurse can counsel the client to avoid environmental pollutants, such as smoke, smog, and household dust. The house or apartment must be made as environmentally safe as possible by reducing pollutants, especially in the sleeping area. Carpeting or rugs where dust can hide should be avoided in the bedroom. The house should be humidified in dry winter months and air-conditioned in summer months. A client who resides in an area of heavy pollution could be advised to relocate.

Some clients may have a disorder with an allergenic basis. Such clients should receive allergy treatment, preferably of the provocative dose method. The provocative dose desensitization program treats the client by testing for the optimal dose level of each antigen. Maintenance therapy is calculated by the individual's symptom response provoked by the antigen. When possible, the offending inhalant allergens should be removed from the environment. In mild-to-moderate disease, discontinuing contact with the chronic irritant may be rewarded by a normalization of pulmonary function and a return to health.

3. *Minimizing Bronchoconstriction and Secretions:* Bronchoconstriction and mucus produced by bronchial irritation play a significant role by reducing air flow and alveolar ventilation. The variety of medications used are particularly effective if bronchial narrowing due to smooth-muscle spasm or mucosal edema of chronic bronchitis is still reversible.

Anhydrous theophylline is quite effective and generally well tolerated by clients. The degree of bronchodilation is directly related to the theophylline blood levels. Improvement is characterized by an increase in air flow, a reduction in wheezing, and a subjective feeling of amelioration. Side effects of theophylline, such as nausea, vomiting, and heartburn, are usually decreased by lowering the dosage. Turbuteline, a sympathomimetic amine, is a beta receptor antagonist and avoids the palpitations induced by alpha receptor drugs such as ephedrine. Nebulizers with a variety of bronchodilators are popular because of administrative ease and rapid onset, but they should generally be avoided because of overdosage problems. These medications are pharmacologically active in the cardiovascular system. They increase heart rate and cardiac oxygen requirements. Overdosage can cause death by ventricular arrhythmia.

If clients are well hydrated, sputum elimination will normally not be a problem. Hence stressing fluid intake is important. Expectorants may be required if sputa are thick and tenacious or when the client is in an infection phase. Glyceryl quaiacolate or SSKI (Saturated Solution of Potassium Iodide) 30 cc two to four times daily can serve as effective expectorant agents. SSKI should be avoided in clients with tuberculosis.

Cromolyn disodium (Intal and Aarane) is a relatively new drug found to be helpful to asthmatics. The drug is in powdered form and is inhaled into the lungs through a special nebulizer from one to four times daily. The drug inhibits the effects of histamine's destruction of mast cells, thereby preventing attacks. Like medication for the treatment of hypertension, this drug must be taken routinely and is not to be used for the acute phase of the asthma attack.

Cough suppressants such as codeine and dextromethorphan and drying agents such as antihistamines should be avoided. These drugs tend to cause retention of mucus and to increase air-flow resistance. Corticoste-roids in large doses should be used only after physician evaluation.

The primary aim of management must be to arrest chronic lung disease in its early stages. This strategy not only will diminish disability but may prevent the awesome complications of bronchogenic cancer.

LUNG CANCER

Pathophysiology

Any consideration of pulmonary diseases seen in an elderly population must include lung neoplasms. Longevity increases the chances for exposure to suspected predisposing factors such as cigarette smoking, air pollutants, ionizing radiation, and a number of industrial hazards, such as asbestos.

Squamous, or epidermoid, cell carcinoma is the neoplasm most frequently seen in lung cancer. The pulmonary structures involved in 90 percent of cases are the bronchi (Robbins 1974). The pathological changes usually originate in the region of the hilus of the lung and the first, second, and third order of the bronchi. Focal thickening of bronchial mucosa is seen in the early developmental stages. The neoplasm can obstruct the airway by occluding the passageway or through a metastatic process in the thoracic cavity, thereby creating external pressure on lung parenchyma, other airway structures, and blood vessels and nerves within the chest. The symptoms presented depend on the extent of the tumor growth and on the structures involved.

In the United States cancer ranks as the second leading cause of death for all ages.

333

The incidence of lung cancer is second only to gastrointestinal neoplasm. The ratio of male to female victims in older clients still reflects that of twenty years ago (six men to one woman). This fact suggests that older women have not increased their smoking habits (Ross 1976). However, these figures have dramatically changed for middle-aged women, as shown by the marked increase in lung cancer in this group. Cigarette smoking is the primary cause of lung cancer (Zimmerman 1976); when cigarette smoke is associated with asbestos dust and radioactive substances, the carcinogenic effects are enhanced (Seidman et al. 1976).

There are no 5-year survivors among clients over 65 years of age with lung cancer, and only 24 percent of this age group presents with localized, resectable lesions (Petty 1976). One-half to two-thirds of such clients will be dead in 6 to 18 months after resection.

Nursing Assessment

Early disease is usually asymptomatic and initial findings may be confusing. These findings are most often localized to the chest but may be extrathoracic, indicating metastases or a paraneoplastic syndrome, which can imitate an endocrinopathy or mimic a primary neurological disorder.

Subjective Findings. Complaints localized to the chest are not specific; they only indicate pulmonary disease and require further study. Highly suspicious signs include dyspnea out of proportion to the client's age and general condition; weight loss; a chronic cough lasting over 1 week, particularly in the absence of infection; or a change in cough pattern in a client with chronic pulmonary disease. A client who exhibits wheezing of recent onset may have partial bronchial obstruction. Hemoptysis in clients over 40 years of age may be due to erosion of pulmonary blood vessels caused by a tumor.

The localization or extension of the tumor may cause a variety of findings. Involvement of the carina causes early, severe dyspnea. Pain, a late complaint, usually indicates extension to the pleura or chest wall, while phrenic nerve involvement causes pain in the affected shoulder.

Objective Findings. Lymph node enlargement in the supraclavicular or scalene nodes may be the primary findings, or the client may present with an asymptomatic pleural effusion. Horner's syndrome indicates invasion of the stellate ganglion and is found with a Pancoast tumor, which is located at the lung apex. Aphonia or dysphonia are found with invasion of the recurrent laryngeal nerve in the superior mediastinum.

Metastatic disease may cause presenting complaints, including extrathoracic bone pain, vertebral collapse, headache, evidence of intracranial tumor, or Addison's disease due to metastatic destruction of the suprarenal glands. Paraneoplastic findings may consist of pulmonary osteoarthropathy with clubbing or endocrinopathies imitating hyperparathyroidism, Cushing's syndrome, or myasthenia gravis (Weiss 1977). Other syndromes appear as cerebellar disease, peripheral neuropathies, or lower motor neuron palsies.

Diagnostics

All clients with the symptoms described above—particularly those with weight loss, hemoptysis, and clubbing—should have a chest x-ray, which will usually reveal some lesion either in the lung periphery or mediastinum. Unfortunately, by the time the lesion becomes visible, 90 percent of clients will die of their disease (Armstrong and Bragg 1975).

Nursing Management

Clients with lesions clearly should be referred to a physician for further evaluation. The nurse can continue to coordinate care and to offer supportive counseling to the client and family. This kind of management provides the continuum of care so often neglected in the oncological victim.

Frequently, particularly in the older client, pulmonary function may be so poor that surgical resection may not be possible. In such cases palliation is the only possible course. Intensive cooperation among all members of the health team will be required to alleviate pain and infection by providing appropriate emotional support as well as palliative medication. Close rapport should be maintained between the client and family with the purpose of sustaining the client's sense of well-being and promoting optimal functioning.

Until better diagnostic and therapeutic techniques become available, prevention through reduction of cigarette smoking and industrial irritants will require encouragement and a concerted effort of education through health instruction, films, and educational material.

SUMMARY

Respiratory problems in the elderly need careful assessment and monitoring by the gerontological nurse. Measures for the promotion of health and prevention of illness are provided to the client and family through careful instruction regarding medications, exercise, and nutrition. Newly diagnosed or acute situations need prompt referral to the physician for further evaluation and attention.

REFERENCES

American Cancer Society. 1976. *Cancer Facts and Figures.* New York.

ANDERSON, F. 1976. *The Practical Management of the Elderly.* Oxford: Blackwell Scientific Publications.

ARMSTRONG, J. D., and D. G. BRAGG. 1975. "Radiology in Lung Cancer: Problems and Prospects." *A Cancer Journal for Clinicians* 25:242–57.

BURNSIDE, I., ed. 1976. *Nursing and the Aged.* New York: McGraw-Hill.

CAPELL, P., and D. CASE. 1976. *Ambulatory Care Manual for Nurse Practitioners.* Philadelphia: J. B. Lippincott.

COULTER, P. P. 1974. "Physical and Muscular Reconditioning." In Christopherson, Coulter, and Wolanin, eds., *Rehabilitation Nursing Prospects and Applications.* New York: McGraw-Hill.

DIRSCHEL, K. 1973. "Respiration in Emphysema Patients." *Nursing Clinics of North America* 8(4):618–19.

"Follow-up on Legionnaires Disease." 1977. *Morbidity Mortality Weekly Reports* 26:43.

———. 1977. *Morbidity Mortality Weekly Reports* 26:111.

FREEMAN, E. 1973. "The Respiratory System." In J. C. Brocklehurst, ed., *Textbook of Geriatric Medicine and Gerontology.* London: Churchill Livingstone.

GILLUS, D. and I. ALYN. 1976. *Patient Assessment and Management by the Nurse Practitioner.* Philadelphia: W. B. Saunders

GUYTON, A. C. 1976. *Textbook of Medical Physiology.* Philadelphia: W. B. Saunders.

HINSHAW, H. C. 1969. *Diseases of the Chest.* Philadelphia: W. B. Saunders.

HOWELL, J. B. L. 1971. "Airway Obstruction." In P. B. Beeson and W. McDermott, eds., *Cecil-Loeb Textbook of Medicine,* 13th ed. Philadelphia: W. B. Saunders.

HYDE, L., et al. 1965. "Cell-Type and the Natural History of Lung Cancer." *Journal of the American Medical Association* 193:52–54.

JONES, D. A., C. F. DUNBAR, and M. M. JIROVIC. 1978. *Medical Surgical Nursing: A Conceptual Approach.* New York: McGraw-Hill.

KNOWLES, J. H. 1962. "Chronic Bronchitis and Emphysema." In T. R. Harrison, ed., *Principles of Internal Medicine,* 4th ed. New York: McGraw-Hill.

LATTIMER, G., and L. V. RHODES. 1978. "Legionnaires Disease: Clinical Findings and One Year Follow-up." *Journal of the American Medical Association* 240:1169–71.

McDERMOTT, W. 1971. "Pneumonia." In P. A. Beeson and W. McDermott, eds., *Cecil-Loeb Textbook of Medicine,* 13th ed. Philadelphia: W. B. Saunders.

PETTY, T. L. 1976. "Chronic Respiratory Diseases." In F. U. Steinberg, ed., *Cowdry's The Care of the Geriatric Patient,* 5th ed. St. Louis: C. V. Mosby.

"Pulmonary Terms and Symbols: A Report of the ACCP–ATS Joint Committee on Pulmonary Nomenclature." 1975. *Chest* 67(5):583–93.

REICHEL, W. 1978. "Pulmonary Problems in the Elderly." In W. Reichel, ed., *Clinical Aspects of Aging.* Baltimore: Williams Wilkins.

"Respiratory Diseases: Task Force Report on Problems, Research Approaches, Needs." 1972. DHEW Publication No. (NIH) 73–432. Washington, D.C.: U.S. Government Printing Office.

ROBBINS, S. L. 1974. *Pathological Basis of Disease.* Philadelphia: W. B. Saunders.

ROSS, W. M. 1976. "How to Deal with Bronchogenic Carcinoma in the Elderly." *Geriatrics* 31:107–10.

RUNYAN, J. 1975. *Primary Care Guide.* New York: Harper and Row.

SEIDMAN, H., E. SILVERBERG, and A. I. HOLLEB. 1976. "Cancer Statistics 1976: A Comparison of White and Black Populations." *A Cancer Journal for Clinicians* 26:2–29.

SPEIR, W. A., JR. 1976. "Outpatient Management of Chronic Bronchitis and Emphysema." *Geriatrics* 31:47–80.

STARK, J. E. 1975. "Diseases of the Respiratory Tract and Infectious Diseases." In H. P. von Hahn, *Practical Geriatrics.* New York and Basel: S. Karger, A.G.

TIMARIS, P. S. 1972. *Developmental Physiology and Aging.* New York: Macmillan.

WANDERER, M. J. 1978. "Acute Respiratory Illness." In C. J. Leitch and R. V. Tinker, *Primary Care.* Philadelphia: F. A. Davis.

WEISS, R. 1977. "Small Cell Carcinoma: The Different Type of Lung Cancer." *Geriatrics* 32:75–79.

WINTROBE, M. M., ed. 1974. *Harrison's Principles of Internal Medicine.* New York: McGraw-Hill.

ZIMMERMAN, S. 1976. "Nursing the Patient with Lung Cancer." In B. Peterson and C. Kellogg, eds., *Current Practice in Oncologic Nursing.* St. Louis: C. V. Mosby.

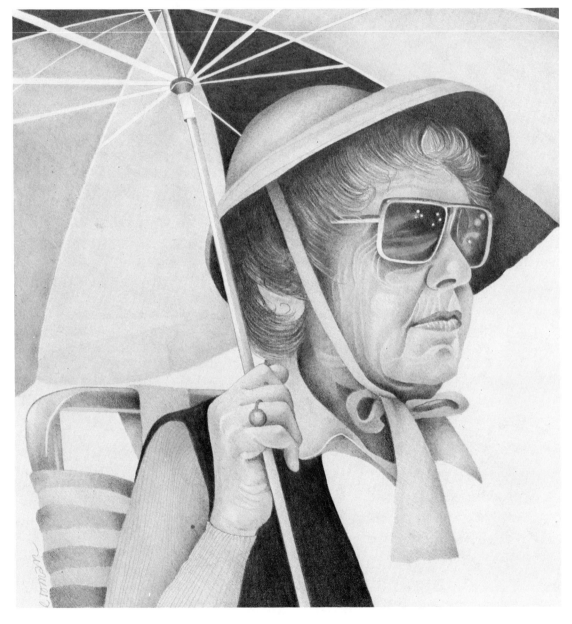

Chapter 12

THE ELDERLY CLIENT WITH A DERMATOLOGICAL PROBLEM

The skin is composed of dermis and epidermis, which participate in a wide variety of pathological disorders that appear as lesions. The skin, or integument, is the most visible and largest organ of the body. Its primary function is to protect the internal organs from the environment. The skin also has an important role in temperature regulation and, in humans, is responsible for a daily obligatory water loss, which can be considerable when perspiration occurs.

SKIN DISORDERS

Pathophysiology

Skin Responses to Infection and Disease. The skin is frequently involved in host responses to infection; in fact, skin lesions often help establish the diagnosis before the etiologic agent is identified. Skin responses to infection are multiple—for example, jaundice is seen in infectious hepatitis; a diffuse cutaneous lesion caused by hyperemia and vascular dilation, in scarlet fever; and vesicular skin lesions, in chicken pox and small pox.

Because of the rich vascular bed in skin papillae and in subpapillary connective tissue layers, skin changes color and thus gives clues about systemic as well as localized problems. The pallor of anemia and of the arteriolar spasm of Raynaud's disease is a good example of how the skin serves to indicate diseases. As another example, serious local circulatory obstruction is often detected by asking the client to elevate the hand and arm above the heart and by observing whether the pallor of the extremity persists for longer than 5 seconds when the hand is lowered to heart level. A permanent change in skin color can, of course, be symptomatic of generalized poor circulation due to ineffective heart action. In addition, skin temperature, which is dependent upon blood flow in dermal blood vessels, can be a barometer for cardiac problems. Edema, from any of several causes, can also affect skin temperature.

Age-Related Changes in the Skin. With advancing years, the upper layers of skin, or epidermis, undergo changes such as a diminution of epidermal depth or thickness. Such thinning is due to diminished activity of basal layer cells, which results in a decrease in the number of cell layers, or atrophy. Individual epidermal cells also undergo change with age; they tend to separate from each other and at times form keratin, an insoluble protein, within the germinal layer. Keratin formation leads to scaling, hyperkeratosis, and water loss, all of which can cause pruritic eczema.

The deeper layers, or dermal tissue, also exhibit age changes—for example, the numbers of mast cells decrease with age. Mast cells appear to be related to tissue repair. Collagen fibers show a degeneration of individual fibers and a loss of network or bundle arrangement. This loss is thought to explain why aged skin loses its elasticity. The nerve endings, or receptors serving cutaneous sensation for touch, pressure, heat, cold, and pain, can also be affected.

Changes in skin appendages such as hair, glands, and nails are seen in the aged. Graying of hair occurs as pigment is lost from the cortex of the hair follicle. Sebaceous and sweat glands undergo atrophy, while the rate of growth slows in finger- and toenails. The nails become brittle, ridged, and distorted. Further, loss of elasticity and fat leads to decreased thickness and diminished resistance to trauma,

which cause disturbances of cutaneous integrity and a decrease in the speed of healing. These latter processes, while not specific to the aged skin, occur more frequently in older age than during the younger periods of life (Pillsbury 1975). Older skin also responds differently to cutaneous sensation because of changes in central nervous system perception, leading to pruritus of the aged (Young 1971), while increased vascular fragility allows easy bruising (Rockstein 1975).

Nursing Assessment

Any classification of skin disease is at best arbitrary; this discussion is limited to conditions commonly found in the older adult. More complete discussions can be found in texts devoted to dermatology, some of which are listed in the references.

The assessment of skin disease requires a skillfully elicited history. The nurse must consider the type of sensation described by the client, infectious contact, climactic conditions, occupational exposure, allergenic origins, and any form of treatment applied by the client.

When examining the client, the nurse must evaluate the lesions and their evolution through various stages. The nurse should note the location and pattern of the lesions as well as their form, distribution on the body, shape, geographic arrangement or configuration, surface characteristics, consistency, moisture, color, and dominant hue.

Lesions That Are Usually Pruritic: Nursing Assessment

Dermatitis. The lesions of nummular dermatitis or lichen simplex tend to recur and are either localized or generalized. The *localized* lesions are distributed at the back of the neck, the extensor surfaces of the forearms, the low back, and the anterior tibial surface. The lesions are linear scratch marks and lead to linear lichenification.

The nurse can differentiate this type of dermatitis from stasis dermatitis, as the latter is usually associated with edema of the lower extremities. Contact dermatitis is less frequently found in the elderly (Pillsbury 1975).

Generalized autosensitization is associated with pinhead-size red lesions. The pinhead lesions always appear after scratching and may spread to form nummular, confluent red plaques.

Winter Eczema. Winter eczema is composed of two types of lesions that appear in the winter, when central heating dries the skin: one is a dry, fissured lesion that weeps when rubbed; the other is a papular lesion that appears on the exterior of the thighs and upper extremities.

Seborrheic Dermatitis. Seborrheic dermatitis consists of an erythematous rash of the forehead and face that is often but not always pruritic. Findings include dandruff in the hair and a fine scale on the brows.

Pruritus Ani and Vulvae. Lesions from pruritus ani and vulvae form a diffuse redness with linear scratches in the perineum. The lesions result from poor hygiene, chafing caused by trapped moisture from nylon pantyhose, and obesity. The nurse must examine for pinworms, trichomoniasis, syphilis, Paget's skin disease, moniliasis, kraurosis vulvae, nonspecific vaginitis, and contact dermatitis.

Nummular Eczema. Nummular eczema is composed of large, annular red lesions, which suddenly appear on the skin. They are usually secondary to other conditions such as poison ivy, stasis dermatitis, and atopic or winter eczema (Pillsbury 1975).

Lesions Due to Infection: Nursing Assessment

Viral Infections. *Herpes zoster (shingles)* consists of a burning, painful area of skin, usually confined to a dermatome. The pain often precedes the eruption, which consists of a cluster of small bullae that usually group around the surface points of the primary branches of the involved nerve. The lesions may become necrotic and edematous. Postherpetic pain is more common in the elderly. This neuralgia may continue for months or years after the eruption heals. It often leads to depression and, when severe enough, suicide. The responsible virus is identical to chicken pox virus, but clients are only minimally contagious. Clients with lymphoma and Hodgkin's disease are particularly susceptible to this illness.

Bacterial Infections. *Staphylococcal infections* cause boils and carbuncles. Generalized furunculosis (boils), if recurrent, requires a search for diabetes.

Streptococcal infections are most commonly found as a cellulitis, often with pus or honey-colored crusts. They often are secondary to other chronic skin disorders associated with fissuring, such as athlete's foot, folliculitis, or chronic dermatitis. The onset is sudden; the area is warm, red, and plaquelike, and systemic findings such as fever or toxicity are usually present.

Fungal Infections. The older client may suffer from *athlete's foot* and *intertrigo*. Any skin fold where moisture collects can develop these lesions. They are often found as a diffuse erythema of the groin; in women they may be found under the breasts. When the fungus infects the nail—onychomycosis—the resultant hyper- and dyskeratosis require a differentiation from psoriasis.

Yeast infections of the vulva, groin, and glans penis cause an erythematous lesion with a white exudate. These lesions are not unusual in debilitated clients and in those with uncontrolled diabetes mellitus.

Bullous Lesions: Nursing Assessment

Some bullous lesions are caused by sensitivity to medication or contactants; rarely, they are the first indication of lymphoma. They are difficult to diagnose and treat and are best referred to a dermatologist.

Skin Tumors: Nursing Assessment

Skin tumors are hypertrophic lesions of the dermis or epidermis and are often easily identified by inspection and palpation. Any doubt as to their nature requires referral to a dermatologist for diagnosis and possible biopsy. Tumors are classified as benign, potentially malignant, and malignant. The last must be quickly referred to a dermatologist, as cure requires early and complete surgical removal.

Benign Tumors. *Moles* are circumscribed pigmented macules, papules, or nodules composed of clusters of nevus cells.

Lentigines are flat, uniformly pigmented, brown-to-black nevi found in the elderly. Although the freckle tends to fade when not exposed to sunlight, the lentigo shows no sign of such change. Lentigines are found in scattered distribution on the body.

Warts are sharply demarcated, rough surfaced, round or irregular, firm, and of varying color. They range in size from 2 to 10 mm in diameter. These hyperkeratotic lesions are found at points of trauma, such as the elbows and fingers. Plantar (foot) warts may be painful and may require surgical excision. The nurse must differentiate warts from callouses, which are usually smooth.

Seborrheic (sebaceous) adenomas are localized in the face. They are slow growing and vary from 1 to 5 mm in size, have a yellow tinge, are shiny and raised, and may have an irregular edge with a central umbilication. These adenomas must be differentiated from basal cell carcinoma and should be referred to a dermatologist or surgeon if any doubt exists about their nature.

Potentially Malignant Tumors. Tumors with malignant potential may be followed, but if any signs of malignancy appear, such as fullness in the epidermis, bleeding, or crusting, they must be referred to a physician for biopsy and removal. Referral should be made if the nurse has any question about their nature.

Seborrheic keratoses (seborrheic warts, senile warts) are slow-growing, superficial epithelial lesions that vary in size and are pigmented. While usually verrucous looking, they may consist of smooth, round or oval papules; have a stuck-on appearance; and exhibit a waxy scaling or crusted surface. Localized in sebaceous areas (face, neck, and upper chest), these lesions are greasy and dark, but they present with lighter pigmentation and are dry in areas of low sebaceous gland activity. Seborrheic keratoses are cosmetically embarrassing and can be confused with small basal cell epitheliomas (Tindall 1978). Although these lesions are not considered premalignant, they may occasionally show signs of degeneration.

Actinic keratoses are found in skin exposed to sunlight and are more common in persons with an occupational history of sunlight exposure (sailors, fishermen, construction workers). They are commonly found on the face, the ear, and the dorsum of the hands. These flat, gray, scaling lesions may also be wartlike, with a color ranging from yellow to brown to black and a horny appearance. Such lesions have malignant potential and should be referred to a dermatologist.

Malignant Tumors. A variety of primary malignancies of the skin may be found, such as basal cell epitheliomas, squamous cell carcinomas, and melanomas. Other systemic cancers, such as Hodgkin's lymphoma, can also have skin manifestations. All these lesions should be referred to a dermatologist for diagnosis and treatment.

The basal cell tumor is the most common skin malignancy and varies from a shiny, firm nodule to an ulcerated, crusted lesion. It may appear as a flat, scarlike, indurated plaque or as a lesion difficult to differentiate from psoriasis or localized dermatitis. The advanced lesion typically has a pearly border with telangiectasia and a small central ulcer (Tindall 1978).

Squamous cell tumors usually appear later in life than the basal variety. A squamous cell tumor can evolve from a preexisting le-

sion, such as actinic keratosis or leukoplakia, but may lack the pearly border; or it can develop in normal tissue. The lesion begins as a red papule or plaque with a scaly or crusted surface and can evolve into a nodular or warty lesion. Squamous cell tumors most often occur on the lower half of the face, with the lips serving as the dividing line; basal cell tumors commonly appear on the upper half of the face (Tindall 1978).

The gerontological nurse can help the elderly adapt to the aging process by encouraging them to accept age-related physical changes and to maintain a good physical appearance; elderly clients need a positive self-image and meaningful activities to develop a sense of well-being.

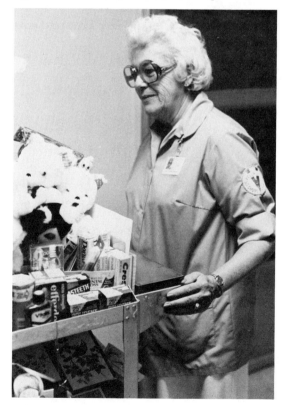

Nursing Management

Health Education and Counseling. Nurses have an obligation to educate clients in the primary prevention of skin cancer. This concern should be primary for those persons who, by virtue of occupation or avocation, are overexposed to the sun's radiation or who have migrated to warmer climates. Many of the elderly consider the sun's warm rays a welcome solace. They naïvely expose their aging skin to dehydration and solar radiation, thereby intensifying age changes and pathological skin conditions.

While inspecting the client's skin, the nurse can discuss the importance of self-inspection, personal hygiene for maintenance of healthy skin, and protection from sun exposure and trauma.

The triad of problems the client with a dermatological condition presents with includes disfigurement, pruritus, and discomfort. Disfigurement can create embarrassment and lead to or compound the client's lowered self-esteem. The empathetic nurse can do a great deal by using a warm, accepting approach. In addition to promoting the client's verbalization of feelings, the nurse should show no hesitation in examining or touching affected areas, although gloves should be worn if infection is suspected.

The gerontological nurse should be aware that emotional stress exacerbates many dermatological conditions. Stress influences the autonomic nervous system, which can cause vasoconstriction in the distal capillaries of skin vessels. The nurse should help clients understand that stress affects skin conditions and should teach clients how to cope with and reduce this stress.

Treatment. The management of skin disease is often based on empirical judgment relating more to the nurse's preferences than to any hard and fast rules. The appearance rather than the etiology of the lesion frequently determines the form of preparation employed. A good rule of thumb is to use wet dressings on dry lesions and dry applications on wet ones. Since the inflamed skin is quite sensitive, the nurse should treat it at first with low concentrations of medication and increase the strength as the lesions improve.

Clients must always receive careful instruction on how and when to apply medication as well as on the quantities to apply. The client must be instructed to contact the nurse if therapy seems to worsen the condition. Any medication may give rise to a skin reaction that will complicate the lesions in treatment.

Pruritic Lesions: Treatment. *Dermatitis* often stems from frequent soap-and-water bathing, which is poorly tolerated by the fragile skin of the elderly and leads to the common problems of drying and eczema. As a general rule, the elimination of soap; the sparing use of bland soaps, such as Basis Soap; or the substitution of nonsoap detergents must be encouraged. The addition of a bath oil, such as Alpha Keri, to the water and the use of an emollient cream, such as Eucrin, Keri lotion, or Nivea, may suffice in mild cases (Sauer 1966). Clients must be instructed to use extra caution to avoid slipping and falling.

The more complex cases should also be treated with topical corticosteroids. These drugs are preferred for the oozing, pruritic, inflamed skin; by reducing the itch, they eliminate the scratching that maintains the eczema. Lotions are used for dry lesions

(Triamcinalone 0.025%, cream, 60 g dissolved in distilled water 0.5 liters), which should be applied to the involved areas four times daily. The dry, scaling rash is best handled with cream, such as Triamcinalone 0.025%, applied sparingly four times daily. Scaling lesions such as seborrheic dermatitis may be helped by the additional use of antidandruff shampoos once or twice weekly.

Infectious complications, revealed by pus or honey-colored crusts, will require the use of systemic antibiotics. A culture and sensitivity test should be taken. Then the treatment may be initiated with a broad-spectrum antibiotic such as erythromycin (Pillsbury 1975).

Pruritus ani is often precipitated by poor anal hygiene or by diarrhea or constipation. Treatment requires control and elimination of these conditions. Pinworms—ova and parasites—should be checked for and, if present, treated appropriately. The diarrhea or constipation must be adequately evaluated and corrected (see chapter 16, on gastrointestinal problems). Diabetes mellitus should be controlled.

Warm sitzbaths, 20 minutes four times daily for 10 days, will reduce itching. The anal area must be carefully cleansed with hot water and cotton after the bowel movement. The region must be patted, not rubbed, dry. Bowel stimulants such as laxatives, caffeine, and alcohol should be avoided. Corticosteroid creams (Triamcinalone 0.025%) should be applied after each sitzbath. Resistant cases should be referred to a proctologist or gastroenterologist.

Pruritus vulvae is often a more difficult problem. A complete gynecological examination, including Pap smear, sampling of any discharge for culture and sensitivity, hanging drop for trichomoniasis, and smear and culture for gonorrhea, should be performed. A urinalysis should be obtained and a search made for diabetes mellitus. Although yeast vaginitis is unusual, it may occur in diabetics, in older clients, and in persons using estrogens. Senile vaginitis, leading to tissue contraction and vaginal mucosal fragility, may cause severe pruritus.

Specific infections should be treated with an appropriate systemic antibiotic. Metroniazide (Flagyl) tablets will resolve trichomoniasis and its discharge. Sexual intercourse should be refrained from during treatment, and the client's sexual partner should also be treated. Yeast vaginitis is an occasional complication of this treatment and is easily managed with an acidifying douche (lactic acid, 2 tablespoons per quart of water).

Control of diabetes mellitus helps to control inflammation; the removal of a retained foreign body (often a pessary) may be necessary. Atrophic vaginitis may require the use of low-dosage hormonal therapy, such as Dienestrol cream 0.01% nightly, or systemic estrogen tablets, diethylstilbesterol 0.1 to 2.5 mg daily 5 days a week. These hormones should be cycled and used sparingly. (See chapter 17, on genitourinary disorders.) Another frequent cause of candidiasis is the use of pantyhose with nylon undergarments. These items cause trapping of moisture, which can be corrected by eliminating nylon and substituting cotton.

Poor response to therapy becomes obvious within two weeks and should be referred to a physician. All clients with tumors or suspicious Pap smears should immediately be referred to a physician. Clients with lichen simplex or nummular dermatitis may benefit from mild sedation.

Chlordiazapoxide 5 to 10 mg four times daily or hydroxyzine 10 mg twice daily, 20 mg at bedtime for no longer than one week may be helpful. A sleeping medication such as chloral hydrate 0.5 g at bedtime may be required. Again, the drug should be time limited and only enough pills ordered for that duration.

Nummular dermatitis, a secondary lesion, requires treatment of the primary dermatitis. Additional corticosteroid applications such as Triancinalone cream 0.025% may be applied four times daily.

Skin Infections: Treatment. Because of the lack of any specific therapy, clients with *viral diseases* are best managed by a physician. Herpes zoster may remain painful, and drug addiction may become a problem. The relationship of herpes zoster to a possible underlying cancer makes referral to a physician almost mandatory.

The majority of *bacterial infection* cases are due to streptococcal infections and are treated with oral penicillin "V" 250 to 500 mg four times daily or erythromycin 250 mg four times daily for 10 days. Local treatment for cellulitis consists of warm, wet wrappings, 20 minutes four times daily, with elevation of the limb to decrease the edema. Diuretic therapy (Chlorthiazide 250 mg to 500 mg daily; Furosemide 40 mg to 80 mg daily) is also useful. Discovery of the cause of the edema and its elimination is the most effective treatment.

The most common *fungal infections* are the intertriginous forms of tinea cruris and tinea pedis. These infections respond well to good hygiene and elimination of the sweat and water accumulations of the day. A lotion of salicylic acid 3% in isopropanol

30% four times daily reduces itching, dries the affected area, and causes regression of the lesion. Recurrences may be treated in a similar manner. A variety of topical anti-athlete's foot preparations, such as Tinnactin and Desinex, may be helpful for tinea pedis. Griseofulvin 250 mg twice daily is curative, but clients have no immunity and tend to become reinfected. Infected areas must be kept dry and exposed to air as much as possible. Nylon footwear or undergarments should be avoided.

Skin Tumors: Treatment. The definitive treatment of skin tumors is their removal either by curettage or excision. Clients with these tumors are referred to a dermatologist or surgeon. Benign tumors may be followed unless they present an aesthetic problem, interfere with movements of the body, or are in a frequently traumatized place.

Clients with tumors of malignant potential must be referred to a surgeon as soon as the nurse suspects that the tumors are undergoing malignant degeneration or if they are in a position where they are easily traumatized. Clients with malignant tumors must be referred to a physician.

SUMMARY

Maintenance of a healthful skin condition in the elderly requires some knowledge of dermatology combined with a caring, supportive approach. While teaching good hygiene and skin health promotion measures, the nurse must remain alert to signs of integumentary changes that are the hallmark of pathology.

REFERENCES

BRUNNER, L. S., et al. 1970. *Textbook of Medical Surgical Nursing,* 2nd ed. New York: J. B. Lippincott.

PILLSBURY, D. M. 1975. "Principles of Clinical Diagnosis." In S. I. Moschella, D. M. Pillsbury, and J. J. Hurley, eds., *Dermatology.* Philadelphia: W. B. Saunders.

ROCKSTEIN, M. 1975. "The Biology of Aging in Humans—An Overview." In R. Goldman and M. Rockstein, eds., *The Physiology and Pathology of Human Aging.* New York: Academic Press.

SAUER, G. C. 1966. *Manual of Skin Diseases.* Philadelphia: J. B. Lippincott.

TINDALL, J. P. 1978. "Geriatric Dermatology." In W. Reichel, ed., *Clinical Aspects of Aging.* Baltimore: Williams and Wilkins.

VERBOV, J. 1972. *Skin Diseases in the Elderly.* Philadelphia: J. B. Lippincott.

YOUNG, W. A. 1971. "Skin Disease." In I. Rossman, ed., *Clinical Geriatrics.* Philadelphia: J. B. Lippincott.

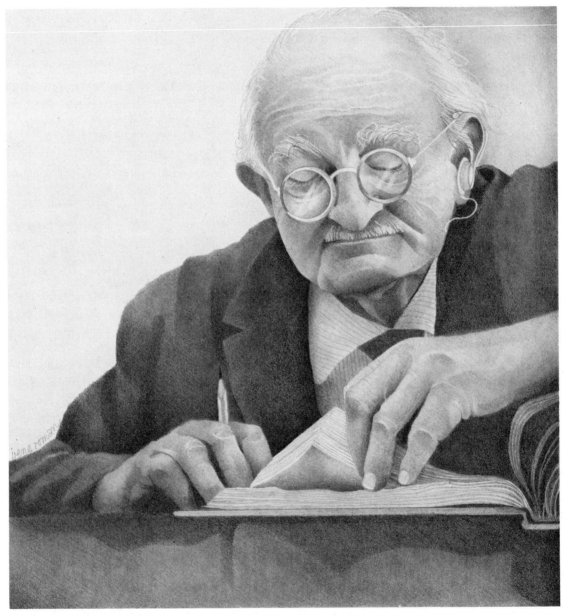

Chapter 13

GERONTOLOGICAL NURSING MANAGEMENT
THE ELDERLY CLIENT WITH A SENSORY VISION OR HEARING PROBLEM

The older adult requires an increased magnitude of stimuli for all sensory perception. Studies do not clearly indicate whether this increased need is due entirely to the aging process.

Decline in visual acuity, in adaptation to darkness, and in accommodation of the lens begins to appear in middle age. In addition to the visual deficit, a marked loss of hearing, especially of sounds in the high frequencies, also occurs among the elderly (Weiss 1959). Melrose, Welsh, and Luterman (1963) discovered a decrease in the ability of the elderly to understand speech, which implies some loss of auditory perception by the central nervous system as well as changes in auditory thresholds.

Corrective glasses and hearing aids maintain adequate social functioning for most elderly individuals; only a small proportion must make a greater adjustment. We must remember that decrements in vi-

sion and hearing may lead to social isolation, which has important psychological and social effects on the elderly individual and thus on the family.

SENSORY VISION PROBLEMS

Pathophysiology of the Eye

Some of the changes of advancing years that affect the eye involve the eyelids. A gradual loss of muscle elasticity and orbital fat may occur, with the development of wrinkling skin and drooping folds of the lids, or dermatochalasis (Vaughen and Asbury 1977). This change can result in ptosis, or drooping of the entire lid. Ptosis can also occur because of excessive weight of the upper lid or because of faulty humoral transmission at the myoneural junction, as in muscular dystrophy or multiple sclerosis. Frank disease processes, as opposed to aging, are involved in the latter two instances.

The lower eyelid may turn inward as a result of degeneration of the facial attachment of the lid (Vaughen and Asbury 1977). When this position change occurs, the eyelashes can rub against and irritate the cornea (trichiasis). In addition, the lower eyelid may sag and become everted as a result of relaxation of the obicularis oculi muscle. Excessive tearing can follow.

Age-associated changes may also occur in the lacrimal apparatus. A decrease in the volume of tear secretion may occur and can cause inflammation of the cornea and conjuctiva.

Aging changes that affect the cornea by "flattening" it can cause astigmatism or alter already present astigmatism: the *axis* of the refractive error is changed, but the *degree* of astigmatism is not greatly affected.

When the normal sclerosis of the lens is extended and intensified, a condition of cataract exists. Fibers in the central lens nucleus become compressed and laminated. Eventually these fiber layers become denatured and coalesce into a homogeneous mass, and the lens becomes diffusely opaque (Schofield 1961). The majority of people over age 70 have a certain degree of opacification. Only when severe visual disability exists is the condition identified as cataract.

The aqueous humor flows through the ligaments supporting the lens and through the pupil of the eye into the anterior chamber. This fluid then leaves the anterior chamber by way of the indocorneal angle into the canal of Schlemm. This canal is in reality a thin-walled vein that encircles the eye and constitutes a drainage vessel for aqueous humor.

Under normal conditions aqueous humor, produced by ciliary body epithelium, flows freely from its source into the anterior chamber to the indocorneal angle and out the canal of Schlemm. When the indocorneal angle becomes blocked with tissue debris or because of tissue sclerosis due to endothelial proliferation and thickening, the aqueous humor is prevented from leaving the anterior chamber. At the same time the ciliary processes are still producing the fluid. The intraocular pressure builds up above the normal range of 10 to 22 mmHg.

The vitreous, occupying the posterior compartment of the eyeball, has the consistency of a gel. All gels degenerate over time; *syneresis* is the name given to this degeneration. As the gel breaks down, fluid-filled cavities can form, leading to detachment from the retina. "Floaters" and "flashing lights" may be described by the client. The opacity caused by "floaters," although annoying, are of no pathological significance and constitute condensation of collagen fibers. The "flashing lights" are caused by abnormal stimulation of the retina (Vaughen and Asbury 1977).

With advancing years, arteriosclerotic changes in retinal blood vessels may result in degenerative changes in retinal tissue. The function of retinal cones, which make color perception and distant and detailed vision possible, may become less effective. The retinal rods, which function best in reduced illumination, may also undergo some functional loss. Senile macular degeneration is another cause of vision loss in the elderly; a fine stippling of pigment is apparent in this disorder. Cystic degeneration can also be caused by vascular disease (Scheie and Albert 1977).

Retinal pathology is common in clients

with diabetes. A thickening of vascular basement membrane occurs, with subsequent narrowing of the lumen. The result is an interference with the metabolism and nutrition of retinal tissue. Similarly the retina can be affected in clients with hypertension. Retinal hemorrhages and infarcts, and even edema of the optic disc, can appear.

Diseases of the eye should not be managed by the nurse alone; treatment should be administered only under the direction of an ophthalmologist. Therefore, management plans only for conjunctivitis and glaucoma are included in this chapter.

Nursing Assessment

Visual acuity should be assessed by using the Snellen Chart. With one eye covered, the individual is asked to read the smallest print possible. Visual fields are also checked with one eye covered. (Both tests are repeated for the other eye.) The external eye should be assessed too, with special attention paid to the cornea and pupil.

The ophthalmoscopic examination will determine opacities and the condition of the fundus and may reveal evidence of increased intraocular pressure. Tonometric testing for glaucoma is necessary if increased tension is evident during the intraocular examination. This testing should be done routinely in clients over 40. Newer techniques using compressed air directed against the eye are replacing the tonometer.

PINGUECULA AND PTERYGIUM

Two common conditions affecting the conjunctiva are pinguecula and pteryg-ium. *Pinguecula* is a subconjunctival degeneration close to the medial and lateral sides of the cornea. Creamy triangular plaques, with their base at the limbus, develop (usually on the nasal side). Etiology is unknown and no specific treatment has been developed. *Pterygium* is a degenerative condition of the conjunctival area. The condition develops from the limbus and extends toward the center of the cornea, forming a triangular zone of opacification. This zone presents an area of vascularization from the conjunctiva. Treatment requires surgical excision by an ophthalmologist if it interferes with vision.

ENTROPION AND ECTROPION

The elderly are susceptible to malpositions of the lids. *Entropion* is a condition in which the lashes are turned inward and irritate the eye because the margin of the eyelids is turned backward. Conjunctivitis, corneal abrasion, and ulceration also may occur, resulting in interference with vision because of opacities. Definitive treatment of entropion often requires a plastic operation on the lid. Taping the lid open may temporarily prevent further damage.

If the lower lid everts and exposes the conjunctiva along its entire length or falls away from the eyeball, the result is a constant escape of tears onto the face. This condition is called *ectropion*. Corrective treatment is surgical. Temporary relief is obtained by taping the lid shut.

VITREOUS DETACHMENT

Vitreous detachment is seen frequently in those over 60 years of age. It usually appears as a dark ring in the area of the disc.

Although the condition itself has little clinical significance, it should be followed, as it can be a forerunner of retinal detachment.

CONJUNCTIVITIS

Conjunctivitis is an inflammation of the conjunctival lining of the eyelids and bulbar portion of the eye. Typically the vessels of the conjunctiva become inflamed and injected. Etiology may be allergic, viral, or bacterial. In conjunctivitis the inflammation originates from the fornix. This condition must be differentiated from ciliary flush, which emerges from the limbus area. The cornea is clear and unaffected in conjunctivitis, while ciliary flush is a more serious condition and does involve the cornea. Some forms of keratoconjunctivitis are of viral origin and are highly contagious; they present with multiple fine spots on the cornea, which may slightly hamper vision (Newton 1978).

Nursing Assessment

The nurse should note the degree and pattern of injection. In acute uveitis injection emanates from the limbus. With keratoconjunctivitis a conjunctival injection occurs. When infected with herpes simplex, the eye may develop a dendritic ulcer. Discharges should be noted as serous, mucoid, purulent, or a combination of these conditions. Smears and cultures of drainage are necessary only if symptoms do not subside in one week. *Allergic* conjunctivitis presents with severe itching, mild injection, and slight discharge, and the condition is binocular. *Viral* conjunctivitis presents with copious tearing and little, if any, injection, and the condition is usually monocular. *Bacterial* conjunctivitis presents with peripheral hyperemia and purulent discharge with burning and itching. Historical evidence for allergies should be elicited. The cornea should be examined with fluorescein dye to check for ulcers or abrasions.

Nursing Management

For the client with an allergic condition, some symptomatic relief may be accomplished by antihistamines. The client should be referred to an allergist if the symptoms persist. Viral conjunctivitis is resistant to treatment and usually runs a course of 14 to 21 days. Warm compresses two or four times daily may give symptomatic relief. If close follow-up supervision is provided, the nurse may elect to have the client use a steroid eyedrop every 3 or 4 hours while awake, for a few days. This treatment will only suppress symptoms and provide comfort. However, if a dendritic ulcer is present, steroids should not be used and the client should immediately be referred to an ophthalmologist for treatment. The client with bacterial conjunctivitis should be instructed to apply warm compresses two or four times daily, and a common ocular antibiotic drop may be ordered. In all cases if symptoms persist, the client should be referred to an ophthalmologist (Newton 1978).

SUBCONJUNCTIVAL HEMORRHAGE

Subconjunctival hemorrhage presents as a painless, bright red blood spot on the sclera of the eye. It varies in size and is usually the result of trauma. However, it can also occur as a result either of straining at stool or of sustained coughing. The nurse should reassure the client that the hemorrhage will be reabsorbed in approximately

2 weeks; no specific treatment for this disorder is known.

TEMPORAL ARTERITIS (GIANT CELL ARTERITIS)

Temporal arteritis is a serious condition that occurs almost exclusively in the elderly and therefore deserves our consideration. The presenting symptoms include headache, preauricular tenderness, and usually a palpable enlarged temporal artery that may or may not pulsate. Occasionally mandibular pain occurs upon mastication. Usually present are lethargy, anorexia, weakness, and weight loss. One-third of clients with temporal arteritis eventually will suffer visual loss secondary to ischemic optic neuropathy. The loss may be precipitous or it may occur over time (Kasper 1978). Clients with suspected temporal arteritis should be referred promptly to an ophthalmologist.

DIABETIC RETINOPATHY

The likelihood of diabetic retinopathy, a complicating aspect of diabetes, increases in proportion to the length of time the client has been a diagnosed diabetic. It is one of the leading causes of blindness in clients under 60 years of age (Patz 1978). The retinopathy is not well correlated with the degree or severity of diabetes. The appearance of new vessel growth in the iris can lead to secondary glaucoma.

Nursing Assessment

Most often the client with diabetic retinopathy has a long history of diabetes, which may or may not be well monitored by a physician. Funduscopic examination reveals retinal changes not unlike hypertensive retinopathy. These retinal changes include the presence of microaneurysms; regular, small hemorrhages; and multiple yellow-white exudates. Tonometry should be performed on the client with retinal changes. The nurse should refer the client to an ophthalmologist if the client has not had a recent evaluation.

GLAUCOMA

Narrow-angle glaucoma presents with severe pain in or around the eye, which may be referred to the brow, temple, and cheek (Jackson 1957); blurred vision; and nausea and vomiting. Objective findings show an intensely congested eye, an elevated intraocular pressure, a hazy cornea, and a dilated pupil with poor reaction, if any, to stimulus. The eyeball is tender to touch, and the eye feels stony hard. Funduscopic examination may reveal evidence of increased intraocular tension by cupping of discs.

In *open-angle* glaucoma, clients have few subjective complaints. A dull headache may be present. Attacks occur more commonly in the winter and at night than at other times. The client has blurred vision and perceives a rainbow or halo effect around lights. Objective findings may show increased intraocular pressure during the attack. Funduscopic examination may reveal an atrophic, cupped disc. Intraocular pressures are highest late at night or early in the morning because of diurnal variations (Kasper 1978). Visual field defects are also present.

Nursing Management

In an acute attack of narrow-angle glaucoma, emergency administration of 1 or 2 drops of 1% pilocarpine and referral to an ophthalmologist are essential to limit visual loss. Treatment includes carbonic anhydrase inhibitors to reduce formation of aqueous solution, or urea or glycerin to increase osmotic tension in the circulating blood and to draw fluid from the hypertensive eye (Kornzweig 1971, p. 231). Surgery may be necessary to prevent further episodes.

Glaucoma needs to be discovered prior to irreversible changes such as loss of vision. The acute cases usually bring the individual to the physician, but chronic, wide-angle glaucoma leads to loss of vision before discovery. Only through regular, periodic measurement of intraocular pressure can this condition be discovered early. As the primary care provider, the nurse practitioner should be responsible for this screening process. Tonometric and funduscopic examination should be considered part of a complete data base and will greatly assist

in the early screening of glaucoma sufferers (Schwartz 1978).

CATARACT

The most common cause of cataract is old age. The lens becomes opaque. Most persons over age 70 present with some degree of cataract. Senile cataract is always bilateral, but the opacity in one eye usually is more advanced than that in the other eye. Removal of the cataract usually brings return of sight. Because of the absence of the lens, glasses are necessary to compensate for loss of accommodation. The latest mode of treatment includes replacement by an artificial lens or the use of contact lenses (Jaffe 1978).

Clients with cataract frequently complain of visual deterioration (fog, haze, and glaring from lights). Funduscopic examination reveals partial or complete loss of red reflex. Interruptions of the red reflex may

The gerontological nurse can help the elderly adapt to the aging process by encouraging a full range of appropriate recreational activities; elderly clients need to participate in mentally stimulating social activities despite, for example, their decline in sensory acuity.

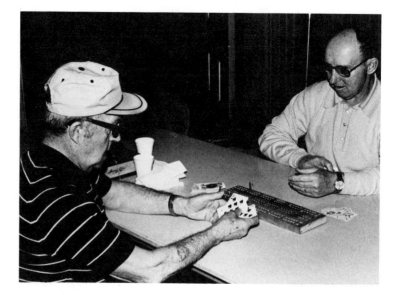

appear as either streaks or spokes of opacity on the periphery or as a central haze interfering with visualization of the retina on deep examination. The outer eye is completely normal.

Diabetic clients develop cataracts at an earlier age. Management of cataract in the aged diabetic is not different from management of cataract in the aged nondiabetic. Treatment is primarily surgical, and clients should be referred to an ophthalmologist for evaluation and follow-up. Because of the possibility of diabetic retinopathy behind the cataract, the results of surgery may be disappointing.

Nursing Management of the Client with a Visual Deficit

The nurse's primary role lies in screening and preventing further visual impairment. For the visually handicapped person, the nurse becomes the counselor in assisting the client and family to deal with the handicap. The family of a blind person may be apt to cast the client in a helpless role. The nurse must intercede and counsel on the importance of the client's maintaining as great a degree of independence as possible. Cane training should begin early for the visually handicapped. Visual aids, such as soft night lights, should be used. The individual should be encouraged to increase usage of senses other than vision. Talking records and large-print books can be obtained from the public library. The client should be encouraged to seek assistance from the American Foundation for the Blind.

Visual aides extend to large telephone-dial numbers, brailled watches and clocks, magnifying glasses, and telescopic devices.

A wide variety of social contact aides in the form of games and individual therapy aids from the American Foundation are also available (Hess and Day 1977). *An Introduction to Working with the Aging Person Who Is Visually Handicapped* is a handy resource guide that the nurse can obtain from the American Foundation for the Blind (1977).

The nurse can assist the client and family by suggesting the importance of not moving familiar objects and furniture in the client's living domain. Medications can be color coded and instructions written in large print. Color schemes can also be employed in the home to provide as great a degree of independence as possible. Fluorescent tapes can be applied around electric outlets, light switches, door handles, and keyholes. For the totally blind client, tactile clues can be used. Materials of different consistency, such as felt, linen, fur, and sandpaper, can be taped to medication-bottle caps (Kart, Metress, and Metress 1978).

The client's interest and motivation in adapting to this handicap will be somewhat determined by the degree of the handicap and its speed of onset. For most elderly, with the exception of those with such disorders as retinal detachment, the sensory handicap develops over time, allowing for a period of adaptation. The degree of the person's adaptability will determine whether the adaptation will be healthy or limited. Unfortunately both the client and nurse may belittle the necessity for health teaching and counseling either because the handicap is not perceived as a priority problem or because its course is so insidious that the handicap does not appear significant. Thus the nurse may miss an opportunity to learn new techniques

355

from the handicapped person. Many sensorially deprived individuals are warehouses of information on how to cope with the handicap and are quite willing to share this information with an interested listener. Furthermore, the client may profit from the nurse's interest and knowledge. Even when the client does not readily perceive the need for this information, a time will come when it will be used, with grateful remembrance of the care provider.

SENSORY HEARING PROBLEMS

Hearing impairment is more common than visual impairment in the elderly (Rubin 1971, p. 247). Hearing loss in the elderly may be secondary to a systemic disease such as Paget's. Hearing impairment for sounds in the higher frequencies and even for speech can be demonstrated in most individuals over age 50 (Bergman et al. 1976). Presbycusis (hearing impairment of age) can be caused by acoustical trauma, genetic factors, and circulatory impairment. Presbycusis is often a mixed neurosensory loss that may or may not be accompanied by speech discrimination loss. For assessment of diseases of the ear see chapter 6, unit 4. The nurse should distinguish between conductive and sensory defects, as the type of defect will influence treatment.

Pathophysiology of the Ear

Two types of deafness occur: *conduction* deafness, due to impaired transmission of sound waves in the middle ear, and *nerve* deafness, due to damage either to the organ of Corti of the cochlea or inner ear or to the auditory nerve.

In conduction deafness the small ossicles in the middle ear may be either destroyed or immobilized by fibrosis or calcification. Conduction impairment may also be present if the tympanic membrane is severely scarred and thickened as a result of frequent attacks of otitis media or tympanitis. This type of hearing impairment may also be caused by a ruptured membrane.

In some cases of nerve deafness in the aged, degenerative changes occur in the inner ear or cochlea. Noise pollution is a prime suspect for this sensory loss. Some cases of deafness with cochlea or auditory nerve damage may be the result of extreme and constant noise attendant to a present or former occupation, such as one involving the use of jackhammers and riveting tools or work around airplanes. Nerve deafness can also be hereditary or it can be caused by medullary tumors or hemorrhage.

Nursing Management of the Client with a Hearing Deficit

A sensory hearing loss can cause profound problems for the elderly. This sensory deficit can compound other health problems by distorting reality, creating social isolation, and alienating the elderly person from necessary contact with the environment. The problem, when not recognized and corrected or alleviated, can lead to unnecessary early institutionalization. The elderly person, hard of hearing and living alone, is further isolated. Depression and paranoid ideation are common severe emotional consequences of the diminished social contacts and other problems due to hearing loss.

Especially problematic for the nurse may be the client who denies the hearing deficit or who accepts it as a normal process of aging. Excellent counseling skills are requisites for managing such a client. The use of an amplification aid may be helpful. However, a prescription for a hearing aid should be given only after *a thorough evaluation is obtained from an audiologist.* Far too often the elderly have obtained hearing aids from salesmen interested in a profit. The elderly person may continue to have auditory perceptual problems. The hearing aid is then relegated to a drawer, and the depressed individual is left with the feeling of having been victimized. The nurse should counsel the client about these possibilities, but offer hope by explaining that other assistance is available in the form of auditory and lipreading training. For the client who can be assisted with a hearing aid, the nurse should remember that auditory and lipreading training may be an additional source of assistance. Sign language can also be taught to the elderly.

Nurses should speak clearly, slowly, and distinctly and face the individual. Since low-frequency tones are usually retained the longest, the nurse should attempt to speak in a deeply toned voice. If touch is used, the nurse should always speak to the individual before touching. Instructions must be kept simple and extraneous noise screened out. The nurse should remember to use stimuli that reach more than one sense—for example, shells can be felt, if not seen; clocks can be heard or seen. Hearing aids should be checked for fit and adjustment. Glasses may need cleaning. To assist in lipreading, the female nurse can wear bright red lipstick when speaking.

The nurse should counsel the client to make an effort to maintain social contacts, although the hearing deficit may be a con-tinuing source of irritation and embarrassment. Inclusion of the family in the counseling process will assist members to understand and help the client.

In working with the client who has a hearing deficit, the nurse must be able to read the client's reaction. An under-reaction may indicate that the client does not understand what is being said.

Often elderly clients have mixed neuro-sensory losses affecting both vision and hearing. The importance of cognitive stimuli and sustained social contact cannot be overemphasized for such clients.

SUMMARY

The majority of health problems affecting the sensory organs require medical referral and management. The gerontological nurse provides an invaluable service as the health educator and counselor for the elderly client and the family. A well-informed and alert nurse can prevent further deterioration of sensory organs by early recognition and continued cooperation with the medical specialist.

REFERENCES

American Foundation for the Blind. 1977. *An Introduction to Working with the Aging Person Who Is Visually Handicapped,* 2nd ed. New York.

BERGMAN, M., et al. 1976. "Age Related Decrement in Hearing for Speech." *Journal of Gerontology* 31:533–38.

BOURNE, G. H. 1961. *Structural Aspects of Aging.* New York: Hafner Publishing.

BURNSIDE, I. M. 1976. *Nursing and the Aged.* New York: McGraw-Hill.

357

BUTLER, R. N., and M. LEWIS. 1973. *Aging and Mental Health: Positive Psychosocial Approaches.* St. Louis: C. V. Mosby.

HESS, P., and C. DAY. 1977. *Understanding the Aging Patient.* Bowie, Md.: Robert J. Brady.

HOFSTETTER, H. W. 1944. "A Comparison of Decane's and Donder's Tables of the Amplitude of Accommodation." *American Journal of Optometry and Archives of American Academy of Optometry* 21:345–63.

JACKSON, C. R. S. 1957. *The Eye in General Practice.* London: E. and S. Livingstone.

JAFFE, N. S. 1978. "Current Concepts in Ophthalmology: Cataract Surgery—A Modern Attitude towards a Technologic Explosion." *New England Journal of Medicine* 299:235–37.

KART, G., E. S. METRESS, and J. F. METRESS. 1978. *Aging and Health.* Menlo Park, Calif.: Addison-Wesley.

KASPER, R. 1978. "Eye Problems in the Aged." In W. Reichel, ed., *Clinical Aspects of Aging.* Baltimore: Williams and Wilkins.

KORNZWEIG, A. 1971. "The Eye in Old Age." In I. Rossman, ed., *Clinical Geriatrics.* Philadelphia: J. B. Lippincott.

MELROSE, J., O. L. WELSH, and D. LUTERMAN. 1963. "Auditory Responses in Selected Elderly Men." *Journal of Gerontology* 18:267–70.

NEWTON, D. S. 1978. "Eye Disorders." In C. J. Leitch and R. V. Tinker, eds., *Primary Care.* Philadelphia: F. A. Davis.

PATZ, A. 1978. "Current Concepts in Ophthalmology: Retinal Vascular Diseases." *New England Journal of Medicine* 298:1451–54.

PRIOR, J., and J. SILBERSTEIN. 1973. *Physical Diagnosis,* 4th ed. St. Louis: C. V. Mosby.

RUBIN, R. 1971. "Aging and Hearing." In I. Rossman, ed., *Clinical Geriatrics.* Philadelphia: J. B. Lippincott.

SCHEIE, H. G., and D. M. ALBERT. 1977. *Textbook of Ophthalmology.* Philadelphia: W. B. Saunders.

SCHOFIELD, P. B. 1961. "Aging Changes in the Eye." In G. H. Bourne, ed., *Structural Aspects of Aging.* New York: Hafner Publishing.

SCHWARTZ, B. 1978. "Current Concepts in Ophthalmology: The Glaucomas." *New England Journal of Medicine* 299:182–84.

VAUGHEN, D. and T. ASBURY. 1977. *General Ophthalmology.* Los Altos, Calif. Lange Publications.

WEISS, A. 1959. "Sensory Functions." In J. E. Birren, ed., *Handbook of Aging and the Individual.* Chicago: University of Chicago Press.

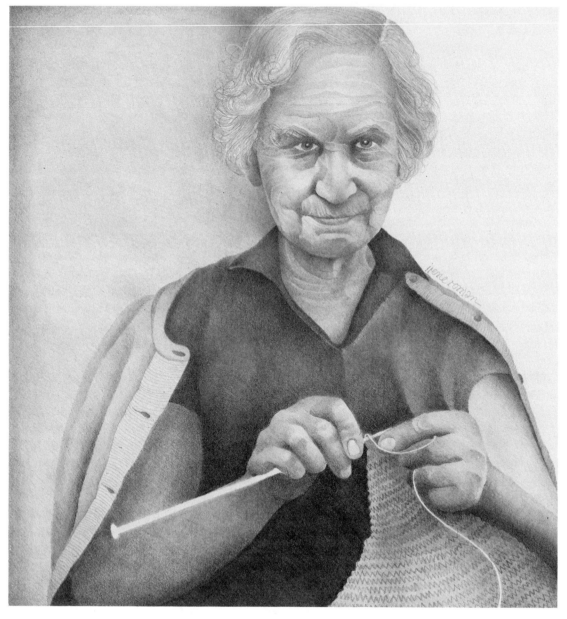

Chapter 14

GERONTOLOGICAL NURSING MANAGEMENT

THE ELDERLY CLIENT WITH A MUSCULOSKELETAL PROBLEM

Musculoskeletal problems, especially the arthritic disorders, usually first appear in middle life and then progress slowly as the individual ages. Discomfort and pain are the most common complaints. This chapter discusses several of the arthropathies seen in the elderly client.

DEGENERATIVE JOINT DISEASE

Pathophysiology

Degenerative arthritis, a degenerative joint disease, is also called *osteoarthritis* or *hypertrophic arthritis*. Osteoarthritis is an inflammatory disorder of movable joints and is characterized by deteriorations, bone hypertrophy, abrasion of articular cartilage, and formation of new growth or bony spurs on the joint surfaces. Only 15 percent of men and 25 percent of women over the age of 60 present with symptoms, although his-

tological changes of osteoarthritis are universal after the second decade of life and radiological evidence is present in those over 50 years of age (Grob 1978, p. 261). Obesity, postural defects, mechanical defects, and occupations that involve weight bearing are recognized as aggravating factors.

Before we discuss the pathological changes in diarthric joints, reviewing the structure of the knee as an example of a freely movable joint will be helpful. The bones of the knee joint include the distal end of the femur, the proximal end of the tibia, and the patella, or kneecap. Although the patella is an essential part of the knee, this discussion of osteoarthritis is concerned only with the articulating surfaces of the femur and tibia. The ends of these two bones are intimately enclosed in an articular capsule, which is attached near each of their articular surfaces. Muscles, tendons, and fascia add to the strength of the capsule and hence the joint. The capsule has an outer fibrous and an inner synovial membrane that covers all bony surfaces not covered by articular cartilage. The synovial membrane encloses a cavity filled with fluid secreted by the membrane itself. Synovial fluid serves to lubricate the joint and to nourish the articular cartilage at the ends of the femur and tibia.

Pathological changes in diarthritic joints are an expression of physiological aging. Postmortem examination has shown that even in the first and second decades of life these changes have begun. The translucent, resilient, bluish-white cartilage begins to appear more opaque, firmer, yellowish, and less elastic (Bourne 1961, p. 30). As the individual ages, surface defects appear on the articular surface of the cartilage; dehydration and softening of cartilage are followed by separation of collagenous fibers, with the result that fissures and clefts develop. With destruction of articular cartilage, underlying, or subchondral, bone is exposed. Irritation of the perichondrium and periosteum causes the proliferation of cells at joint margins. Extensive hypertrophy produces bony outgrowths, or spur formation—hence the term *osteoarthritis*. When bony spurs of two or more articulating bones project into the joint and come in contact with one another, they cause considerable pain and limitation of motion.

The pathological changes that affect the diarthritic knee joint also affect the spine. The changes are similar because fibrocartilaginous discs exist between each vertebra, just as cartilage is present in the knee joint, and because the spinal column, like the knee, is extensively involved in almost all physical activities. The cartilaginous discs undergo degenerative changes and hypertrophic spur formation, and lysis develops at the edges of adjacent vertebrae. Again, pain and limitation of motion accompany these advanced pathological changes. The extent of degeneration is variable: some individuals exhibit more arthritic changes at age 35 than others do at 60 (Harvey 1967, p. 1411).

Nursing Assessment

Subjective Findings. In evaluating clients with degenerative joint disease (DJD), the nurse must realize that subjective complaints correlate poorly with the degree of objective findings. Clients with advanced articular changes may have few complaints, while others with marked objective findings may have minimal objective evidence of disease.

People with DJD are usually middle aged or elderly. The affected joints are those that have been subjected to trauma in the past or that undergo weight bearing. The exception is the frequent involvement of the distal interphalangeal articulation of the hands, which is more commonly found in women. The most common subjective complaint is stiffness on initial movement after sitting. This stiffness is rapidly relieved by further movement. Another is pain with motion, which is relieved by rest.

Objective Findings. Commonly the joint appears normal. Objective findings may include swelling, creaking, grating, and crepitus on palpation. Evidence of inflammation, such as warmth or redness, is rare. Constitutional symptoms of anorexia, anemia, or fever are not found. Tenderness limited to the joint and its capsule may be found. Articular enlargement usually feels firm, as joint effusion is often minimal and rapidly resolved by a few days' rest.

Hand involvement is usually limited to the distal interphalangeal joints of the fingers. Typically one finds Heberden's nodes, which may be tender. These cartilaginous and bony enlargements are localized to the dorsal and lateral aspects of the joint. They are often associated with small, gelatinous, synovial cysts on the dorsum of the joint or just proximal to it. Advanced changes of the phalangeal joints include flexion and lateral deformity. Occasionally the proximal interphalangeal joints are involved (Bouchard's nodes).

Diagnostics

Laboratory studies are normal. X-rays show joint narrowing, sharpening of articular margins and interarticular structures, bony sclerosis, osteophytes, and marginal lipping and bone cysts (Grob 1978, p. 263).

Nursing Management

Health Education and Counseling. The nurse should establish a reasonable program of rest and activity for all clients who have an arthritic problem. Activities should be planned with the intention of promoting the maintenance of limber joints. The client should be reminded that pain experienced during exercise is not significant when it is transitory. The client and significant other must be told why exercises are essential. *Yoga for Your Leisure Years* by Eve Diskin (1978) is an excellent book that can be used by clients. This book stresses moderation of effort with continued stretching of sluggish muscles. It is a paperback, published in large, readable print, and contains many photos of older adults performing the exercises.

Precipitating factors should be noted. Apinal curvatures may be corrected by bracing or appropriate lifts on the shortened side. These devices may be fitted by an orthopedic surgeon. Obese clients present a particularly refractory problem, since they are usually aware that obesity contributes to their problem. The nurse should evaluate whether the obese individual truly understands the dynamics of the condition and determine whether prolonged counseling to change eating habits will be successful. Pain frequently leads the client to be so inactive as to contribute further to muscular atrophy. Clients should be advised against excessive exercise, but also told that excessive rest is detrimental. A firm mattress is indicated, especially for clients with spinal involvement or back pain. Clients should be instructed not to place a pillow under the knee, as the bending of the knee invariably leads to flexion deformity.

Cervical pain may be helped by a gentle range of motion exercises. Stretching exercises and rest usually prove efficacious for clients who have spondylosis. For those who are unrelieved by such measures, traction may be helpful. A simple towel splint or Thomas collar may be used for those who have cervical spondylosis.

The nurse should note bodily postural habits and counsel the client on maintenance of good posture. A home visit will be necessary to determine whether furniture is available to promote needed postural support when sitting.

A chair should (1) have armrests to assist in rising, (2) be deep enough so that thighs

363

are supported but circulation is not impaired at the popliteal spaces, (3) be high enough to permit feet to rest on the floor, and (4) have the seat level or tilted slightly forward to promote minimum flexion of hips and knees.

Elevating a chair's height by several inches will increase comfort when sitting and provide leverage on arising. Railing in the bathroom for shower, tub, and toilet will promote stability and assist in rising. Sometimes raising the height of the toilet seat is indicated (Shafer et al. 1971, p. 84).

Management is aimed at symptomatic relief. The nurse should recommend heat, preferably moist, to the joint, as this treatment relieves aching and stiffness. Long applications have decreased effectiveness. Several applications of 20 to 30 minutes each are usually the best. Painful Heberden's nodes are helped by paraffin dips at 43°C to 48°C (110° to 120°F) or by warm baths.

Treatment. The purpose of medication is for analgesia and anti-inflammatory activity. The most effective medication is a salicylate. The most commonly used is aspirin 600 to 900 mg four times daily with meals and at bedtime, to minimize gastric intolerance. An adequate trial requires 5 days to 1 week of treatment; the nurse must warn the client to use the aspirin as prescribed and not just for pain relief. If salicylates are poorly tolerated, which seems common in clients with a history of peptic ulcers, ibuprofen 300 to 400 mg two or four times daily may be tried. This medication has fewer gastrointestinal side effects. Phenylbutazone is sometimes helpful when salicylates fail (Robinson 1971).

Indomethacin given with supper and at bedtime, 50 to 150 mg daily, may be helpful. Phenylbutazone and indomethacin may induce severe gastric irritation, ulceration, and bleeding as well as bone marrow depression. In such cases the dosage should be decreased or the medication eliminated as quickly as possible. Systemic corticosteroids should rarely be used in degenerative joint disease.

Evaluation of Care. Clients suffering from severely symptomatic joints and not responding to nursing management should be referred to an orthopedic surgeon or rheumatologist. Intraarticular injections may provide prolonged relief (Moskowitz 1972). A variety of surgical procedures are available. Occasionally osteotomy or the prosthetic replacement of a symptomatic joint may improve symptoms and slow the disease process sufficiently to warrant the intervention.

RHEUMATOID ARTHRITIS (ATROPHIC ARTHRITIS)

Pathophysiology

Rheumatoid arthritis, in contrast to localized degenerative arthritis, is a chronic systemic inflammatory disease of connective tissue. It consists of inflammatory changes of connective tissue and a symmetrical polyarthritis with joint destruction. Although many organs can be affected, the major disabling effect is seen when inflammation occurs in the synovial membrane of articulating joints. After the disease becomes established, a bisymmetrical effect tends to occur—for example, if the synovial membrane of one ankle joint is affected, the other will also tend to become inflamed.

Rheumatoid arthritis occurs in people between 20 and 80 years of age, with a peak incidence at 35 to 45 years. Therefore, the large majority of rheumatoid arthritics will be diagnosed by the time they reach age 50. The disease is two to three times more common in women than in men (Ragan 1972).

Although the exact cause is not known, two theories have been advanced to explain the cause of rheumatoid arthritis. The first theory implicates microorganisms such as *streptococci, staphylococci,* and *diphthneroids* as the cause of the initial synovitis (Robbins 1974, p. 1467).

The second theory proposes an immunologic cause. This theory is supported by the presence of hypergammaglobulinemia in most individuals with rheumatoid arthritis. Specifically "an antibody against immunoglobulin (IgG), known as rheumatoid (RF) factor, can be demonstrated in the serum of 85 to 90 percent of these cases" (Robbins 1974, p. 1467). In fact, the serum titer of RF has been shown to be proportional to the severity of the disease. The immunologic theory goes on to suggest that phagocytic cells of the synovial membrane engulf the RF antigen-antibody complex; when the phagocytic cell dies, it releases a biochemical, lysosomal acid hydrolase, which causes an inflammatory response in the synovial membrane. In either case, synovitis develops. Initially the synovial membrane of small joints in the hands and feet become involved. In advanced rheumatoid arthritis large joints, such as the knees and elbows, are affected.

The first response of the synovial membrane is that it becomes thickened and edematous. Synovial cells proliferate, invade the interior of the joint, and adhere to the surface of articular cartilage. The synovial membrane extension is called a *pannus.* Because the pannus covers and invades the articular cartilage, this tissue is deprived of its nutrition and is destroyed. This destruction can also occur in subchondral bone. In addition, joint motion can traumatize the pannus, causing it to bleed into the synovial space. This bleeding is followed by the formation of fibrin clots and granular tissue. All of these responses can ultimately lead to obliteration of the synovial space and permanent ankylosis of the affected joint. The joints become enlarged, deformed, and tender, with pain accompanying joint motion. Rheumatoid arthritis is not confined to diarthroidal joints; it frequently affects the upper portion of the vertebral column.

Nursing Assessment

Findings are both general and localized; they vary in severity independently in the same client over time and from person to person.

Subjective Findings. The earliest subjective complaints consist of fatigue, weakness, weight loss, and numbness and tingling of the hands and feet. These vague findings are often precipitated by an emotional strain or an acute infection. Joint complaints consist of pain and stiffness. The pain occurs with use, is relieved by rest, and is often out of proportion to the degree of joint swelling. Stiffness is most common in the morning; clients frequently require 30 to 60 minutes to limber up. One or many joints may be involved. Pain and stiffness may occur acutely with fever or have a slowly progressive course involving multiple articulations. Muscle aching without joint involvement also may be present.

Objective Findings. The objective findings consist of a low-grade fever, anemia, and weight loss. The hands may be reddened on the thenar and hypothenar eminences ("liver palms").

Articular involvement is usually migratory and progressive. Eventually the small articulations of the hands and feet become involved. The objective findings of joint involvement are swelling, warmth, and tenderness. Once these symptoms occur, they persist for several weeks while other joints also become involved. The swelling may be fluctuant because of increased intraarticular fluid or it may be firm because of a thickened synovium and periarticular capsule. Tenderness is limited to the joint and its capsule. Redness may also be present.

Limitation of joint motion is initially due to pain, later to capsular fibrosis and muscle shortening. Eventually limitation is due to an increasing fibrous ankylosis of the articular cartilage. Rarely, in the later stages bony ankylosis may occur. Skin atrophy over the affected joints causes a smooth, shiny appearance.

Other findings include pallor and a chronically ill appearance. Clients with rheumatoid arthritis often appear undernourished. Splenomegaly with or without adenopathy may be found. Tachycardia, fever, and pedal edema also may be present.

The clinical course consists of cycles of exacerbations and remissions. The former are progressive, with new joint involvement and further functional loss in joints previously attacked. Remissions may be long; during remission clients may be relatively comfortable. Remissions are longer and more common at the onset of illness. Initially the disease may appear monoarticular, but once it is established, it is almost always symmetrical. Other organ systems may be involved and cause vasculitis, myositis, or anemia.

Diagnostics

Laboratory tests usually reveal a normochromic, normocytic anemia. However, if the hemoglobin is below 10 g per 100 ml, another etiology should be sought (Robinson 1972). Evidence of inflammation includes an accelerated erythrocyte sedimentation rate and a protein electrophoretic pattern of decreased albumin and increased alpha-2 and gamma globulins. The latex fixation test for rheumatoid factor is positive in 65 to 95 percent of clients (Vaughn et al. 1968). The antinuclear antibody (ANA) and anti-DNA are usually negative. X-ray changes are nonspecific and of little help in the early phase of illness.

Differentiating rheumatoid arthritis from other articular problems requires careful evaluation of the client as well as use of laboratory aids. A blood uric acid level will differentiate rheumatoid arthritis from gout. However, low-dose salicylates may raise uric acid blood levels, which must be considered. Lupus erythematosis may begin exactly like rheumatoid ar-

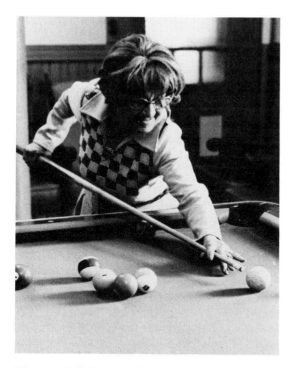

The gerontological nurse can help the elderly adapt to the aging process by recommending physical exercises and activities that help maintain mobility; elderly clients are more likely to carry out therapeutic exercise when they understand the benefits of the exercise and enjoy the activity as well.

thritis. A positive serum ANA or anti-DNA test is strong evidence for this disorder.

Nursing Management

Management of the rheumatoid arthritic is performed in conjunction with an orthopedic surgeon or rheumatologist. The primary goal of treatment is to obtain a remission and prolong it for as long as possible. The choices of therapy are confusing both to the client and to the nurse. Given the absence of a known etiology and the natural course of remissions and exacerba-

tions, knowing which modes of therapy are more effective is difficult.

Goals of Rheumatoid Arthritis Therapy
To inhibit the inflammatory response and its symptoms
To preserve function
To prevent joint deformity
To restore function by repairing existent deformity

Since the course of the illness is often long and discouraging, the client may suffer severe economic and social pressures, sometimes in search of a quick, miraculous cure. The nurse must establish close rapport with the client to improve morale during the symptomatic periods and to prevent excessive optimism during the period of remission. Assessment of needs is based on the client's functional ability and not on the medical diagnosis or the client's age. Education regarding drugs, their toxicity, and how to take them is needed because complications occur even with simple medications like aspirin.

PAGET'S DISEASE (OSTEITIS DEFORMANS)

Pathophysiology

Paget's disease, a disorder of unknown etiology, is a chronic progressive disease characterized by softening, enlargement, and bowing of the bones. It is more common in men and rarely seen before age 40. The characteristic problem is excessive bone resorption and deposition, leading to a sclerosis. The disorder is characterized by deformities of both flat and long bones.

367

Common sites are sacrum, spine, skull, pelvis, and lumbar vertebrae. The femur, tibia, and clavicle also are often involved. It is a local, asymmetrical disease.

The deformities of Paget's disease are due to the softening, destruction, and resorption of normal bone, accompanied by replacement with Paget bone, which is architecturally and biochemically abnormal, and with fibrous tissue. The bulk of the replacement tissue exceeds the original bone tissue; hence enlargement occurs. However, because this tissue not only is soft and porous but also contains wide osteoid seams, it becomes deformed when subjected to weight bearing. In the vertebral column, Paget bone is compressed, and kyphosis, scoliosis, and lordosis can result. Pain frequently accompanies bone compression and enlargement.

Nursing Assessment

Subjective Findings. The most common subjective complaint is deep, aching pain, aggravated by weight bearing. Headaches, dizziness, hearing loss, and other unusual disturbances may also occur.

Objective Findings. Objective findings include bowing and elongation of the tibia and femur. Advanced changes include enlargement of the upper portion of the skull, with engorged temporal arteries. The head is often held so that the chin is in the sternal notch.

Diagnostics

Laboratory findings include primarily an elevated serum alkaline phosphatase and urine hydroxyproline. Serum calcium and phosphorous levels are normal. X-ray findings are often diagnostic but must be distinguished from those due to metastases from a breast or prostatic cancer.

Increased pain and a further rise in alkaline phosphatase may indicate a fracture or a sarcoma.

Nursing Management

The nurse should be aware that some pain may be due to osteoporotic joints and that this discomfort will continue regardless of treatment. Therefore, the client with chronic symptomatic pain should be advised accordingly. Bed rest is dangerous because it mobilizes calcium. Aspirin 900 to 1,500 mg four times daily may be helpful.

Severely painful and symptomatic disease can be treated with Calcitonin Salmon, a synthetic calcitonin that decreases bone resorption and arrests the disease. Initial dosage is 100 MRC units administered subcutaneously daily. Elevated alkaline phosphatase levels should return to normal within 2 months, but pain relief may require up to 6 months of treatment. Secondary treatment failure may occur in up to 60 percent of these treated clients (DeRose et al. 1974). Etidronate disodium (Didronel) is the first oral medication for treatment of clients suffering from Paget's disease. The drug diminishes bone resorption and new bone formation. It relieves bone pain, improves healing, and reduces the elevated cardiac output. In excessive dosage it may increase pain and cause fractures. The recommended daily dosage is 5 mg per kg of body weight with water or juice. Treatment, instituted after consultation with a physician, should not exceed 6 months (Abramowicz 1978).

368

OSTEOPOROSIS

Pathophysiology

Osteoporosis is still of unknown origin. This disease consists of a decrease in bone mass and an increase in bone porosity. In animals calcium deficiency has been demonstrated to cause osteoporosis. Classically osteoporosis occurs in postmenopausal women and in older members of either sex. The peak incidence is after age 50. It is readily distinguished from secondary osteoporosis and iatrogenic disease due to steroid administration.

Nursing Assessment

Osteoporotic pain frequently does not appear until a fracture occurs. Vertebral compression fractures can occur as a result of minor trauma, such as lifting a window. Compression of dorsal and lumbar vertebrae leads to a loss of height, kyphosis, and back pain. Clients incur fractures particularly of the proximal femur and distal radius. Fortunately only one-third of cases of vertebral collapse are symptomatic. The kyphosis and vertebral collapse increase the downward angle of the ribs and cause the formation of typical horizontal skin folds across the chest and abdomen. Occasionally the lower ribs may override the pelvis, leading to bilateral flank pain, eased by hyperextending the back. Back pain may be sharp and localized to a specific area of the spine or it may be diffuse, indicating extension and recurrent vertebral collapse. Typically these fractures occur with minimal trauma. They usually heal normally.

Diagnostics

X-rays reveal osteoporosis with a thin cervical bone and vertebral collapse. Rarely, the back pain may precede x-ray evidence of fracture for a few weeks (Heaney 1971). These changes are nonspecific and also are found in hyperparathyroidism and multiple myeloma.

Laboratory studies are normal. Serum calcium, phosphorous, as well as alkaline phosphatase are normal.

A diagnosis of multiple myeloma should be excluded in all cases of symptomatic osteoporosis, a high sedimentation rate often being the initial clue. Blood electrophoresis, which will reveal a monoclonal globulin spike in myeloma, should be ordered. Urine should be tested for the presence of Bence-Jones protein, which is found in the client with multiple myeloma.

Other causes to consider in diagnostic studies include Cushing's syndrome and iatrogenically induced bone resorption due to chronic steroid administration.

Nursing Management

Health Education and Counseling. Care must be taken in even the nonsymptomatic elderly to prevent falls, since the more brittle the bones become, the more susceptible they are to fracture. Not uncommonly those of advanced age develop fractures unrelated to trauma such as the "sitdown fracture" of the pelvis.

Intake of dietary calcium is believed to be an efficacious prophylaxis for osteoporosis. One quart of skim or whole milk per day will supply the client with 400 U of vitamin D and over 1 g of calcium. Trea-

369

ment is aimed at symptomatic relief as well as at reversal of bone loss.

Since a collapsed vertebral fracture requires complete bed rest and analgesia, the nurse must take precautions to counteract the constipatory effects of such treatment. Bed rest is prescribed for 3 weeks, after which the client should be fitted with a lightweight corset with steel ribs. Graduated activity is encouraged for the next 8 weeks, after which the corset should be discarded. The client should be instructed on performing abdominal and back exercises, which should be maintained over the client's lifetime (Barzel 1978, p. 281). Emotional support to counteract apathy and a feeling of helplessness is essential.

Treatment. Other therapy includes calcium supplements on the order of 2 g calcium daily, either in high-calcium foods or as calcium gluconate or lactate or calcium diphosphate 0.5 g tablets taken as 1 g three times daily with vitamin D 1,000 U. Calcium replenishment is highly variable; in a number of clients individual response may vary over time.

Estrogens with or without androgens rapidly decrease pain and may play a beneficial role. They are given as conjugated equine estrogen 1.25 to 2.5 mg daily with methyltestosterone 5 to 20 mg daily. Estrogens should be cycled to prevent vaginal bleeding. Testosterone and other androgens may cause hepatic toxicity. Recent studies using fluoride seem to be promising (Hanson and Roos 1976). Secondary osteoporosis is reversed by treatment of the primary illness.

OSTEOMALACIA

Osteomalacia, while rare in this country, can occur in older people residing in northern climates with little sunlight. The bones become decalcified. Osteomalacia may be due to adult rickets or to a variety of disorders of the bone associated with hypocalcemia and hypophosphatemia.

The disease can occur in clients with chronic renal failure. It involves a deficiency of the most active form of vitamin D, which the kidney metabolizes. This deficiency, in turn, leads to impaired absorption of calcium from the intestinal tract. The end result is that mineralization of bone is impaired and the epiphyseal growth plates are closed (Reifenstein 1974, p. 1969).

Nursing Assessment

Osteomalacia should be suspected in clients who have a history of peptic ulcer, partial gastrectomy, renal disease, or functional colon. Osteoporosis is more common in clients with an alcoholic history (Saville and Heaney 1975, p. 368). Assessment frequently finds a lactose malabsorption syndrome or nutritional deficiency of dairy products high in calcium. A thorough dietary history will determine the adequacy of a diet rich in vitamin D. In addition many elderly clients lead such a withdrawn life that they are deprived of sunlight. They often have a history of generalized, unrelenting bone pain (Barzel 1978, p. 282).

Diagnostics

The differential lab diagnosis for osteomalacia shows a low serum calcium or low phosphorous and above-normal alkaline phosphatase. A 24-hour urine test will reveal below-normal calcium excretion.

Nursing Management

Management of osteomalacia is relatively simple if the cause is nutritional and solar (vitamin D) deficiencies. For such clients a quart of milk a day may suffice. For clients who have a vitamin D malabsorption syndrome, the nurse should prescribe 50,000 to 100,000 U of vitamin D per day. Medication dosage is begun low for 2 to 3 weeks before loading doses are prescribed. The withdrawn client must receive counseling and follow-up home visits. Osteomalacia secondary to Fanconi syndrome is treated with both phosphate replacement and vitamin D. The chronic use of laxatives must be discouraged. Clients with constipation are encouraged to increase dietary fiber and fluids. Psyllium hydrophilic mucilloid (Metamucil and others) may be helpful (see chapter 16).

POLYMYALGIA RHEUMATICA

Polymyalgia rheumatica (PMR), unlike rheumatic heart disease (RHD), primarily affects women over the age of 55. It is of unknown etiology and is included in this chapter because of its symptom presentation. Because 40 percent of clients have associated giant cell arteritis, a number of authorities consider it a manifestation of systemic arteritis (Hahn 1976, p. 26). Other clients eventually develop rheumatic heart disease, systemic lupus erythematosis, polymyositis, temporal arteritis, rheumatoid arthritis, or polyarteritis nodosa, making the problem a candidate for an autoimmune disorder (Grob 1978, p. 257).

Nursing Assessment

The lack of correlation between subjective and objective findings frequently leads to the labeling of clients as suffering from a psychoneurotic problem.

Subjective Findings. Subjective complaints include severe pain in the neck, shoulder girdle, upper arms, and thighs, which is associated with stiffness and may be of abrupt or insidious onset. Usually a low-grade fever is present, with weakness anorexia and easy fatigability. Some clients may also complain of temporal headache, transient visual loss, claudication of the jaw, or pain in the tongue on chewing.

Objective Findings. The physical examination does not reveal any significant findings. Clients have little or no muscle wasting and weakness; however, they are reluctant to perform muscle-strength testing in girdle areas. Due to pain on palpation, muscle tenderness may be found. Superficial arteries of the head or neck may be enlarged and tender.

Diagnostics

Laboratory tests are normal except for the sedimentation rate, which is elevated. A variable degree of anemia may be present with hematocrit reading as low as 25% (Rodman 1973, p. 66). A protein electrophoresis and bone marrow study may be necessary to exclude multiple myeloma. Serum enzymes are normal, as is electromyography. Because of the potential for the serious complication of temporal arteritis, Hahn recommends that all clients with a diagnosis of PMR be referred to a rheumatologist for consideration of temporal artery biopsy and to an ophthalmologist for funduscopic assessment (Hahn 1976, p. 26).

Nursing Management

Counseling. The focus of care for clients with PMR involves emotional support and relief of symptoms. Because of the protracted nature (several months to two years) of the problem, emotional stress is compounded. Clients should be reassured that the condition is treatable.

Treatment. When the temporal artery biopsy is negative and no symptoms suggesting temporal arteritis are present, a trial dose of 15 to 20 mg of prednisone will usually produce diagnostic relief in 48 hours. If relief is not obtained, a 2-week course of 20 to 60 mg of prednisone is attempted. Should this therapy not relieve symptoms, the client most likely does not have PMR. This initial loading dose is quickly tapered to 10 mg of prednisone for several months. Therapy continues with smaller intermittent doses over a variable period of time that is usually not more than six months.

SUMMARY

Musculoskeletal problems in the elderly are problems for which the gerontological nurse practitioner can render invaluable assistance, particularly because the common complaints include pain and problems of positioning and mobility.

REFERENCES

ABRAMOWICZ, M., ed. 1978. *The Medical Letter on Drugs and Therapeutics* 20(18):78–79.

BARZEL, U. S. 1978. "Common Metabolic Disorders of the Skeleton in Aging." In W. Reichel, ed., *Clinical Aspects of Aging.* Baltimore: Williams and Wilkins.

BAYLES, T. B. 1972. "Salicylate Therapy for Rheumatoid Arthritis." In J. I. Hollander, ed., *Arthritis and Allied Conditions.* Philadelphia: Lea and Febiger.

BERG, C., and L. HANEBUTH. 1977. "Paget's Disease: A Challenge in Nursing Care." *Journal of Gerontological Nursing* 3(3):27–30.

BOURNE, G. H. 1961. *Structural Aspects of Aging.* New York: Haefner.

DeROSE, J., et al. 1974. "Response of Paget's Disease to Porcine and Salmon Calcitonins." *The American Journal of Medicine* 56:858–66.

DISKIN, E. 1978. *Yoga for Your Leisure Years.* New York: Warner Books.

ENGELMAN, E. P. 1972. "Conservative Management of Rheumatoid Arthritis." In J. I. Hollander, ed., *Arthritis and Allied Conditions.* Philadelphia: Lea and Febiger.

FREMONT-SMITH, K., and T. B. BAYLES. 1965. "Salicylate Therapy in Rheumatoid Arthritis." *Journal of the American Medical Association* 192:1133–36.

GROB, D. 1978. "Common Disorders of Muscle in the Aged." In W. Reichel, ed., *Clinical Aspects of Aging.* Baltimore: Williams and Wilkins.

HAHN, B. A. 1976. "Arthritis, Bursitis, and Bone Disease." In F. U. Steinberg, ed, *Cowdry's The Care of the Geriatric Patient.* St. Louis: C. V. Mosby.

HANSON, T., and B. ROOS. 1976. "Effect of Combined Therapy with Sodium Fluoride, Calcium, and Vitamin D on the Lumbar Spine in Osteoporosis." *American Journal of Roentgenology, Radium Therapy, and Nuclear Medicine* 126:1294–96.

HARVEY, A. M. 1967. "Diseases of the Connective Tissue (the Collagen Diseases)." In P. B. Beeson and W. McDermott, eds., *Cecil-Loeb Textbook of Medicine,* 12 ed. Philadelphia: W. B. Saunders.

HEANEY, R. P. 1971. "The Osteoporosis." In P. D. Beeson and W. McDermott, eds., *Cecil-Loeb Textbook of Medicine.* Philadelphia: W. B. Saunders.

MOSKOWITZ, R. W. 1972. "Treatment of Osteoarthritis." In J. I. Hollander and D. J. McCarty, eds., *Arthritis and Allied Conditions.* Philadelphia: Lea and Febiger.

RAGAN, C. 1972. "The Clinical Picture of Rheumatoid Arthritis." In J. I. Hollander, ed., *Arthritis and Allied Conditions.* Philadelphia: Lea and Febiger.

REIFENSTEIN, E., JR. 1974. "Metabolic Disorders of the Bone." In M. M. Wintrobe, ed., *Harrison's Principles of Internal Medicine.* New York: McGraw-Hill.

ROBBINS, S. 1974. *Pathologic Basis of Disease.* Philadelphia: W. B. Saunders.

ROBINSON, W. D. 1971. "Diseases of Joints." In P. B. Beeson and W. McDermott, eds., *Cecil-Loeb Textbook of Medicine.* Philadelphia: W. B. Saunders.

RODMAN, G., ed. 1973. *Primer on the Rheumatic Diseases,* 7th ed. New York: The Arthritis Foundation.

SAVILLE, P. D., and R. P. HEANEY. 1975. "Osteoporosis." In H.P. von Han, ed., *Practical Geriatrics.* New York and Basel: S. Karger, A.G.

SHAFER, K. N., et al. 1971. *Medical-Surgical Nursing.* St. Louis: C. V. Mosby.

SODEMAN, W. A., and SODEMAN, W. A., JR. 1970. *Pathologic Physiology.* Philadelphia: W. B. Saunders.

VAUGHN, J. H., E. S. MORGAN, and R. R. JACON. 1968. "Role of Gamma Globulin Complexes in Rheumatoid Arthritis." *Transactions of the Association of American Physicians.* 81:231–39.

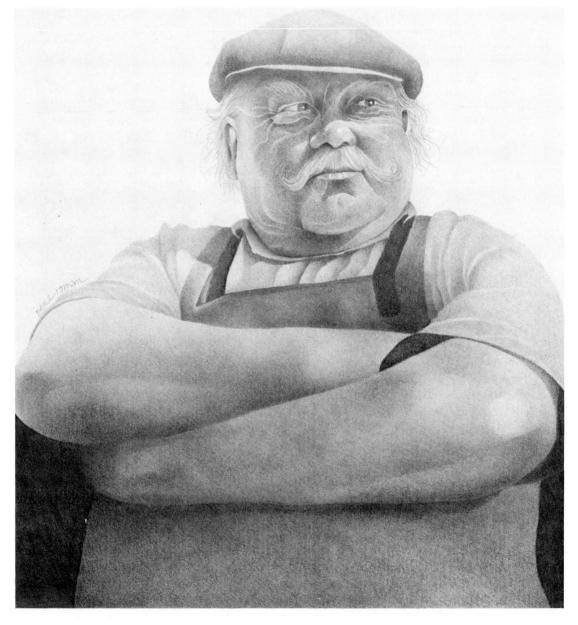

Chapter 15

GERONTOLOGICAL NURSING MANAGEMENT
THE ELDERLY CLIENT WITH AN ENDOCRINE DYSFUNCTION

One of the major endocrine disorders seen in the elderly is diabetes mellitus. A large number of elderly diabetics may have been diagnosed at a younger age; however, a significant proportion of cases arise in later life. Diabetes is a chronic disease of serious proportions that can cause a number of complications. Fortunately the incidence of newly diagnosed diabetes declines in clients over age 65 (Rifkin and Ross 1971). This chapter focuses mainly on the chronic aspects of diabetes. The nature of diagnosis of myxedema and hyperthyroidism in the elderly necessitates a brief overview of thyroid conditions.

DIABETES MELLITUS

Pathophysiology

The exact mechanism involved in the development of diabetes mellitus remains unclear. It is generally considered to be a genetically mediated, chronic metabolic disorder characterized by an absence of, or a deficiency in, the production of insulin. Diabetes mellitus can also be caused by a metabolic disorder in insulin utilization. Some diabetics produce adequate or even excessive amounts of insulin but are unable to use it because of an inborn error or active inhibition of the insulin molecule. Current research is focusing on autoimmunity and virus-mediated trigger mechanisms in juvenile-onset diabetes. In any case, the end result is the same: carbohydrate metabolism is deranged, which in turn results in an abnormally high metabolism of fats and proteins. These metabolic disorders are manifested by glycosuria and an increase in blood glucose levels.

In addition to glycosuria and an increased blood sugar level, diabetes mellitus is usually accompanied by secondary effects. Susceptibility to atherosclerosis of coronary, renal, and cerebral vessels increases. The chronic diabetic usually exhibits elevated plasma lipid levels, which probably play a significant role in the genesis of atherosclerosis. Microangiopathy, or small-vessel disease, is also a complication of diabetes. Most commonly these pathological changes occur in the retinal and renal blood vessels. Vascular changes begin at an earlier age in the diabetic than in the nondiabetic person.

Certain variables such as environmental factors, obesity, physical stress, and pregnancy can precipitate the disorder in those who have a predisposition to the disease. In the obese client with normal blood sugar, insulin levels are high. However, this problem can be corrected by a return to normal weight. Studies have shown that the juvenile-onset diabetic has an absolute or nearly absolute failure of beta cells to produce insulin. In adult-onset diabetics the pathology is less well defined. Some of the hypotheses proposed for diabetes mellitus include (1) failure or delayed release of insulin, (2) biologically ineffective insulin, and (3) release of some factor, as yet unidentified, that acts as an antagonist to the insulin produced.

Regardless of whether the diabetes is of juvenile or adult onset, the morphological pathology found in the pancreas is indistinguishable in the two types. In the islets of Langerhans, the insulin-producing beta cells exhibit abnormalities. In addition, the islets themselves show morphological changes such as intracellular hyaline degeneration and fibrosis of the capsule and stroma. In adult-onset diabetes the basement membranes of blood vessels adjacent to the beta cells are thickened. However,

researchers have found no evidence that this thickening acts as a barrier to the secretory process of the beta cell (Robbins 1974).

Insulin functions as a "carrier" for glucose as it crosses cell membranes for use by fibroblasts and muscle and fat cells. The absolute or relative lack of insulin, therefore, deprives cells of energy-rich glucose. The outlook for diabetics can depend, in large measure, on the time of onset of the disease; the prognosis is better for adult-onset clients than for juvenile-onset clients.

Nursing Assessment

Subjective Findings. In the older client diabetes mellitus usually takes an insidious form. The typical situation presents as unsuspected hyperglycemia during routine testing or while the origin of one or several of the complications of diabetes, such as vascular, ocular, and dermatological problems or neuropathies, is being investigated. A mild fatigue may be present. Another important suggestive complaint, in men, is a recently acquired primary impotence or absence of early morning erections. Generalized pruritus in both sexes and vulval pruritus in women should bring one to consider diabetes mellitus, as should balanitis in men.

Occasionally the nurse will be confronted with the classic symptoms of polyuria and polydipsia, weight loss, and dehydration. Even more uncommonly, a rapidly developing ketoacidosis and coma are the initial findings of diabetes in the older client. Excessive appetite, thirst, and urinary frequency indicate glycosuria and impending ketoacidosis. Fatigue and generalized weakness suggest poor control in the known diabetic. However, in others these symptoms may also be due to an endocrine disorder, hematologic problem, or infection. Rapid weight loss, more common in the young, may also be found in the older diabetic client in association with insulin dependence and severe glycosuria.

Objective Findings. The objective findings are equally nonspecific. However, when correlated with the subjective complaints, they become highly suggestive of the diagnosis. These findings may be due to the diabetes itself or may be manifestations of complications. Signs include a chronically ill and fatigued appearance or loosened skin, which is evidence of weight loss. In the lower extremities thinning of the skin and atrophy of subcutaneous tissue with plantar redness of the feet are often found. Xanthelasma of the eyelids, flat xanthomas of the upper trunk, and necrobiosis lipoidica diabeticorum (raised erythematous plaques evolving to white atrophic areas with dilated purple veins) are found at any age. Signs of the complications are more common. Vulvovaginitis and balanitis were mentioned above. Staphylostreptococcal skin infections are frequent and dangerous in the diabetic. Septic ulcers of the feet are often associated with diabetic peripheral neuropathy or with evidence of peripheral vascular disease. Cataracts and diabetic retinopathy have often been described. Diabetic retinopathy is classified in five stages: (1) microaneurysms with or without punctate hemorrhages or exudates; (2) dot or blot hemorrhages and waxy exudates; (3) venous sclerosis, newly formed vessels, massive hemorrhages, retinitis proliferans, and retinal detachment; (4) retinal destruction; and (5) hypertensive retinopathy (Ballan-

tyne 1964). Generalized arteriosclerosis and angina pectoris are common.

The neuropathy of diabetes may present as an involvement of single or multiple peripheral or cranial nerves. Findings may include paresis of ocular movement, wasting of small hand muscles, incomplete bladder emptying, or impotence, as well as other peripheral sensory changes (Williams 1978). The prominent findings are in the lower extremities, with painful sensations aggravated by walking and an early loss of vibration and position sense (Dyck 1971). Patellar and achilles tendon reflexes may be diminished or absent. Temperature sensation is diminished. Autonomic nervous system involvement causes a profuse, watery diarrhea that often awakens the client or causes fecal incontinence at night. Other complications include renal infection, diabetic nephropathy with massive proteinuria and edema, and generalized atherosclerosis with arteriosclerotic heart disease.

Diagnostics

In the diagnosis of diabetes mellitus, most endocrinologists place emphasis on the demonstration of an abnormal hyperglycemia. Fasting levels of the blood (serum or plasma) sugar above 130 mg per 100 ml or blood sugar levels above 200 mg per 100 ml 2 hours after the ingestion of 50 gm of glucose are diagnostic. The older client will often have normal fasting levels. The abnormalities usually appear at the 2-hour point.

Older persons have consistently been found to have an altered carbohydrate metabolism, evidenced by a declining glucose tolerance change. Because of this aging process, diagnosis of diabetes for most older

377

adults must not be based on the same laboratory norms seen in the younger or middle-aged adult.

Because of the older client's difficulties in handling postprandial blood sugar levels, many clinicians will have a blood sugar determination drawn 2 hours after ingestion of 100 g of the flavored glucose solution or 2 hours after the ingestion of a highly sweetened meal. However, some endocrinologists do not agree with this technique because they feel that those who have an altered metabolism due to aging and who are unable to handle a glucose load do not necessarily have diabetes (Levin 1976, p. 137). Because of the confusing laboratory picture of older clients, some authorities subscribe to the use of normograms, which are percentile ranks for 2-hour glucose values at any age. Therefore, the individual is judged against values from the peer age group. This technique, however, cannot determine which percentile rank indicates that an individual has diabetes and which percentile rank represents the altered effect on glucose tolerance due to aging (Williams 1978, p. 327). Random blood levels of over 180 mg per 100 ml are also indicative of diabetes, provided that the client is not ill (Anderson 1976).

The oral glucose tolerance test should be reserved for clients suspected to have diabetes but in whom the criteria mentioned above have not been found. Accurate testing requires that the client be well nourished to avoid the false positive results of "starvation diabetes." For 3 days prior to the test, clients should be prepared with diets containing at least 150 g and preferably 250 g carbohydrates (Rifkin and Ross 1971). In addition the client should be active and not seriously ill, to avoid false posi-

tive test results. A complete analysis of the test may be found in the report of the Committee on Statistics of the American Diabetes Association (American Diabetes Association 1969).

Because of the conflicting data available on laboratory confirmation of diabetes in the older client, caution should be exercised in labeling the older client a diabetic on the sole basis of glucose intolerance (Williams 1978).

Nursing Management

Treatment. Once the diagnosis has been made, treatment should be kept simple. The habits of a lifetime are difficult to change; only those that conflict with diabetic control or pose potential complications should be interfered with. Good management requires lowering of blood sugar levels in order to (1) prevent worsening of the disease; (2) avoid the development of ketoacidosis, lactic acidosis, or hypoglycemia; and (3) delay the development of complications and, if possible, diminish or eliminate them. Control is accomplished through a combination of diet, exercise, and medication. Good skin care and body hygiene must also be employed to prevent complications. Considerable evidence shows that controlling the hyperglycemia will prevent the long-term complications of neuropathy, retinopathy, nephropathy, and arteriosclerosis (Lauvaux 1976). "The burden of proof is upon those who maintain that diabetes control using the above measures is without effect" (Cahill et al. 1976).

The vast majority of elderly clients are controlled by *diet*. Those who are overweight, who have few or no symptoms, and

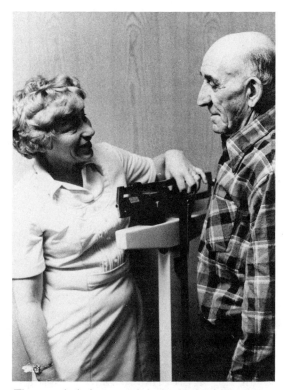

The gerontological nurse can help the elderly adapt to the aging process by developing good relationships with them during health checkups; elderly clients need one-to-one, personalized communication to understand the most effective ways to promote and maintain their health.

in whom blood sugar levels are not excessively high at the time of diagnosis (e.g., 300 mg per 100 ml) usually can be controlled without medication. Food preferences must be respected, as these have ethnic and social connotations, and the nurse must be flexible so that client compliance is obtained. Bread, rice, spaghetti, and corn are equally good sources of carbohydrates and are well tolerated in reasonable amounts. Fruits containing simple sugars can help satisfy a desire for sweets. Caloric restriction is essential for the obese client.

Other clients must receive sufficient calories to maintain normal body weight. Adequate amounts of high-quality protein must be provided, at least 1 g per kilogram of normal body weight. Carbohydrate needs are 3 to 5 g per kilogram of body weight and fat from 1 to 2 g per kilogram of body weight. The total daily basal caloric need approximates 25 calories per kilogram (11 calories per pound of normal body weight). This ratio represents the total caloric need for a new diabetic until the diabetes is controlled. Writing out the dietary recommendations is important. Once control is achieved, nonobese clients may have their diet increased 20 percent for sedentary work, 25 percent for moderate work, and 30 percent for strenuous activity. Further caloric adjustments may be made in relation to observed changes in the client's weight.

A sustained program of *regular daily exercise* can do much toward achieving diabetic control. An exercise program for the diabetic should involve mild forms of exercise, such as swimming and walking. A daily 30 minutes of vigorous walking will help the obese client lose weight. By following this regimen, the moderately obese individual will average a 20-pound weight loss per year (Williams 1978).

For a small number of clients, insulin therapy is not indicated but strict adherence to diet does not achieve the desired control of symptomatic hyperglycemia. Such clients should be allowed the choice of an oral agent, with full knowledge of the possible complications. *Oral hypoglycemic agents* are divided into two types: the sulfonureas, derivatives of sulfonamides, and the biguanides. Recent controversy has sharply limited the use of these agents.

379

Studies have demonstrated that their use may be associated with an increased incidence of cardiovascular complications and death (Report of the Committee for the Assessment of Biometric Aspects of Controlled Trials of Hypoglycemic Agents 1975). In particular, the biguanides (phenformin HCL) potentiate lactic acidosis and are associated with high mortality. Biguanides should not be used to treat diabetes mellitus (Conley and Loewenstein 1976; UGDP 1971a; UGDP 1971b).

Sulfonureas are classified according to their duration of action. They all stimulate insulin production by the beta cells of the pancreas and are of no value in the treatment of insulin-dependent diabetic clients. The sulfonureas may produce hypoglycemia with all its attendant dangers. Phenylbutazone, sulfa drugs, salicylates, and bishydroxycoumarin potentiate the action of sulfonureas and can cause prolonged hypoglycemia. Alcohol, in the presence of sulfonureas, can cause an antabuse reaction with severe vomiting and collapse. All sulfonureas require 1 week to create a stable effect on blood sugar levels.

Tolbutamide (Orinase) is the most commonly used of the group. It is short acting, with a peak effect in 4 to 6 hours. The usual dosage is 500 mg to 3 g daily in divided doses. Chlorpropamide (Diabinese) is the longest acting preparation, with an effect lasting over 24 hours. The usual dosage is 125 to 750 mg daily in divided doses. Other preparations such as acetohexamide and tolazamide are intermediate in activity. The usual technique is to administer a daily dosage of medication before breakfast and monitor the blood sugar levels in 1 week. If more medication is required, a second daily dosage is given before supper.

The next additional, or third, dosage increase is given before breakfast and the next one before supper. Any further augmentation is given before lunch. Should blood sugar not be controlled with the maximum dosage of 4 tablets per day, a trial with another oral agent or a switch to insulin will be necessary. Occasionally clients not responding to tolbutamide will respond to a longer acting preparation.

Insulin exists in regular or crystalline short-acting form or in a variety of slower acting preparations with a longer duration of activity (see table 15.1). All preparations exist in a variety of strengths. The current tendency is to use an internationally standard strength of 100 U per ml. This preparation has the added advantage of being measurable in any standard l-ml syringe (0.1 ml = 10 U insulin). Regardless of the strength employed, the client must be given the appropriately marked syringe. Other concentrations are 40, 80, and 500 U per ml. The danger of insulin administration is a hypoglycemic reaction that, in the elderly, can lead to brain injury and death. Insulin shock may resemble either a stroke with unilateral focal neurological findings or a form of dementia indistinguishable from chronic brain syndrome. Therefore, the client should use only as much insulin as necessary. Blood levels should be maintained between 150 to 200 mg per 100 ml. To minimize the danger of hypoglycemia, urine sugars should show 1 or 2 plus at least once daily. In clients with a tendency toward hypoglycemia, glucosuria is acceptable if the blood sugar levels are low and if the urines are negative at least once each day. Changes in insulin dosage require 3 days before a stable effect on blood glucose is seen. Absolute indications for insulin

TABLE 15.1
Action of Various Insulin Preparations

Preparation	Approximate Time of Onset	Time of Peak Effect	Approximate Duration of Action	Usual Time of Administration	Time of Highest Risk of Hypoglycemia
Short Acting				20–30 min.	Before lunch
Regular	1 hour	2–4 hours	6 hours	before	
Crystalline	1 hour	2–6 hours	8 hours	breakfast	
Semilente	1 hour	6–10 hours	14 hours		
Intermediate Acting				1 hour	Before supper
Globin	2 hours	6–12 hours	24 hours	before	
NPH	2 hours	8–14 hours	24 hours	breakfast	
Lente	2 hours		24 hours		
Long Acting				½–1 hour	Between
PZI	6–7 hours	12–24 hours	30–36 hours	before	midnight and
Ultralente	7 hours	12–24 hours	36 hours	breakfast	breakfast

therapy are a history of ketoacidosis, persistent polyuria, polydypsia, and weight loss or relentless diabetic neuropathy.

Short-acting preparations are classified as regular, crystalline, or semilente insulin. They have a rapid onset of action, and the action is of short duration (table 15.1). These preparations are particularly suited for the treatment of ketoacidosis or for use in clients with acute hypermetabolic and unstable conditions, such as those that occur in severe infections, during and after surgery, or immediately after acute infarction or stroke. Short-acting preparations offer high flexibility in exchange for the necessity of multiple daily injections. When used to cover glucosuria in older clients, the dosage should be kept low: 5 U administered for 3+ and 10 U for 4+ (Rifkin and Ross 1971).

Longer acting preparations are usually classified as intermediate and prolonged (table 15.1). Globin, NPH, and lente insulins are intermediate in type. The 7 A.M. dose has its maximum effect between 1 P.M. and 9 P.M. PZI and ultralente insulins have prolonged action. A 7 A.M. dose of these insulins has peak activity between 7 P.M. and 7 A.M. the next morning. These preparations have the advantage of requiring one or, rarely, two daily injections. The choice of preparation usually depends on the time of day of maximum hyperglycemia as well as on the clinician's familiarity with the preparation. Rapid-acting preparations may be used in combination with a longer acting one, thus modifying the timing of the hypoglycemic effects of both. The decision to begin insulin therapy as well as the choice of preparation are best left to a physician.

Health Education and Counseling. The client and significant other(s) should know the type of diet and medication that the

381

client needs. If insulin is used, the client and a responsible significant other should be taught how to measure and administer this potent drug as well as to recognize symptoms of insulin shock and diabetic coma. Teaching should include sterile injection technique, choice of sites, and care of materials. The same persons should be taught how and when to test the urine for sugar. The newer paper testing materials require minimal equipment and time. The client must not urinate directly on the test paper, as this washes off the enzyme and causes false negative reactions. Urine for testing should be obtained by having the client void, waiting 15 minutes, and then having the client void again. The second specimen, a good representative of current blood sugar levels, is then tested. Clients using insulin should test four times daily not only to monitor their degree of glucosuria, but also to be aware of any impending hypoglycemia. The latter is established by the presence of a persistently negative urine sugar. These clients should be instructed to report either persistent glycosuria or persistently negative urines and will certainly require evaluation for either diet or insulin adjustment. Clients treated only with diet or with diet and oral hypoglycemic agents should strive for consistently negative urine tests. Once stabilized, they may be permitted to test their urines two to three times weekly, preferably 2 hours after their largest meal of the day. They must be advised that persistent glucosuria is sufficient reason to contact the nurse.

Health instructions include general hygiene, with particular attention to the care of the feet. An ingrown, improperly cut toenail or a neglected cut can lead to septic ulceration, gangrene, and amputation. For treatment of peripheral vascular lesions, see chapter 10, on cardiovascular problems.

Diabetic clients who have progressive visual loss due to retinopathy require special attention. See chapter 13, on sensory vision losses. Additionally two special publications are printed by the American Foundation for the Blind that focus on self-care techniques but also will assist the nurse in caring for clients: *Devices for Visually Impaired Diabetics* and *Blindness and Diabetics*.

THYROID PROBLEMS

Pathophysiology

Although the frequency of thyroid disease does not increase with age, its diagnosis becomes more difficult. This endocrinopathy affects almost every body system, causing findings that are easily confused with other, more common problems of the aged. Thyroid disease may be secondary to pituitary disease or primary due to abnormal function of the thyroid gland itself.

The two lateral lobes of the thyroid gland normally flank the larynx and trachea and are connected ventrally by the isthmus. Histologically the thyroid gland is composed of spheroidal sacs, the walls of which are composed of cuboidal cells. The active, circulating hormone produced by these cells is tri-iodothyronine (T3) and thyroxine (T4) (Robbins 1974, p. 480).

Acquired hypothyroidism (myxedema) in the adult is the result of a deficiency of circulating thyroid hormone. The pathological changes vary. In some cases the size of the gland is reduced; the atrophied gland may also be fibrotic. In other cases the gland may be enlarged and exhibit extensive cellular destruction (Peery and Miller, 1971, p. 724). In all cases the production of thyroid hormone is impaired, the level of the circulating hormone is reduced, and the rate of cellular metabolism falls below normal. As a further consequence a generalized increase in interstitial edema occurs. The accumulation of fluid in the skin is reflected in the individual's physical appearance. When the cardiac interstitium is edematous, normal cardiac function is affected.

ADULT HYPOTHYROIDISM (MYXEDEMA)

Myxedema is the most common thyroid problem in the aged, but because of the difficulty in diagnosing it, the disorder often goes undetected (Asch and Greenblatt 1978). In addition, the presentation of hypothyroidism is quite similar to hyperparathyroidism, which, like myxedema, frequently goes undiagnosed in the elderly.

Myxedema is seven times more frequent in women than in men. It may occur as a late result of untreated Hashimoto's thyroiditis (chronic thyroiditis) or after treatment for hyperthyroidism with surgery or radioactive iodine. Myxedema progresses slowly, with progressive changes in appearance and mentation. Secondary failure is due to hypopituitarism and presents with other endocrine diseases such as hypoadrenalism.

Nursing Assessment

Subjective Findings. The most frequent subjective complaints are decreased tolerance to cold, lethargy, and constipation. Occasionally muscle weakness, pain, stiffness, and loss of sense of smell or nasal stuffiness may be prominent. Answers to questions are slow and often inappropriate. Hallucinations and depression (Anderson 1976) and even overt insanity (myxedema madness) may occur (Rawson et al. 1964). Careful assessment for myxedema is essential in all clients who present with an acute brain syndrome.

Objective Findings. Objective findings include lifeless, dry hair; coarse, dry, and thickened skin; and prominent lips and nostrils. The eyebrows are sparse, with loss of the outer third margin. The eyelids are often puffy and the tongue is thickened. Many of these findings are of little use in the very old, in whom hair loss and puffy features are normal. The heart may be enlarged and a pericardial effusion may be present; congestive heart failure, bradycardia, and angina pectoris may also be found (Rawson et al. 1964). The voice is often husky and weak. Constipation and even evidence of intestinal ileus may be present; abdominal examination may show ascites. A striking finding is the slow relaxation phase on examination of the deep tendon reflexes. This finding is most apparent in the ankle jerk in younger patients. Myxedema coma may also develop.

Diagnostics

Clinical diagnosis of thyroid disease is confirmed by abnormalities of serum thyroxine (T4), tri-iodothyronine resin uptake (T3 uptake), free thyroxine iodine (FTI), radioactive iodine uptake (RAI), and thyroid scanning. Blood levels of thyroid stim-

383

ulating hormone (TSH) may also be measured; suppression tests of this hormone can aid in distinguishing between primary and secondary disease.

Laboratory studies often reveal normochromic, normocytic anemia. A low T4, T3, and FTI are diagnostic; RAI uptake is very low. In primary disease TSH levels are elevated; in secondary disease the levels are low. When myxedema is due to thyroiditis, the anticytoplasmic antibody complement fixation test or tanned red-cell agglutination test (TRC) will be strongly positive (DeGroot 1971).

Nursing Management

Treatment. Treatment requires hormone replacement therapy. Thyroid extract has been criticized as undependable and should be avoided. Today, however, synthetic substitutes for pure thyroxine (T4) are both dependable and inexpensive. The usual practice in treating clients with advanced disease is to begin with small doses and then increase them slowly in order not to precipitate an episode of thyroid storm. One can give thyroxine 0.025 mg daily for 7 days, increase this to 0.05 mg for 2 weeks, and then increase the dose every 2 weeks to a maintenance dose of 0.2 to 0.3 mg daily. The client is euthyroid when plasma levels of T4 and TSH (if higher initially) are normal. Normal levels may occur prior to return of clinical euthyroidism.

Developing or increasing angina pectoris or the appearance of congestive heart failure may require a slowing of the schedule or a lower than optimal maintenance dose. Myxedema coma requires hospitalization and close physician surveillance.

Health Education and Counseling. When counseling the newly diagnosed hypothyroid client and, if possible, the family, the nurse should keep in mind that body image may be a major concern. The changes in skin, hair, and facial appearance as well as problems of weight gain may cause great alarm, frustration, or depression. The individual and family should be reassured that these changes are manifestations of the problem and should reverse gradually with thyroid hormone replacement. They should also know that cold intolerance is not imaginary and that chilling should be avoided. The client who has been subject to psychoses, depression, or changes in personality and behavior may have alienated himself or herself from the family. The family should be informed that such behavior is a manifestation of the disorder.

The client must be given the amount of time required to carry out activities of daily living. Because of the time required to accomplish tasks, family or friends are apt to step in and assist or do things for the client. This behavior is to be discouraged, as self-sufficiency is important for all elderly people. Because of intolerance to cold, familial conflicts relating to differences in environmental temperatures may arise. The client should be instructed to dress warmly and add clothes as necessary.

Special skin care is indicated because of drying. Soap should be avoided and creams and emollients applied freely. Constipation is most frequently a concomitant problem and must be treated by the addition of dietary bulk (see chapter 16).

The client, although appearing apathetic and indifferent, may be very upset by this condition and will begin to express feelings of anger, depression, or frustration as therapy progresses. Sexuality may be of considerable concern to the man with a hypothyroid condition, as impotence can be a major problem.

HYPERTHYROIDISM

Nursing Assessment

Subjective Findings. Hyperthyroidism in the elderly client can frequently present with cardiovascular symptoms, such as angina pectoris, atrial fibrillation, congestive failure, and arteriosclerotic parkinsonism, and with gastrointestinal disorders (Asch and Greenblatt 1978). Other symptoms such as depression, lability, and confusion are often mislabeled as chronic brain syndrome.

When the disorder presents overtly, diagnosis is not difficult. Weakness, fatigue, weight loss, tremulousness, increased cold tolerance (or decreased heat tolerance) are not difficult findings to relate to hyperthyroidism. Less obvious is a history of diarrhea, particularly in a client who presents with diabetes of recent onset, and complaints of apathy or lethargy (Thomas et al. 1976).

Objective Findings. Classic objective findings include a warm, damp, smooth, fine skin with evidence of excessive perspiration. The eyes have a peculiar stare, as if in anger or fear. A decrease in blinking occurs or a frank bulging exophthalmos may be evident. A mass in the neck may be palpable or it may be nondiscernible as it plunges behind the sternum. Tachycardia

or atrial fibrillation may be present and associated with severe, intractable heart failure. Muscle weakness in the quadriceps of the thighs may prevent the client from stepping up onto a chair. The hand often has a rapid tremor, fine in the young and course in the aged, which may be demonstrated by asking the client to extend the arm and hand with the fingers extended. The tongue will also have a fine tremor if extended from the mouth.

Diagnostics

Laboratory tests reveal the increased T4, T3, FTI, and RAI uptake. In certain cases the level of T4 is normal, but the level of T3 (by radioimmunoassay) is elevated. Scanning will reveal the hidden enlarged gland. In questionable cases a T3 suppression test may be performed. The client is given triiodothyronine 50 to 100 mcg (μg) daily for 7 to 10 days. On the last day plasma T4 level is measured again and the RAI uptake is repeated. In normal clients the T4 should fall to very low levels, and the RAI uptake is suppressed to 50 percent or less of that prior to suppression. Persistent high levels of T4 and nonsuppressible RAI uptake confirm the diagnosis of hyperthyroidism.

Nursing Management

Treatment. Treatment requires decreasing the hormone production of the gland. This decrease is accomplished surgically by removing a portion of the gland or medically either by administering sufficient radioactive iodine to destroy a portion of the gland or by using medication to suppress hormone production. Surgery is rarely per-

385

formed in the older client in the absence of thyroid cancer. Antithyroid treatment requires up to 2 years of oral therapy and has a considerable recurrence rate. The administration of radioactive iodine (I^{131}) is the preferred treatment; its only untoward effect is a rather high rate of hypothyroidism as a long-term aftereffect. The calculation of the dose is based on the estimated size of the gland and its activity. This calculation should be done under the surveillance of a physician licensed to administer radioactive iodine. Since radioactive iodine requires up to 1 year for its full effect, clients often require supplemental antithyroid therapy for 3 to 6 months after the radioactive iodine dose is administered.

The antithyroid agents are either propylthiouracil or methimazole. Both of these agents can cause a skin rash, agranulocytosis, or neutropenia; any or all of these effects require that the individual drug employed be stopped and the other used instead. The usual dosage of propylthiouracil is 100 mg; that of methimazole is 10 mg. These drugs are administered every 6 or 8 hours in most cases. Since the duration of action of the medication is short, the dose must be taken on schedule.

Untreated or partially treated clients have a high risk of entering into a thyroid storm. In these cases severe tachycardia, fever, agitation, and weakness occur. Thyroid storm is a dangerous, life-threatening complication and is best treated by a physician in a hospital.

Health Education and Counseling. The client with a hyperthyroid condition needs an accepting, empathetic listener. The client with irrepressible mood swings and irritability often feels that these are routed in neuroticism. Usually family and friends have become exasperated by the client's behavior, thereby compounding feelings of anxiety and loneliness. The gerontological nurse counsels both client and family and informs them that the excessive sensitivity and irritability are part of the disorder. The client is told to avoid emotionally stressful situations and to take frequent small rests to conserve energy resources. Some clients can be helped by involving them in a community class to promote occupational therapy at home.

Health teaching includes instructing the client to be more careful about body hygiene because of increased perspiration. Dietary intake is increased to promote weight gain, which can be problematic if the client lives alone or suffers from anorexia. The underweight client should be instructed to eat more frequently until weight gain is restored to normal.

SUMMARY

The gerontological nurse can offer a significant health-provider relationship to the client with an endocrine problem. Support, health education, and counseling assume primary significance in these illnesses. For a majority of cases, health care management can be effectively provided by a nurse practitioner in collaboration with a physician. The nurse must be alert to seeking out the underlying symptomatic cause, thereby assisting in early diagnosis and initiation of management. Effective management can prevent or ameliorate disabling complications and maintain health.

REFERENCES

American Diabetes Association, Committee on Statistics. 1969. "Standardization of the Oral Glucose Tolerance Test." *Diabetes* 18:299.

American Foundation for the Blind. *Devices for Visually Impaired Diabetics.* 15 West 16 Street, New York, NY, 10011.

_____. *Blindness and Diabetics.* 15 West 16 Street, New York, NY, 10011.

ANDERSON, F. 1976. *Practical Management of the Elderly.* Oxford: Blackwell Scientific Publications.

ASCH, R., and R. B. GREENBLATT. 1978. "Geriatric Endocrinology." In W. Reichel, ed., *Clinical Aspects of Aging.* Baltimore: Williams and Wilkins.

BALLANTYNE, A. J. 1964. "Diabetes Mellitus." In G. G. Duncan, ed., *Diseases of Metabolism,* 5th ed. Philadelphia: W. B. Saunders.

CAHILL, G. F., D. D. ETZWIKEE, and N. FREINKEL. 1976. "Control and Diabetes." *New England Journal of Medicine* 294:1004–05.

CONLEY, L. A., and J. E. LOEWENSTEIN. 1976. "Phenformin and Lactic Acidosis." *Journal of the American Medical Association* 235:1575–78.

DeGROOT, L. J. 1971. "Diseases of the Thyroid." In P. B. Beeson and W. McDermott, eds., *Cecil-Loeb Textbook of Medicine.* Philadelphia: W. B. Saunders.

DYCK, P. J. 1971. "Diseases of Nerve Roots, Plexuses, and Peripheral Nerves." In P. J. Beeson and W. McDermott, eds., *Cecil-Loeb Textbook of Medicine.* Philadelphia: W. B. Saunders.

LAUVAUX, J. P. 1976. "Le Role de l'Hyperglycemie Chronique dans l'Apparition et le Développement de la Triopathie Diabétique: Neuropathie, Nephropathie, Retinopathie." Postdoctoral thesis. Brussels: Presse Universitaire.

LEVIN, M. 1976. "Diabetes Mellitus." In F. Steinberg, ed., *Cowdry's The Care of the Geriatric Patient.* St. Louis: C. V. Mosby.

PEERY, T., and F. MILLER. 1971. *Pathology.* Boston: Little, Brown.

RAWSON, R. W., M. SONENBERG, and M. L. MONEY. 1964. "Diseases of the Thyroid." In G. G. Duncan, ed., *Diseases of Metabolism,* 5th ed. Philadelphia: W. B. Saunders.

Report of the Committee for the Assessment of Biometric Aspects of Controlled Trials of Hypoglycemic Agents. 1975. "Review of the UGDP Study." *Journal of the American Medical Association* 231:593–608.

RIFKIN, H., and H. ROSS. 1971. "Diabetes in the Elderly." In I. Rossman, ed., *Clinical Geriatrics.* Philadelphia: J. B. Lippincott.

ROBBINS, S. 1974. *Pathological Basis of Disease.* Philadelphia: W. B. Saunders.

SHAFER, K. N., et al. 1971. *Medical Surgical Nursing,* 5th ed. St. Louis: C. V. Mosby.

THOMAS, F. B., E. I. MAZZAFERRI, and T. S. SKILLMAN. 1976. "Apathetic Thyrotoxicosis: A Distinct Clinical and Laboratory Entity." *American Journal of Medicine* 72:967–69.

University Group Diabetes Program (UGDP). 1971a. "A Study of the Effects of Hypoglycemic Agents on Vascular Complications in Patients with Adult Onset Diabetes. II: Mortality Results." *Diabetes* 19 (Supplement 2): 787–830.

_____. 1971b. "A Study of the Effects of Hypoglycemic Agents on Vascular Complications in Patients with Adult Onset Diabetes. IV: A Preliminary Report on Phenformin Results." *Journal of the American Medical Association* 2171:784–87.

WILLIAMS, T. F. 1978. "Diabetes Mellitus in Older People." In W. Reichel, ed., *Clinical Aspects of Aging.* Baltimore: Williams and Wilkins.

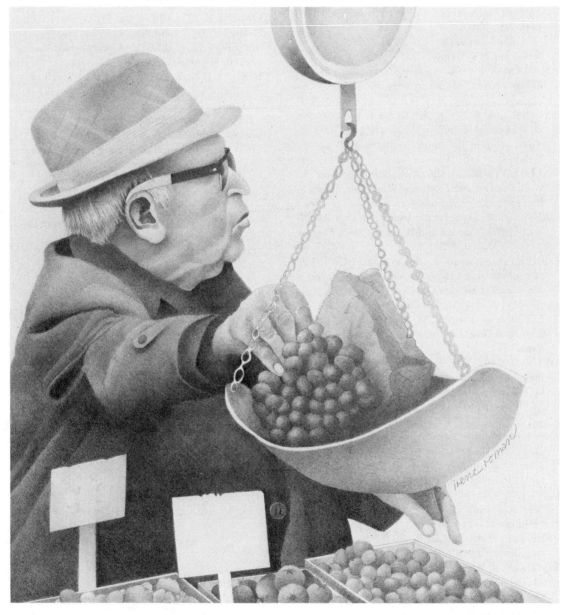

Chapter 16

GERONTOLOGICAL NURSING MANAGEMENT

THE ELDERLY CLIENT WITH A GASTROINTESTINAL PROBLEM

The aging process, through its effect on the vascular and neurological systems, may disrupt gastrointestinal function, thus causing diminished absorption and altered motility. Gastrointestinal disturbances account for the most frequent and troublesome group of disorders in the aging client. They range from simple dyspepsia to carcinomatous conditions. Certain diseases, such as gastrointestinal cancer, appear with increasing frequency after middle age. This chapter proceeds from the major problematic conditions of the buccal cavity to those of the lower gastrointestinal tract as they occur in the elderly client.

GASTROINTESTINAL DISORDERS

Pathophysiology

The alimentary, or gastrointestinal, tract can be said to be a long, muscular tube beginning at the lips and ending at the anus. The thickness and arrangement of the smooth-muscle layers vary with the sections of the tract. However, the general plan reveals a tube lined with epithelial tissue, or mucous membrane, containing many secretory and absorptive cells and covered on the outside with areolar connective tissue, or adventitia. The mucous layer is connected to the external muscular layer by loose connective tissue called the *submucosa*. This loose, pliable layer contains blood vessels and nerves that supply the three other layers of the tube. It also contains the secretory portions of many glands, such as the enzyme-secretive glands of Lieberkuhn of the small intestines. As each gastrointestinal problem is considered here, the histology will need to be further examined for a better understanding of the pathophysiology.

According to Andrew (1961, pp. 64–69), changes in the alimentary tract due to biological aging can be found throughout the tract. In the mouth salivary glands atrophy, and as a result the amount of saliva and the concentration of its enzymes are decreased. The ability to discriminate taste also declines because of a decrease in the size and number of tastebuds. Muscular layers of the oropharynx also have been shown to undergo atrophy, leading to difficulty in swallowing for some of the elderly.

In the stomach the mucosa thins out and the volume of hydrochloric acid and gastric enzymes markedly declines. The atrophic stomach is also subject to the development of carcinoma and benign gastric polyps. Not much has been done to demonstrate age changes in the small intestines; however, both the muscular layers and the mucosa are generally believed to undergo atrophy. Functionally this atrophy has been shown to diminish the absorptive capacity of the small intestine. Such diminution would be of concern in the nutrition of the older individual. Another age change is the weakening of the smooth-muscle layers in the colon. The incidence of diverticulosis is known to increase markedly with aging.

Problems of the stomach seen in the elderly (although not limited to them) include flatulence, dyspepsia, hernias, ulcers, and neoplasms. Gastric flatulence is frequently incorrectly labeled as indigestion by its sufferers. Most often the cause of the distension is swallowed air, anxiety, poor eating habits, or gastric pathology, all of which aggravate the condition. Regardless of the cause, gastric flatulence is a source of discomfort and embarrassment to the individual (Robbins 1974, p. 904).

ORAL CAVITY DISORDERS

The gastrointestinal system begins in the oral cavity. Here the breakdown of foods and the digestive processes begin. Mastication plays a small but important role in supplying the body with needed nutrients. It also plays a cultural role in the social activity involved in eating. Teeth are seen as an element of attractiveness and health.

Common oral problems of the elderly are edentulousness and ill-fitting dentures. The percentage of edentulous persons, most of whom wear dentures, increases with age (Kart, Metress, and Metress 1978). Periodontal disease accounts for the major oral problems in persons over age 40. Factors contributing to the development of periodontal disease include malnutrition, poor oral hygiene, xerostomia, diminishing sensation, and malocclusions. Causes of xerostomia include both atrophy of the salivary ducts and iatrogenic drugs, such as the thiazides and antacids, which are widely used by elderly clients. Calculus (tartar) is a major factor in the development of periodontitis. Buildup of calculus creates a reservoir of infection with little or no symptoms initially. As the disease progresses, gums become hypertrophic and bleed easily, and alveolar bony structure resorbs, thereby loosening teeth.

Parotitis, another oral problem, is usually caused by the *staphylococcus* organism. Parotitis occurs more frequently in elderly clients who are in a debilitated state and in those who are edentulous. The edentulous client has a reduced ability to masticate. Mastication of solid foods is usually avoided, and the client resorts to soft or liquid foods. This diet reduces parotid gland function and increases susceptibility to infection. The susceptibility is compounded when oral hygiene is poor, thereby establishing a locus for bacterial growth.

Cancer of the oral cavity accounts for 5 percent of all cancers in the United States and mostly affects men over 50 years of age. The greatest proportion of lip and oral cavity neoplasms are of the squamous cell type. Leukoplakia is considered a premalignant lesion and is characterized by white thickened patches on the tongue or buccal mucosa. Causes may be attributed to ill-fitting dentures and to tobacco usage.

Nursing Assessment

The importance of assessing the oral cavity cannot be overstressed. This area is perhaps the most neglected one in the assessment of elderly clients, second only to gynecological examination in female residents in long-term care facilities. Examining the oral cavity of a client who has unpleasant-smelling breath or who is drooling may be aesthetically displeasing. However, for a thorough assessment of the elderly client, the nurse must smell the breath and palpate the oral cavity. Additionally the client must remove partial or full dentures. To learn the condition of the gums, fit of dentures, and status of oral hygiene requires but a few questions and a few seconds for examination. The presence of stones in salivary ducts usually cannot be detected without a fingertip examination. Palpation is also required to detect the degree of swelling in parotitis.

Nursing Management

Health Education and Counseling. The nurse's most important role again lies in primary prevention. Correct oral hygiene must be stressed even if clients lack teeth. Those unable to eat with their dentures can be encouraged to wear them most of the day for cosmetic and morale purposes. Frequently clients can use either an upper or a lower denture, whichever fits better, to assist in mastication. The fitting of dentures for clients with retracted gingiva is costly and time-consuming. Further, geriatrician dentists, who enjoy working with the elderly or have the expertise and patience for it, are few. The nurse should refer clients who can afford the procedure to dentists with the necessary qualifications. Unless the clients are motivated highly enough to wear the dentures frequently, they need a support system to remind them to do so.

Periodontal disease is receiving more consideration now by dentists than it has in the past. For the client who has teeth, regular dental checkups and prophylactic measures should be stressed. Often the elderly may neglect attending to dental visits because of limited income and the absence of dental care insurance. The nurse can stress the importance of good oral hygiene and at least occasional dental visits. Regular visits are mandatory for clients who use tobacco. A client who is worried about the possibility of losing teeth may be able to rearrange budgetary priorities to provide for the visits.

The problem of shrinking gums is compounded by bone resorption in the elderly. Clients should be instructed to clean dentures and soak them overnight, thereby reducing constant pressure on the gingiva. They should also be instructed to massage their gums each morning and evening to stimulate circulation. To assist xerostomial clients, fluids should be increased to moisten the mouth. Edentulous clients should be encouraged to eat finely cut solid foods and to make an extra effort to masticate solid food.

Treatment. The client suffering from parotitis should be treated with an appropriate antibiotic and mouthwashes four times daily. Either cold or warm compresses can be applied externally to reduce discomfort. Acetomenophen may be ordered for pain, or codeine for severe discomfort.

Any client with leukoplakia, other lesions, or suspected neoplasm should be referred to a dentist or oral surgeon for biopsy.

ESOPHAGEAL DISORDERS

The esophagus is a tubular organ whose primary purpose is to transport ingested material from the mouth to the stomach. The esophagus passes through the thoracic cavity, where it is affected by pressure changes induced by respiration. The existence of an anatomical sphincter closing the pharyngeal orifice and a physiological intrinsic sphincter closing the gastric end permits normal esophageal function in spite of pressure variations. The act of swallowing relaxes the upper sphincter, permitting the entry of the bolus of food or liquid and thus initiating the phenomenon of peristalsis. Shortly following deglutition and prior to the arrival of the peristaltic wave, the sphincter relaxes, permitting passage of the bolus (Hightower 1969; Pope 1973; Ingelfinger 1958). The upper sphincter prevents aspiration of swallowed food from the pharynx. The lower sphincter serves to pre-

vent esophageal reflux of gastric contents (Ingelfinger 1958). One study (Eckardt and LeCompte 1977) has shown that ganglion cells decrease with aging. This change slows esophageal transport. Thus clinical problems relate to esophageal function: gastric reflux causes reflux peptic esophagitis, whereas obstructive phenomena are induced by rings, strictures, and tumors.

DIAPHRAGMATIC HERNIA (HIATAL HERNIA)

The incidence of a diaphragmatic hiatal hernia increases sharply with age and is found in 67 percent of persons over 60 (Strauss 1971). Bockus (1974) believes that small hiatal hernias are physiological in late life, probably because of the loss of fat tissue and the reduction of elastic tissue in the dome of the diaphragm. These changes result in the relaxation and displacement of the muscular tissue of the hiatus. Frequently hiatal hernias occur in obese elderly women. Other factors in the development of hiatal hernias include esophagitis and intraabdominal operations, such as vagotomy or subtotal gastrectomy.

Nursing Assessment

Most hiatal hernias are asymptomatic and are found as incidental radiological findings during examination for an unrelated problem. Indeed, special techniques may be required to demonstrate the herniation (Wolf and Guglielma 1956); the controversy still rages over whether these hernias have any real significance (Botha 1975; Pope 1973; Bockus 1974).

The rarer paraesophageal hiatal hernia may cause complaints of fullness and pain after eating, which are related to entrapment of the stomach above the diaphragm. When complicated by volvulus, the hernia will cause severe postprandial pain, vomiting, and even hematemesis.

Nursing Management

The nurse will have to counsel the obese client. Long-standing obesity may be rooted in deep psychological problems or may be related to an increased number of fat cells due to excessive alimentation during the childhood growth years (Guyton 1976). In either situation management requires sustained, lifelong effort by the client. The nurse should urge the client to seek help in an established obesity-control group that stresses learning new eating habits while maintaining a peer support system.

For complaints related to diaphragmatic entrapment due to the paraesophageal hernia, some physicians recommend surgical repair because of the risk of volvulus and gastric infarction (Hill and Tobias 1968). Older clients who are unable to tolerate this surgery must be encouraged to eat small, frequent meals; to avoid tight clothing; and to sleep in a semirecumbent position.

Coffee, alcohol, and tea should be avoided. The regular use of postprandial antacids has been found helpful for clients who have chronic dyspepsia. Clients who exhibit a degree of renal impairment must exercise caution in the use of antacids containing calcium or magnesium. Antacids containing calcium carbonate should be avoided because they increase gastric production and tend to cause constipation, a condition already present in many elderly clients. Clients should be instructed to

avoid snacking at bedtime. Antispasmodics and anticholinergics should be avoided because they enhance esophageal reflux and may aggravate symptoms secondary to glaucoma and prostatism.

Clients with chalasia or reflux have complaints related to peptic digestion of the distal esophagus. Such clients have heartburn and suffer from reflux peptic esophagitis, which is discussed in the next section.

REFLUX PEPTIC ESOPHAGITIS

Loss of competence of the lower esophageal sphincter permits the reflux of contents into the distal esophagus. These contents, along with their pepsin and acid or bile and duodenal contents, may remain in the esophagus for prolonged periods (Haddad 1970), thereby causing a digestive irritation to the sensitive mucosa. This irritation may or may not be associated with an esophageal hiatal hernia (Cohen and Harris 1971).

In its initial phases esophagitis causes acute inflammation and ulceration of the mucosa. In the chronic phase chronic inflammatory changes occur and ulceration extends beyond the mucosa and penetrates deeply into the esophageal tissue. Hyperplasia and thickening of the mucosa are also seen (Sandry 1972). The changes due to esophagitis can lead to upper gastrointestinal hemorrhage and esophageal stricture.

Nursing Assessment

Subjective Findings. Clients with reflux esophagitis complain of pain, usually described as a burning sensation or heartburn and usually felt in the low retrosternal area.

393

It may radiate to the epigastrium, to the interscapular area of the upper back, to the upper chest, and even down both arms. The pain may have two components associated with swallowing: heartburn and a painful sensation. The retrosternal burning or pain usually occurs very quickly after eating, particularly if the client bends over or lies down. It is frequently provoked by the ingestion of very hot or cold liquids, citrus juices, alcohol, or hot coffee. Heartburn frequently occurs at night, awakening the client. This nocturnal episode is often associated with a sour taste in the mouth or even with finding the pillow wet with gastric juice. Similar regurgitation of gastric contents may occur if the client bends over to pick up something or lies down very shortly after eating. Odynophagia (painful swallowing) may be related to the ingestion of solids, such as steak, or may occur with anything, even saliva. Odynophagia often occurs episodically for days or weeks and is usually associated with an exacerbation of the other symptoms, particularly dysphagia in the distal esophagus. The distinguishing character of the dysphagia is that it is always worse for solids than for liquids, and the firmer the food the greater the difficulty. When the clients ingest food, it becomes trapped in the esophagus or slowly descends into the stomach. Women may have a history of heartburn that occurred during the last trimester of pregnancy. Clients often have a history of weight gain either prior to or associated with the onset or exacerbation of symptoms.

The most common complication of peptic esophagitis is the formation of a *distal esophageal ulcer*. This ulcer is usually painful, and the pain is often felt in the back and in the interscapular area. The next most common complication is *stricture for-mation* (Palmer 1968). Clients with this disorder complain of dysphagia, which usually becomes progressively more severe and eventually prevents the ingestion of all solid food. Bleeding may occur. Bleeding most often presents as an occult blood loss with iron-lack anemia and a hemocult stool test that is positive. Occasionally frank melena or hematemesis may occur, requiring hospitalization and transfusion.

Objective Findings. The physical examination is rarely of any help. Obesity may be present or, in cases with strictures, malnutrition-induced weight loss may be found. Reflux esophagitis has approximately a 25 percent association with duodenal ulcer (Palmer 1971).

Diagnostics

Laboratory studies are of limited value in the diagnosis of reflux esophagitis. A hematocrit and hemoglobin test may reveal the presence of an anemia; a stool examination for occult blood may be positive.

Radiological examination may be diagnostic. However, the acute ulcerations are usually flat and easily missed by an uninformed radiologist. In most cases diagnostic findings consisting of motor and mucosal abnormalities require that the radiologist be notified of the clinical suspicions. In the advanced case the diagnosis is usually apparent. Findings are more evident when a penetrating ulceration or stricture is present. In the event of a stricture or ulcer, an endoscopist must rule out the possibility of cancer.

If the x-ray examination is negative, the client should be referred to a gastroenterologist for further examination. Esophagoscopy and biopsy, esophageal motility tests, and pH studies, as well as an acid perfusion test, may be required.

Nursing Management

The management of a client with reflux esophagitis is based upon the prevention of reflux and the treatment of the esophagitis. Reflux is managed by avoiding the factors that increase it and by diminishing the irritating nature of the refluxed material.

Health Education and Counseling. Clients are instructed to avoid wearing tight belts and garments that increase intra-abdominal pressure and to avoid lying down after meals. They are generally advised to avoid eating for at least 2 hours or, in more severe cases, up to 4 hours before retiring. No dietary restrictions are imposed except in very symptomatic cases, in which clients are advised to avoid caffeine-containing beverages and alcohol. Those who are overweight should reduce. In addition, to prevent reflux, the head of the bed should be raised 4 to 6 inches, which can be accomplished by placing 6-inch-high 4-by-4-inch blocks under the legs at the head of the bed.

Treatment. The main thrust of therapy until now has been to use intensive antacid therapy. Adequate doses of non-calcium-containing antacids (Maalox 45 ml, Mylanta II 30 ml) 1 hour and 3 hours after each meal and at bedtime should be given to the symptomatic client for an 8-week period. Diarrhea can be controlled by using a preparation with more aluminum hydroxide (Amphogel 45 ml) at bedtime in place of the other preparations. Anticholinergics decrease the pressure and competence of the lower sphincter and should be avoided.

More recently Cimetidine, an H2 histamine-blocking agent, has been shown to prevent gastric acid secretion and to increase intragastric pH. The usual dosage is 300 mg before meals and at bedtime for 8 weeks. This medication has proven more effective than antacids in the treatment of reflux esophagitis. However, improperly used, it has been known to cause rapid exacerbation of duodenal ulcer (Grossman 1976). Therefore, it should be used only if the diagnosis is certain and probably only with medical consultation and when other methods are ineffective.

The client with severe reflux esophagitis, particularly if it is complicated by penetrating ulcer, hemorrhage, or stricture, should be managed by a gastroenterologist. These clients require hospitalization, close medical supervision, and intensive, often very specialized, treatment. The client who has a stricture requires frequent esophageal dilations by a trained specialist. Management is carried out in collaboration with a physician who directs the medical regimen. Surgery becomes a consideration in severe, complicated esophagitis.

ESOPHAGEAL RINGS

Intermittent and recurrent episodes of otherwise asymptomatic dysphagia characterize the presence of an esophageal ring. The intermittent nature distinguishes this disorder from other esophageal conditions.

Nursing Assessment

Clients, usually 50 to 70 years old, who have an esophageal ring will suddenly develop esophageal obstruction during the course of a meal when a piece of meat or bread becomes stuck in the lower esophagus. Not infrequently this food can be regurgitated, and the client can then continue eating without further difficulty. But sometimes a piece of meat may become impacted in the esophagus, and the client will require hospitalization and esophagoscopy. At endoscopy the esophagus is cleared and usually no other pathology is seen. The upper G.I. x-ray is also usually normal. This chain of events may recur several times, and the client becomes labeled a psychosomatic. However, if the radiologist is informed of the clinical consideration, an appropriate x-ray study employing the Valsalva maneuver is performed, and as the barium bolus passes through the distended lower esophagus, the lower esophageal ring is demonstrated. Another technique is to have the client swallow an unchewed barium-soaked marshmallow, which will be trapped by the ring and then will dissolve at body temperature (MacMahon et al. 1958; Goyal et al. 1970).

Rarely, clients with iron-deficiency anemia may complain of dysphagia. Examination may reveal spooning of the nails, leukoplakia of the oropharynx, and a normal barium-swallow esophageal study. These clients may have the Plummer-Vinson syndrome, which is an iron-deficiency anemia with dysphagia due to an associated esophageal web (a ring in the upper esophagus). Iron-deficiency anemia is described in chapter 18, on hematological problems.

Nursing Management

The nurse should advise clients to masticate food thoroughly and slowly. Those in whom symptoms recur frequently should be referred to a gastroenterologist or a thoracic surgeon for esophagoscopy and dilation of the ring. Surgery is rarely necessary.

In cases of acute obstruction due to a meat bolus (but only after consultation with a physician), a solution of meat tenderizer may be used to treat the acute episode, provided that an x-ray does not reveal the presence of bone spicules in the meat. The client sips 15 to 30 ml of the solution every 30 minutes. The bolus will usually pass within 2 to 3 hours (Pope 1973). Esophageal webs require dilation by a trained medical specialist.

ESOPHAGEAL DIVERTICULA

Esophageal diverticula are usually asymptomatic except for the hypopharyngeal pouch, known as *Zenker's diverticulum*. This disorder usually occurs in clients over 60 years of age.

Nursing Assessment

Clients with esophageal diverticula complain initially of persistent soreness, excessive mucus, and the presence of something caught in the throat when they are swallowing. Cough and hoarseness are common. Food and mucus may be regurgitated at night or after meals. Dysphagia is progressive. Eventually complete obstruction due to compression of the esophagus by the large extramural mass occurs. The diagnosis is usually made by x-ray, either a plain film of the neck or barium x-ray studies of the pharynx and esophagus.

Nursing Management

Treatment of Zenker's diverticulum is surgical; clients should be referred to a thoracic surgeon. Attempts to temporize include thorough chewing of bland, low-residue food and drinking large amounts of water after each meal to flush out the pouch. Esophageal dilation by a physician may give some relief.

ESOPHAGEAL TUMORS

Esophageal tumors may be benign or malignant. The most common benign tumor is the leiomyoma. It is rarely symptomatic but is usually an incidental finding during an upper G.I. series. Clients with such tumors should always be referred to a gastroenterologist for further evaluation. A thoracic surgeon may be required to evaluate the necessity for surgery.

The most common malignant esophageal tumor is the carcinoma, which represents 4 percent of all fatal human cancers. It has an incidence of 5.8 per 100,000 cases annually in the United States for whites and 20.5 per 100,000 for nonwhites. It is unusual before age 40 and has a peak incidence between ages 60 and 70 (Pope 1973).

Nursing Assessment

Progressive and unrelenting dysphagia is the single most common complaint. It is frequently insidious; clients learn to chew their food carefully and to take small bites to avoid any difficulty. Usually by the time the clients are seen and examined, they are markedly malnourished. Pain, either substernal or radiating posteriorly into the back and interscapular area, usually means extension of the tumor. Occasionally pneumonia due to aspiration may force the client to seek health care attention. Barium-swallow, upper G.I. x-rays will usually reveal the tumor. These clients should be referred to an experienced endoscopist who will obtain tissues and cytology to permit evaluation for further therapy.

Nursing Management

Radical surgery is excluded in the majority of cases, particularly in clients with obvious metastatic disease or other severe illnesses and in most clients over age 75 (Nakayama 1974). This restriction will exclude 80 percent of clients with esophageal tumors (Ellis et al. 1959; Gunnlangsoon et al. 1970). Radiation therapy may induce effective temporary palliation. In other clients a trained specialist will perform an esophageal dilation and pass a large-bore, hollow, plastic (50 Fr) tube. This treatment may permit adequate palliation. It allows the client to eat and prevents the aspiration of esophageal mucus and saliva. Since cure is rare, the nurse should help the client understand the choices of treatment. The medical management should be directed by a physician. The nurse can best help these unfortunate clients by providing them and their families with psychological support, which is most essential in this situation.

GASTRODUODENAL DISORDERS

The stomach and duodenum appear to function as a single physiological unit. A variety of interrelated feedback mechanisms control pyloric activity as well as gastric and duodenal secretion and pH. In peptic disease the pathology appears to be intertwined, so that secretions from the

397

duodenum, abnormally present in the stomach, injure cells, while gastric secretion in the duodenum plays the same role in causing mucosal injury in that organ. Peptic disease appears to increase with age, as do gastritis and gastric malignancy.

CHRONIC ATROPHIC GASTRITIS AND GASTRIC ATROPHY

The incidence of chronic gastritis increases with age (Cornet et al. 1964; Chisholm 1976). The course of events appears to be a superficial gastritis, followed by an atrophic gastritis, followed by a stage of gastric atrophy. The etiology is obscure. Foods, alcohol, and coffee might be capable of causing acute gastritis, but authorities generally agree that these factors play no role whatsoever in the development of chronic disease. Two possible causes are under investigation: reflux of bile and the presence of certain autoantibodies. Reflux of bile from the duodenum eventually injures the gastric mucosa. This recurrent injury finally leads to atrophic gastritis and eventually gastric atrophy (Siurala and Taewast 1958; Lambling et al. 1969). On the other hand, autoantibodies to intrinsic factor (IF) and to gastric parietal cell cytoplasm have been discovered in the blood of clients with gastric atrophy (Jeffries et al. 1962; Taylor et al. 1962; Jeffries and Sleisinger 1965). Unfortunately, neither theory has been proven or fits all the known facts. Gastric atrophy has been associated with chronic iron-deficiency anemia and also with pernicious anemia.

Nursing Assessment

Except for symptomatic anemia, subjective and objective findings are few. The client usually has a history of chronic dyspepsia and diffuse abdominal discomfort. The diagnosis is usually raised by an astute radiologist during an evaluation for anemia or for nonspecific gastrointestinal symptoms. The diagnosis requires endoscopy and biopsy.

Nursing Management

Other than the treatment for the specific anemia, no therapy exists for atrophic gastritis or atrophy. The achlorhydria is not to be treated by the addition of acid. Nonspecific digestive complaints are best treated symptomatically and by allowing the client to avoid foods that seem to worsen the symptoms. For these clients the nurse can provide reassurance, which is usually the most effective therapy. The treatments of pernicious anemia and iron-lack anemia are discussed in chapter 18, on hematological problems.

PEPTIC ULCERS

Pathophysiology

Before discussing the subject of peptic ulcers, it would be helpful to consider the mechanism of hydrochloric acid synthesis and secretion by the parietal cells of the fundus and body of the stomach. These large fundal cells are located within the gastric gland, which also contains cells that secrete mucus, gastric enzymes, and intrinsic factor. In the distal end, or antrum, of the stomach are certain epithelial cells that secrete a hormone called *gastrin*. These cells respond to several types of stimulus, including vagal nerve stimulation, distension of the antrum by food, and particular ingested substances like calcium ions (Grossman 1976), alcohol, caffeine, and digestive products of proteins (Jensen 1976, p. 849). When gastrin is secreted, it enters the blood stream, travels to the gastric glands, and stimulates parietal cells, which respond by secreting hydrochloric acid.

Normally the mucosa of the various segments of the alimentary tract are protected both by the presence of a thick layer of alkaline, acid-binding mucus and by the ability of mucosal cells to regenerate. When "an imbalance [exists] between the aggressive action of acid-peptic secretions and the defensive forces that protect the normal mucosa, a peptic ulcer can develop" (Robbins 1974, p. 918). The diminution of protective mucus, injury to the gastric cell membrane, and a decline in mucosal cell regeneration, rather than excessive hydrochloric acid secretion, are generally held to be the basis for gastric ulceration.

In cases of acute gastric ulcer, the lesion usually involves only the mucosa. In cases of chronic ulcer, the ulceration begins in the mucosa and penetrates through submucosa and the smooth-muscle layers. Eroding blood vessels cause bleeding ulcers and irritation of nerve endings, which are reflected in gastric pain.

Ulcers in the duodenum are thought to be due more to excessive secretion of gastric acid than to loss of protection afforded by mucous cells. In clients with duodenal ulcers, the volume of hydrochloric acid secreted can be twice the normal volume, or 2,000 ml in 24 hours as opposed to 1,000 ml. The depth of the ulcer varies from superficial lesions involving only the mucosa to those that penetrate down to the muscular layers and beyond.

DUODENAL ULCERS

Duodenal ulcer is found at all ages, from infancy to the seventies. The peak incidence for onset is between 40 and 50 years. The usual course of the disease is 25 years (Walker 1973). The etiology is unknown; however, an increased gastric secretory drive mechanism that is not controlled at the normal levels apparently exists. This mechanism results in a higher than normal gastric H+ ion concentration. This highly acidic secretion manages to attack the duodenal mucosa, the pylorus, or the distal gastric antrum, causing peptic ulceration in these areas (Fordtran 1978). Factors that seem to predispose individuals to the development of duodenal ulcer are the use of large amounts of caffeine and alcohol and the use of tobacco (Grossman 1976).

Nursing Assessment

Subjective Findings. The single common symptom of a duodenal ulcer is pain. This pain is visceral and therefore poorly localized, deep in the abdomen, variable in intensity but never cramplike or severe, and described in the vague terms of burning, dull, and aching. The pain is usually localized to the epigastrium and has a well-known pattern. It is not present in the morning or on arising. It occurs 1 to 3 hours after eating and is relieved by the ingestion of milk, protein-rich foods, and antacids or by vomiting. Sometimes the client is awakened by pain 2 to 3 hours after going to sleep. These episodes tend to recur daily while the ulcer is active. The bouts of pain tend to recur periodically in pain "clusters" (Rinaldo et al. 1963). Some clients may complain of weight loss and vomiting, but these symptoms are not helpful diagnostically.

399

Persistent vomiting of copious amounts of gastric contents is usually indicative of pyloric obstruction. Occasionally, undigested food may be recognized. Frequently this vomiting occurs only in the late afternoon or at night.

Sharp, severe pain that can be easily localized usually indicates ulcer penetration or perforation into the peritoneum. Hematemesis indicates blood vessel erosion and hemorrhage. In the elderly this symptom may be the first evidence of peptic ulceration (Kaiser and Rogers 1973).

Objective Findings. The physical examination of the uncomplicated duodenal ulcer is often of little help. Epigastric tenderness, while usually found, is diffuse. A slight succussion splash of the stomach may be present, indicating a delay in gastric emptying. Pinpoint localization of pain, rebound tenderness, and a palpable mass indicate penetration with or without perforation. A rigid abdomen usually indicates a free perforation with peritonitis, particularly with rebound tenderness and absent bowel sounds. A loud, easily elicited succussion splash ordinarily indicates obstruction and gastric stasis.

Diagnostics

The diagnosis is made by means of the upper G.I. series (Belber 1971). If symptoms are present and no ulcer is seen on x-ray, or if a duodenal ulcer is found on x-ray in an asymptomatic client, the client should be referred to a gastroenterologist for consideration of endoscopy.

All clients with evidence of penetration, perforation, obstruction, or hemorrhage should be hospitalized immediately and placed under the care of a physician. Diagnosing a perforation may be difficult because of the elderly client's lower pain sensation; the presenting symptoms of pain tend to be less localized and more diffuse (Berman and Kirsner 1976).

Nursing Management

Treatment. Since duodenal ulcer is a chronic, recurrent disease, treatment must be effective, inexpensive, and easily followed. Only foods and substances specifically known to cause or predispose the mucosa to injury or to increase gastric acid secretion or peptic activity should be avoided. All other aspects of the client's life should be left intact, so that maximum cooperation with treatment is obtained. Aspirin, caffeine, alcohol, Indocin, and calcium salts are known to injure mucosa or increase gastric acid output and will delay healing. The only foods that must be avoided are those containing these substances. (The client may use decaffeinated beverages, such as Sanka or Decaf, but should avoid coffee, tea, and cola drinks.) In addition, the client should avoid alcohol. Once the ulcer is healed, modest amounts of alcohol, just before or with the meal, may be used. Milk and creamed soups are no longer felt to be essential or even desirable. Nighttime snacks are avoided, as these cause increased nocturnal acidity. The client is also told to avoid other foods that persistently cause pain or indigestion.

Until recently the basis of treatment has been the use of antacids, which must be given in sufficient quantity to neutralize the gastric acid produced until the next meal or dose. Liquid preparations have been shown to be most effective; these must be given in large doses (e.g., Mylanta II 30 ml, Maalox 45 ml, Riopan 45 ml) 1 hour and 3 hours after meals and at bedtime to effectively decrease acidity and raise the pH (Fordtran and Collyns 1966). Anticholinergics are expensive. They have limited, if any, usefulness and can cause or precipitate gastric or urinary obstruction and glaucoma in the older client, so they are best avoided. Recently an H2 inhibitor that prevents the secretion of gastric acid has been introduced into the treatment program. Cimetidine 300 mg 30 minutes before meals and at bedtime will suppress acid production for 7 hours. (During its use serum gastrin levels rise, thus predisposing the client for a rapid and severe recurrence if the medication is discontinued too soon.) The usual duration of treatment is 4 to 6 weeks. Antacid supplementation is used for symptoms that should not persist beyond the fourth day (Blackwood et al. 1976).

Health Education and Counseling. Once the ulcer has been healed, clients should be cautioned that a return to their former lifestyle will probably induce a recurrence. They should not resume the use of caffeine, they should use alcohol only in modest amounts before or with meals, and they should attempt to reduce stress and obtain approximately eight hours of rest nightly. They should avoid the use of aspirin and the ingestion of a variety of medications, including corticosteroids, phenylbutazone, indomethacin, and reserpine. The nurse should instruct the client to avoid over-the-counter drugs. All of these drugs have been implicated in causing or perpetuating peptic ulceration or bleeding (Walker 1973).

Evaluation of Care. Clients who fail to respond to treatment with reduction of symptoms within one week or in whom symptoms rapidly recur after completion of a course of therapy, or in whom any complication of ulcer appears while in therapy, should be referred immediately to a gastroenterologist. Clients must be advised that they have a chronic illness and to report the recurrence of symptoms immediately.

GASTRIC ULCERS

In contrast to duodenal ulcers, gastric ulcers are usually associated with decreased levels of gastric acid secretion. Gastric ulcers are more common than duodenal ulcers in the elderly (Berman and Kirsner 1976). Capper (1967) proposed the generally accepted theory that the regurgitation of duodenal contents injures the gastric mucosa. The lesion appears to be due to bile salts and results in an antral gastritis. The functioning parietal cells continue to secrete acid, causing the development of an ulcer at the juxtaparietal-antral junction. The primary problem in the diagnosis of gastric ulcer is to differentiate it from an ulcerating carcinoma.

Nursing Assessment

Subjective Findings. As in cases of duodenal ulcer, pain is the major presenting complaint of clients with gastric ulcer. Again the pain is more diffuse and diminished than in the younger client. It is usually epigastric and midline and is frequently described as dull, nagging, or pressurelike. Often the client describes radiation to the back. The pain usually be-

401

gins 30 minutes to 3 hours after a meal. Most often, eating relieves the pain. Occasionally the ingestion of food aggravates the pain, and clients state that their stomachs feel better empty. Some clients awaken with pain 1 to 2 hours after going to bed. In addition to being relieved by food, the pain is usually relieved by ingestion of an antacid or by vomiting.

Approximately 50 percent of clients with gastric ulcer complain of anorexia or diminished appetite and experience some weight loss. Nausea and vomiting are much more frequent in these clients than in those with duodenal ulcer. The vomiting is always associated with pain and usually relieves it. Water brash, an excessive and sudden salivation, is common in clients with gastric ulcers.

Objective Findings. The physical examination may reveal tenderness in the epigastrium. The presence of a palpable mass is usually consistent with a malignancy. Marked tenderness, rebound tenderness, abdominal guarding, and absence of bowel sounds indicate perforation. Hematemesis and melena are common presenting problems in the elderly. Any of these findings warrants immediate referral to a hospital for examination by a physician.

Diagnostics

An upper G.I. series should reveal the presence of the ulcer, and the radiologist usually will also indicate whether the lesion appears benign. Ninety percent of radiological findings are accurate (Richardson 1973). Complete evaluation includes fiberoptic endoscopy by a physician to visualize the lesion and to obtain biopsies and exfoliative cytology of the lesion and its surroundings. The complete evaluation should permit diagnosis with better than 95 percent accuracy (Dodd and Nelson 1961).

Nursing Management

Treatment. All clients with gastric ulcer should be referred to a gastrointestinal endoscopist for further evaluation. The use of antacids in gastric ulcer is based on the belief that they relieve pain and hasten healing. Many current studies are questioning the actual effect of the antacids in gastric ulcer (Scheurer et al. 1977). Current treatment is to give sufficient quantities of a nonabsorbable, non-calcium-containing liquid antacid (Mylanta II 30 ml; Riopan and Gelusil 45 to 60 ml) 1 and 3 hours after meals and at bedtime. Food and beverages other than water and medication should be avoided at bedtime. The usual bland diet has no place in the current therapy for gastric ulcer. Clients should be advised to avoid caffeine-containing products such as coffee, tea, colas, and chocolate. Alcohol- and aspirin-containing medication should be avoided, as well as other medications known to cause gastric irritation, such as indomethacin, phenylbutazone, and corticosteroids.

Evaluation of Care. Three weeks after the institution of therapy, a repeat upper G.I. x-ray is obtained and should show 50 percent healing. Another upper G.I. x-ray study is again obtained in 6 weeks and should show at least 90 percent healing. If the ulcer is still present, the client must be followed at 6-week intervals until the ulcer is completely healed. If the ulcer does not heal, becomes larger, or begins to show any of the radiological criteria of malignancy, the client must be referred to a physician for definitive surgical therapy. The development of bleeding or complications in treatment also requires immediate referral. Cimetidine has been reported as an.effective treatment of gastric ulcer (see the section on duodenal ulcers).

Health Education and Counseling. Once healing has occurred, clients should be instructed to continue to avoid caffeine, to decrease tobacco use, to avoid the use of alcohol except with meals, to get 8 hours of rest at night, and to avoid bedtime snacks. If the client can be persuaded to follow this advice, recurrence may be avoided.

GASTRIC CANCER

Both benign and malignant tumors can occur in the stomach. The most common gastric tumor in the elderly is a malignant carcinoma. For this reason, and because it is beyond the scope of this text to consider the other less common gastric tumors, only malignant gastric carcinoma is discussed here.

Pathophysiology

The incidence of carcinoma of the stomach is greater after age 40 and increases in each subsequent decade. It is twice as common in males as in females. "This neoplasm occurs four times more often in families of clients with gastric carcinoma. A disproportionate fraction of those afflicted have group A blood" (Robbins 1974, p. 924). Other suspected predisposing factors include certain dietary elements, low vol-

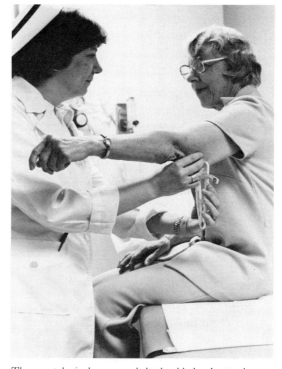

The gerontological nurse can help the elderly adapt to the aging process by monitoring the effects of diet; elderly clients need to understand the importance of diet to their well-being and be encouraged to adapt their cultural patterns and habits to their particular nutritional requirements.

ume or absence of gastric hydrochloric acid, pernicious anemia, gastric atrophy, and gastric polyps.

Carcinoma may appear as a mass or as an infiltration of an ulceration anywhere in the stomach. The ulcerative craters vary in size from a few tenths of an inch to 5 to 7 inches in diameter. On x-ray they may appear perfectly benign or have the malignant characteristics of being heaped up with overhanging edges. Polypoid cancers are characterized by large cauliflower growths that protrude into the lumen of the stomach. Infiltrative carcinoma, on the

403

other hand, may show up as plaquelike lesions called *linitis plastica.* The growth is directed into the many-layered stomach wall, where all layers thicken and become rigid (Robbins 1974, p. 925).

Cancer of the stomach can metastasize to lymphatic nodes in nearby regions and to the liver. The left supraclavicular and scalene nodes can also be seeded. This malignancy frequently spreads to the lungs, brain, and bones. Unfortunately clients usually do not experience the symptoms that characterize this illness until organs other than the stomach become involved.

Nursing Assessment

Subjective Findings. The most frequent initial complaint is weight loss, often associated with a dull, vague, epigastric, midlinj pain, which may be relieved or exacerbated by food or antacid. Nausea and vomiting are frequent, as is anorexia. Symptoms of anemia and pallor may cause the client to seek help. Very rarely does the client come because of the discovery of an abdominal mass. Pain or other complaints due to metastases, such as ascites, back pain, pedal edema, or a pathological fracture, may be the presenting problems. In a small number of clients, the first sign of illness is an acute gastric perforation with peritonitis.

Objective Findings. The physical examination may reveal the presence of a palpable left supraclavicular lymph node (Virchow's node), indicating intraabdominal malignancy with metastases, or an epigastric mass, possibly with an enlarged, hard, irregular liver. On performing a rectal examination, the nurse may discover a hard shelflike projection, or Blumer's shelf, anterior to the rectum. All these findings indicate metastatic disease; in the presence of a gastric ulcer, they are highly indicative of malignancy.

All clients with gastric ulcers or tumors should be referred to a gastroenterologist for evaluation.

Nursing Management

In the absence of evidence of metastases, surgery is the only possible treatment for gastric cancer. Incurable lesions require surgery only for bleeding and obstruction.

A variety of chemotherapy regimens, usually associated with 5 fluorouracil, have been used with variable success.

The medical treatment of these clients should be directed by a physician skilled in oncology. The nurse may continue to coordinate the client's health care. Supportive care by an empathetic nurse is essential for the client with an incurable health problem.

UPPER GASTROINTESTINAL BLEEDING

Bleeding from any point above the ligament of Treitz, at the junction of the duodenum and jejunum, can be associated with upper G.I. bleeding. If hematemesis occurs, the site of bleeding is certain to be in the upper tract. Melena without hematemesis may be from any portion of the tract. The differential considerations in upper tract bleeding include esophageal varices, esophagitis, gastric varices, gastritis, gastric ulcer, benign gastric tumor, and gastric cancer. Duodenal ulcer may be silent in 20 percent of clients; its first manifestation may be an upper gastrointestinal hemorrhage. In the jaundiced client with blood in the stool, carcinoma of the ampulla of Vater must be considered, as well as other causes such as cirrhosis with complicating varices or a gastrointestinal cancer with hepatic metastases.

Nursing Assessment

Subjective Findings. Assessment includes determining the extent of the bleeding and obtaining clues about the source of the bleeding. Frequently no subjective findings appear at the time of bleeding, so questioning should touch on periods preceding the acute illness. A history of indigestion and the frequent use of antacids is significant and may indicate peptic ulceration. Also a history of weight loss may indicate a gastric malignancy, and pain following alcohol or aspirin ingestion may indicate acute erosive gastritis. A prior history of bleeding or peptic disease is also helpful. Finally an adequate history of other illnesses and medications taken for treatment should be obtained.

Objective Findings. Physical examination includes a search for the stigmata of disease. Spider telangiectasia, jaundice, and hepatomegaly or splenomegaly point to cirrhosis and esophageal varices. Evidence of rheumatoid arthritis should point to the use of an anti-inflammatory medication causing gastric ulceration. The nurse should evaluate the extent of hemorrhage by noting the client's pulse, blood pressure, and circulatory status.

Diagnostics

Laboratory studies involve assessment of hemoglobin, hematocrit, white blood cells, and differential. The nurse should also obtain a partial thromboplastin time (PTT), a prothrombin time (PT), a platelet count to evaluate the client for a blood dyscrasia or bleeding diathesis, and liver-function studies to help delineate the etiology.

Nursing Management

Clients with upper gastrointestinal bleeding should be evaluated by a physician in a hospital. The nurse continues to coordinate the client's primary health care.

INTESTINAL DISORDERS

Little evidence exists for altered intestinal absorption due to age. Intestinal surface is probably too extensive for current testing techniques to appreciate any changes. The absorptive changes that do occur are related to vascular problems of aging that decrease blood flow and secondarily decrease the rate of absorption. Constipation, diverticulosis, colonic polyps, and colonic cancer increase in frequency with age.

DIVERTICULOSIS

The natural history of diverticular disease has shown progressively increasing frequency in the Western world. The frequency increases from an incidence of 5 percent at age 50 to 50 percent at age 90 (Parks 1975). Forty percent of persons over age 70 have diverticular disease (Berman and Kirsner 1976). The diverticula are outpouchings of colonic mucosa through the muscular coats to the serosal surface. They tend to retain stool and eventually may perforate, causing an abscess called *acute diverticulitis*. This abscess can lead to peritonitis and intestinal obstruction and require surgical resection to save the client's life.

SPASTIC COLON AND DIVERTICULAR DISORDERS

Nursing Assessment

Subjective Findings. Clients with spastic colon have subjective findings usually associated with the functional or irritable bowel. A common complaint is cramping abdominal pain localized to the lower abdomen in the left lower quadrant. Constipation or alternating constipation and diarrhea may be associated with the pain. Occasionally the pain is localized to the right upper quadrant. Passage of flatus or a bowel movement frequently relieves the pain. This pain will almost never awaken the client.

Clients with spastic diverticulosis may have exactly the same clinical picture. Simple diverticulosis is asymptomatic.

Objective Findings. On examining the client, the nurse finds a tender left lower quadrant and frequently a palpable bowel loop. No evidence of bowel obstruction is found either clinically or by x-ray, and stool is often present in the rectum at rectal examination. Stools are negative for blood, fat, and ova and parasites. A barium-enema x-ray showing diverticulosis almost completes the diagnosis. Sigmoidoscopy should be performed to search for polyps.

Acute diverticulitis is the inflammatory complication of diverticulosis. Perforation and the formation of a pericolic abscess cause pain in the involved area, total con-stipation, anorexia, nausea, and frequently fever and chills.

Physical examination reveals local evidence of bowel perforation with tenderness and rebound tenderness. A mass may be palpated, or signs of generalized peritonitis with a rigid abdomen and absent bowel sounds may be found. Rectal examination may reveal a tender mass.

Diagnostics

Laboratory studies usually reveal an elevated white blood cell count, indicating acute inflammation. Urinalysis should be performed, and pus or blood cells may be found due to extension of the abscess to the bladder. Involvement of the left ureter may cause obstruction of this organ and left hydronephrosis. Urinary infection or fistula may result. Clients with these findings should be referred for cystoscopy.

Nursing Management

The treatment of uncomplicated diverticular disease, functional colon, and irritable bowel syndrome involves the use of a high-roughage diet rich in hemicellulose (Painter, Almeida, and Colburne 1972; Painter and Burkitt 1975). A careful explanation must be given to the client, who will expect the traditional low-residue diet. The addition of 2 tablespoons of natural unprocessed bran daily decreases stool transport time, constipation, and colon segmentation and improves stool evacuation.

Cramping will gradually decrease but can be treated temporarily by means of anticholinergics, such as propantheline bromide (Probanthine) 15 to 30 mg three times daily. This treatment may help to tide the client over the first 4 days. The reward of larger, satisfactory bowel movements usually encourages the client. Unfortunately a general distaste for rough-textured foods can cause the client to neglect treatment. One bowl of All-Bran cereal or 2 tablespoons of Psyllium seeds daily are also helpful. The seeds can be mixed with a fruit juice or water.

Purgatives should be avoided. Clients with acute diverticulitis should be referred directly to a physician. Such clients have a pericolic abscess with intestinal obstruction and usually require hospitalization, antibiotics, and intravenous therapy. Once the client is over the acute episode, treatment for diverticulosis should be instituted and maintained during the client's lifetime. The nurse must advise the client that this health problem is chronic and lifelong.

CONSTIPATION

Because of the enormity of the problem of constipation in the elderly, a separate, brief discussion is warranted. Due to a variety of contributing factors, constipation assumes increasing significance with advancing years. Among these factors are (1) decreased exercise; (2) cultural eating habits; (3) decreased gastrointestinal motility due to vascular changes; (4) low fluid intake; (5) inadequate dentition; (6) decreased muscle tone in the small and large intestine; (7) lowered sensory and motor stimulus to innervate the urge for bowel defecation; (8) the ingestion of drugs that affect gastrointestinal functioning, such as sedatives, tranquilizers, hypnotics, and antihypertensives; and (9) problems of psychogenic origin, such as depression and anxiety. Compounding the problem of con-

stipation is an abuse of laxatives, purgatives, and enemas.

Nursing Assessment

The nurse chiefly relies on a careful history of food ingestion and bowel habits for all elderly clients. Most often no physical signs are found other than slower bowel sounds and hardened, dry stool on rectal examination.

Nursing Management

The chief contribution of the nurse to the client is patient education. As in the client with diverticulosis, dietary habits must be altered to include increased fluids and a high-residue diet. The addition of 2 tablespoons of raw bran daily or a bowl of bran cereal and fiber breads will greatly alleviate the problem. The assistance of stool softeners such as dioctyl sodium sulfasuccinate may be necessary. Mineral oil 15 to 30 ml at bedtime may be helpful until stools are soft and bulky. Laxative use should be avoided when possible.

COLONIC POLYPS

Colonic adenomatous polyps are the premalignant phase of colonic carcinomas (Morson 1962). Once early malignant change appears, the incidence of metastases is only 1 to 5 percent. Invasion raises this incidence dramatically. As these tumors are often silent, efforts to locate them should be part of every client evaluation.

Nursing Assessment

Hematochezia or melena are two of the rare findings of polyps. Occasionally a

407

polyp on a long stalk may be caught by the bowel and cause cramping. Villous adenomas may cause copious, wet diarrhea. Physical examination is generally negative. The nurse should routinely perform a digital rectal examination. Proctoscope examination for polyps should be included, as these tumors are not palpable. The client may be referred to a physician for sigmoidoscopy or fiberoptic colonoscopy. Clients undergoing general evaluation should be placed on a high-residue, meat-free diet for 3 days. Three stool specimens are obtained during the diet period and tested for occult blood. A single positive specimen indicates the need for an air-contrast, barium-enema x-ray in a well-prepared and purged client.

Nursing Management

Clients with rectal bleeding or stools positive for occult blood and in whom a good air-contrast enema reveals polyps should be referred to a colonoscopist for removal of the polyp. Clients with negative air-contrast enemas and positive stools require sigmoidoscopy; if this examination is negative, a complete evaluation of the entire gastrointestinal tract for other lesions is indicated and will require both x-rays and endoscopic evaluation. Polyps should always be removed; this treatment may be performed endoscopically by an experienced colonoscopist. Fiberoptic colonoscopy is well tolerated, with an overall morbidity of 0.42 percent (Berci et al. 1974). After polyp resection, clients should be followed with yearly stool examinations for occult blood and should have an air-contrast barium enema every 3 years to search for a recurrence (Winawer et al. 1976).

COLONIC CANCERS

Pathophysiology

The majority of benign neoplasms of the colon are adenomatous. They appear as a polypoid extension of the mucosa of the colon and can be found in any segment. Over 90 percent of them, however, are found in the rectosigmoid segment (Robbins 1974, p. 962). They are a precursor to malignant carcinoma (Morson 1962).

Carcinoma represents more than 90 percent of the malignant neoplasms of the colon and rectum. About three-fourths of the cases are discovered in people over age 60. A familial tendency for this condition has been identified. Also recognized is the predisposition for carcinoma in patients with adenomas or ulcerative colitis.

Studies have shown that the gross morphology of carcinomas developing on the left side differs from those developing on the right side. A carcinoma of the left side grows in such a way that it encircles the colon and can ultimately cause an obstruction. A carcinoma of the right side tends to form a cauliflowerlike polyp. Both types of carcinoma can penetrate into the bowel wall and metastasize into regional lymph nodes, liver, lungs, and bone.

Colonic cancers are most commonly adenocarcinomatous. They may present as silent tumors of the cecum or ascending colon and cause an iron-deficiency anemia with occult blood in the stools; they cause obstructive symptoms more commonly when they occur in the transverse or descending colon. These tumors are less common in persons eating a high-roughage diet (Painter and Burkitt 1975).

Nursing Assessment

Subjective Findings. Clients may complain of a recent change in bowel habit, with increasing constipation or alternating periods of constipation and diarrhea. Hematochezia may be the presenting complaint; although hemorrhoids may be present, they must not be accepted as the cause until all diagnostic steps have been taken.

Objective Findings. Objective findings may be limited to the presence of fecal blood, or the tumor or a metastatic complication may be palpable. The client may be obviously anemic. Rectal examination may permit palpation of the hard tumor mass.

Diagnostics

Sigmoidoscopy should be requested and will reveal low-lying tumors, while x-ray examination of the colon by barium enema may reveal the higher ones. Referral to a colonoscopist for colonoscopy may be necessary for diagnosis. The fiberoptic endoscope permits examination of the entire colon in 90 percent of persons.

Nursing Management

Management is focused on referral to a surgeon for early surgery. Even tumors that have metastasized often require operation to prevent obstruction or, in rectal lesions, to prevent the tenesmus that renders the final days so miserable in these persons. The nurse must help ease the client through the difficult evaluations and fears regarding treatment. The ideal treatment is the discovery of bowel tumors while they are still adenomatous polyps. With an annual examination of stools for occult blood, the nurse can most benefit the client by early diagnosis and referral.

SUMMARY

The digestive system continues to operate relatively well throughout life. While a certain variety of vascular disorders cause disruption of transport and absorption, the most common problems relate to eating and dietary habits. Over 50 percent of the gastrointestinal complaints of the elderly are found to be of a functional nature with no evident organicity (Sklar 1978). The gerontological nurse should understand that adult clients of all ages require a balanced, nutritive diet with sufficient bulk and the avoidance of excessive irritants such as alcohol.

REFERENCES

ANDREW, W. 1961. "Aging Changes in the Alimentary Tract." In C. H. Bourne, ed., *Structural Aspects of Aging.* New York: Hafner Publishing.

BELBER, J. P. 1971. "Endoscopic Examination of the Duodenal Bulb: A Comparison with X-Ray." *Gastroenterology* 61:55–62.

BERCI, G., et al. 1974. "Complications of Colonoscopy and Polypectomy: Report of the Southern California Society for Gastrointestinal Endoscopy." *Gastroenterology* 67:584–85.

BERMAN, P. M., and J. B. KIRSNER. 1976. "Gastrointestinal Problems." In F. U. Steinberg, ed., *Cowdry's The Care of the Geriatric Patient.* St. Louis: C. V. Mosby.

BLACKWOOD, W. S., et al. 1976. "Cimetidine in Duodenal Ulcer: Controlled Trial." *Lancet* 2:174–76.

BOCKUS, H. L. 1974. "Diaphragmatic Hernia, Esophageal Hiatus Hernia, Eventration and Paralysis of the Diaphragm. Part I: Clinical Analysis." In H. L. Bochus, ed., *Gastroenterology*, 3rd ed. Philadelphia: W. B. Saunders.

BOTHA, G.S.M. 1975. "Radiologic Localization of the Diaphragmatic Hiatus." *Lancet* 1:662–68.

CAPPER, W. M. 1967. "Factors in the Pathogenesis of Gastric Ulcer." *Annals of the Royal College of Surgery* 40:21–25.

CHISHOLM, M. 1976. "Immunology of Gastritis." *Clinical Gastroenterology* 5:419–28.

COHEN, S., and L. D. HARRIS. 1971. "Does Hiatus Hernia Affect the Competence of the Lower Esophageal Sphincter?" *New England Journal of Medicine* 284:1053–58.

CORNET, A., et al. 1964. "La Muqueuse Gastrique chez des Sujets Agés." *Archives des Maladies de l'Appareil Digestif* 53.365–72.

DODD, G., and P. S. NELSON. 1961. "The Combined Radiologic and Gastroscopic Evaluation of Gastric Ulceration." *Radiology* 77:177–85.

ECKARDT, V. I., and P. M. LeCOMPTE. 1977. "Histology of Esophageal Smooth Muscle and Auerbachs Plexus in Elderly Persons." Presented at the Annual Meeting of the American Gastroenterological Association, May 23, Toronto, Canada.

ELLIS, F. H., JR., et al. 1959. "Carcinoma of the Esophagus and Cardia: Results of Treatment 1946 to 1956." *New England Journal of Medicine* 260:351–60.

FORDTRAN, J. S., and J.A.H. COLLYNS. 1966. "Antacid Pharmacology in Duodenal Ulcer." *New England Journal of Medicine* 274:920–27.

FORDTRAN, J. S. 1978. "The Pathogenesis of Peptic Ulcer." In M. H. Sleisinger and J. S. Fordtran, eds., *Gastrointestinal Disease*. Philadelphia: W. B. Saunders.

GOYAL, R. K., J. J. CLANCY, and H. M. SPIRO. 1970. "Lower Esophageal Ring." *New England Journal of Medicine* 282:1298–1302.

GROSSMAN, M. I. 1976. "A New Look at Peptic Ulcer." *Annals of Internal Medicine* 84:57–67.

GUNNLANGSOON, G. H., et al. 1970. "Analysis of the Records of 1,657 Patients with Carcinoma of the Esophagus and Cardia of the Stomach." *Surgery, Gynecology, and Obstetrics* 130:997–1006.

GUYTON, A. C. 1976. *Textbook of Medical Physiology.* Philadelphia: W. B. Saunders.

HADDAD, J. K. 1970. "Relationship of Gastroesophageal Reflux to Yield Sphincter Pressures." *Gastroenterology* 58:175–82.

HIGHTOWER, N. G. 1969. "Applied Physiology of the Esophagus." In *Gastroenterologic Medicine*. Philadelphia: Lea and Febiger.

HILL, L. D., and J. A. TOBIAS. 1968. "Paraesophageal Hernia." *Archives of Surgery of Chicago* 96:735.

INGELFINGER, F. J. 1958. "Esophageal Motility." *Physiological Review* 38:550–53.

JEFFRIES, G. H., D. W. HOSKINS, and M. H. SLEISINGER. 1962. "Antibody to Intrinsic Factor in Serum from Patients with Pernicious Anemia." *Journal of Clinical Investigation* 41:106–15.

JEFFRIES, G. H., and M. H. SLEISINGER. 1965. "Studies of Parietal Cell Antibody in Pernicious Anemia." *Journal of Clinical Investigation* 44:2021–32.

JENSEN, DAVID. 1976. *The Principles of Physiology.* New York: Appleton-Century-Crofts.

KAISER, M. H. and A. I. ROGERS. 1973. "Geriatric Gastroenterology." In J. C. Brocklehurst, ed., *Textbook of Geriatric Medicine and Gerontology.* London: Churchill Livingstone.

KART, C. S., E. S. METRESS, and J. F. METRESS. 1978. *Aging and Health.* Menlo Park, Calif.: Addison-Wesley.

LAMBLING, A., J. R. GOSSET, and D. COLIN. 1969. "Les Dyspepsies et Les Gastrites par Reflux Alcalin Duodeno-Gastrique." *Revue Medicale* (Paris) 10:509–22.

MacMAHON, H. E., R. SCHATZKI, and J. E. GARY. 1958. "Pathology of a Lower Esophageal Ring." *New England Journal of Medicine* 259:1–13.

MASON, J. K. 1963. "Radical Surgical Treatment of Intraoral Carcinoma." *Surgical Clinics of North America* 43:1013–22.

MORSON, B. C. 1963. "The Muscle Abnormality in Diverticular Disease of the Sigmoid Colon." *British Journal of Radiology* 36:385.

MORSON, B. D. 1962. "Precancerous Lesions of the Colon and Rectum." *Journal of the American Medical Association* 170:316–20.

NAKAYAMA, K. 1974. "Part II: Surgical Treatment of Esophageal Malignancy." In H. L. Bockus, ed., *Gastroenterology*, 3rd ed. Philadelphia: W. B. Saunders.

PAINTER, N. S., A. Z. ALMEIDA, and K. W.

COLBOURNE. 1972. "Unprocessed Bran in Treatment of Diverticular Disease of the Colon." *British Medical Journal* 2:137–40.

PAINTER, N. S., and D. P. BURKITT. 1975. "Diverticular Disease of the Colon, a 20th-Century Problem." *Clinical Gastroenterology* 170:316–20.

PALMER, E. D. 1968. "The Hiatus Hernia-Esophagitis-Esophageal Stricture Complex. Twenty-Year Prospective Study." *American Journal of Medicine* 44:566–72.

————. 1971. "Therapy of Hiatal Hernia." In D. Katz and P. Hoffman, eds., *The Esophago-Gastric Junction.* Amsterdam: Exerpta Medica.

PARKS, T. G. 1975. "Natural History of Diverticular Disease of the Colon." *Clinical Gastroenterology* 4:53–70.

POPE, C. E. 1973. "The Esophagus." In M. H. Sleisinger and J. S. Fordtran, eds., *Gastrointestinal Disease.* Philadelphia: W. B. Saunders.

RICHARDSON, C. T. 1973. "Chronic Gastric Ulcer." In M. H. Sleisinger and J. S. Fordtran, eds., *Gastrointestinal Disease.* Philadelphia: W. B. Saunders.

RINALDO, J. A., P. SCHEINOCK, and C. E. RUPE. 1963. "Symptom Diagnosis: A Mathematical Analysis of Epigastric Pain." *Annals of Internal Medicine* 59:145–54.

ROBBINS, S. 1974. *Pathologic Basis of Disease.* Philadelphia: W. B. Saunders.

SANDRY, R. J. 1972. "Pathology of Reflux Esophagitis." In D. B. Skinner et al., eds., *Gastro-esophageal Reflux and Hiatal Hernia.* Boston: Little, Brown.

SCHEURER, U., et al. 1977. "Gastric and Duodenal Ulcer Healing under Placebo Treatment." *Gastroenterology* 72:838–41.

SHATZHI, R. 1932. "Die Hernien des Hiatus Oesophageus." *Deutsch Archive Kliniker Medizin* 173:85.

SIURALA, M., and M. TAEWAST. 1958. "Duodenal Regurgitation and the State of the Gastric Mucosa." *Acta Medica Scandinavica* 153:481–90.

SKLAR, M. 1978. "Gastrointestinal Diseases in the Aged." In W. Reichel, ed., *Clinical Aspects of Aging.* Baltimore: Williams and Wilkins.

STRAUSS, B. 1971. "Disorders of the Digestive System." In I. Rossman, ed., *Clinical Geriatrics.* Philadelphia: J. B. Lippincott.

TAYLOR, K. B., et al. 1962. "Autoimmune Phenomena in Pernicious Anemia: Gastric Antibodies." *British Medical Journal* 1:3147–52.

WALKER, C. O. 1973. "Chronic Duodenal Ulcer." In M. H. Sleisinger and J. S. Fordtran, eds., *Gastrointestinal Disease.* Philadelphia: W. B. Saunders.

WINAWER, S. J., M. MELAMED, and P. SHERLOCK. 1976. "Potential of Endoscopy, Biopsy, and Cytology in the Diagnosis and Management of Patients with Cancer." In P. Sherlock and N. Zamchek, eds., *Clinics in Gastroenterology,* vol. 5, no. 3. Philadelphia: W. B. Saunders.

WINTROBE, M., ed. 1974. *Harrison's Principles of Internal Medicine.* New York: McGraw-Hill.

WOLF, B. S., and J. GUGLIELMA. 1956. "A Method for Roentgen Demonstration of Minimal Hiatal Herniation." *Journal of Mt. Sinai Hospital of New York* 23:738–41.

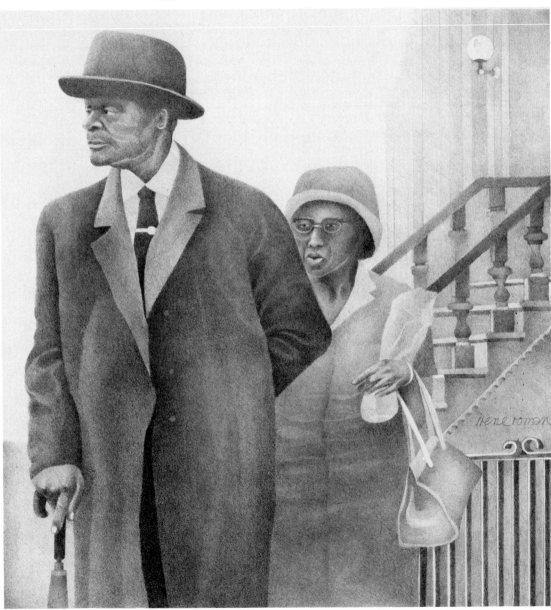

Chapter 17

GERONTOLOGICAL NURSING MANAGEMENT
THE ELDERLY CLIENT WITH A GENITOURINARY/GYNECOLOGICAL PROBLEM

Genitourinary/gynecological problems in the elderly are very common. This chapter discusses a number of urinary problems, prostatic conditions, gynecological problems, and sexual problems.

URINARY INCONTINENCE

Pathophysiology

A brief review of the anatomy and physiology of the bladder will facilitate understanding the pathophysiology of urinary problems.

Anatomy and Physiology of the Bladder. The external wall of the urinary bladder is the *serous peritoneum;* three thick layers of smooth muscle make up the muscular coat of this organ. The middle, circular smooth-muscle layer thickens to form the *internal sphincter* at the proximal end of the urethra. Internally the lining of the bladder is composed of a mucous membrane classified as *transitional epithelium*. When the bladder is empty, this membrane is thrown into folds of layers six to eight cells thick. When the bladder is distended, containing 220 to 300 cm³ of urine, the bladder mucosa thins out and forms layers one or two cells thick. Two slitlike orifices where the two ureters empty into the bladder and the single orifice of the urethra form an internal triangle at the neck, or base, of the hollow organ. This triangle, called the *trigone,* is frequently the locus of infection. At the ureteral orifice the valvelike entry prevents reflux of bladder urine. The thickened middle smooth-muscle layer of the bladder has interlacing fibers that surround the beginning of the urethra and constitute the internal bladder sphincter. Only 2 inches long in the female, the urethra in the male measures about 8 inches. In men the first inch or so of the urethra is surrounded by the prostate gland. The external sphincter is a band of striated muscle fibers surrounding the proximal end of the urethra at the bladder neck (urogenital diaphragm). It is found in both sexes and is under cortical control.

Micturition, the act of emptying the bladder, is a complex mechanism involving interaction of voluntary and involuntary processes. Under normal conditions, when approximately 300 ml of urine have accumulated in the bladder, the bladder wall is stretched. Through a reflex arc mediated in the sacral segments of the spinal cord, the smooth-muscle layers of the bladder wall (detrusor muscle) contract as a unit. The internal sphincter relaxes, and if voluntary control of the external sphincter and perineal muscles is relaxed, micturition occurs. The higher centers prevent micturition by maintaining tonic control of the external sphincter. Muscle tone of the bladder can be diminished in older adults. If this diminution is associated with increased sphincter tone or urethral narrowing, micturition is incomplete. The remaining residual urine can become infected and cause an irritating cystitis.

Incontinence. As voluntary control of micturition requires a normal anatomy, an intact reflex arc, and normal connections between the sacral cord and the higher centers, interference with any of these requirements can lead to urine retention or to incontinence. Injury to the nerves in the cauda equina and sacral plexus prevents normal micturition. Urination occurs only as an overflow from the markedly distended bladder. The flaccid, atonic,

"autonomic neurogenic bladder" is particularly susceptible to infection. This *paradoxical,* or false, incontinence is also found in bladder neck obstruction. The incontinence occurs when intravesical pressure exceeds sphincter pressure (Smith 1975). Injury to the spinal cord above the sacral segments will eliminate all cortical control, which results in an autonomic or "cord bladder." In this case the bladder is spastic and empties completely and frequently in response to distension. If the cortical centers are damaged by hemorrhage or infarction, sensation is retained but voluntary control can be lost. This precipitate urination is due to an "uninhibited neurogenic bladder."

In old age incontinence is generally due to a predisposing factor and a precipitating factor (Brocklehurst et al. 1971). The predisposing factor is often some form of neurogenic bladder disorder, and the precipitating factor is an injury or infection. Clinically, incontinence may be classified into one of four types: (1) *true* incontinence, which occurs with injury to the bladder sphincter, as after prostatectomy or with an acquired neurogenic bladder; (2) *stress* incontinence, which occurs during the act of straining in association with a weakened urethral sphincter or in association with vesical neurogenic disease; (3) *urgency* incontinence, which is usually associated with infection but also occurs in the presence of upper motor-neuron disorders; and (4) *paradoxical,* or false, incontinence, which is associated with bladder neck obstruction or lower motor-neuron disease. The incontinence is either established or transient. If the injury can be treated, the incontinence will cease.

Nursing Assessment

Subjective Findings. The complaints relate either to the precipitating factor (injury or infection) or to the predisposing factor (neurogenic bladder disorder). Infection leads to dysuria, frequency, nocturia, and urgency incontinence. Stress incontinence may occur from coughing, sneezing, laughing, or lifting, but is unusual in the recumbent client. An associated history of other lesions, injuries, or vascular accidents is a significant clue. Subjective findings also vary with the type of neurogenic bladder. The *spastic bladder* is hypertonic because of upper motor-neuron injury with preservation of the sacral reflex arc (injury above the lumbar cord). Urination occurs frequently; as the client is unaware of any bladder sensation, voiding is involuntary, frequent, and scanty. Micturition may be associated with an involuntary spastic movement of the lower extremities. Clients with this problem often complain of sensory loss and spastic paralysis below the level of the lesion.

The *flaccid (atonic or autonomous) bladder* has been liberated from the reflex arc because of injury to the lumbar spine, the cauda equina, or the pelvic nerves. No bladder sensations occur, the client is constantly wet (overflow incontinence), and pressure on the abdomen over the bladder will often cause voiding. Loss of sensation, flaccidity, and loss of muscle control are usually associated with this type of neurogenic bladder.

The *uninhibited neurogenic bladder* is the most common urinary problem in the aged. It is characterized by a cortical motor injury with an intact sensory system and an impaired inhibitor motor system. Clients with uninhibited neurogenic bladder complain of frequency, urgency incontinence, and nocturia. This disorder may be aggravated by hospitalization, a stroke, or confusion, causing total incontinence. The volume of urine is usually small (Brocklehurst et al. 1971). The uninhibited bladder is generally associated with a normal examination. If a stroke has occurred, neurological deficits may be present.

Objective Findings. Objective findings also vary with the cause and complications as well as type of dysfunction. The *spastic* bladder is associated with a normal or increased anal sphincter tone. The bladder is not distended to palpation and percussion. Voiding may be induced by palpation of the lower abdomen and is accompanied by involuntary movements of the lower extremities. Neurological examination reveals a spastic paralysis below the level of the lesion. Babinski's sign may be present.

The *flaccid* bladder is a distended bladder. The neurological examination reveals flaccid paralysis and diminished sensation in the lower extremities. Reflexes are absent or depressed. Pressure over the bladder may induce voiding.

Diagnostics

Laboratory findings are generally nonspecific. Urinalysis, culture, colony count, and—if the colony count is significant (greater than 75,000)—drug sensitivities should be obtained to determine appropriate treatment. Hematuria may indicate a stone, infection, or tumor. Anemia is found in long-standing infection, and uremia in-

415

dicates deteriorating renal function or dehydration.

Abdominal x-rays may reveal calcified stones. X-rays of the spinal column may reveal fractures, metastatic disease, or tumors. The intravenous pyelogram (IVP) outlines the general state of the urinary tract and the size and general condition of the bladder. The bladder is small and trabeculated in spastic disease, large and trabeculated in flaccid disease, and normal in clients with uninhibited vesical problems. Further assessment by means of cystometrograms or voiding cystourethrograms should be supervised by a urologist.

Nursing Management

Counseling. Many elderly people have experienced a lifetime of inculturation in which control of bodily excrement functions is closely tied to social acceptance and a healthy body image. Loss of control brings a concomitant lowering of self-esteem and can cause tremendous anxiety and depression. Counseling should focus on the emotionally disruptive effects of the loss of bladder function.

Treatment. Appropriate treatment and amelioration of incontinence can improve the lot and self-esteem of the older client (Newman 1969). The client with an uninhibited bladder may develop incontinence because of a change in environment. Placing a light at the bedside, providing a bedside commode or urinal, or lighting the way to the bathroom may be sufficient treatment (Brocklehurst 1971). Drugs may induce incontinence: sedatives and tranquilizers diminish awareness, and diuretics increase urinary output. The nurse should think of decreasing the sedative or instructing the client to take the diuretic earlier in the day. Treatment and resolution of a urinary infection may stop the incontinence. Infection is a frequent compounding problem and should be ruled out in all such clients.

A neurogenic bladder may often be retrained. Training should be initiated immediately after the initial phase of the stroke or spinal shock. During this first phase catheterization may be necessary. However, permanent indwelling catheters commonly result in bacteriuria. Intermittent, clean catheterization reduces the incidence of infection (Comarr 1972; Perkash 1974); however, this technique requires frequent nursing attention, and temporary placement of an indwelling catheter may be required if sufficient personnel is lacking.

The spastic neurogenic bladder of large capacity may be retrained if the client is dry for 2 to 3 hours and can precipitate voiding by squeezing the thigh, lower abdomen, or genital organs. A low-capacity bladder requires some type of surgical procedure on the sphincter, a permanent external collection device, or a permanent indwelling catheter.

In an attempt to increase bladder capacity, a trial of medication may be indicated. This treatment has been most useful in clients with less severe problems, such as an uninhibited neurogenic bladder. Anticholinergic quarternary-amines, such as methantheline bromide (Banthine) 50 to 100 mg three to four times daily by mouth or propantheline bromide (Probanthine) 15 to 30 mg three to four times daily by mouth, decrease bladder tone and increase capacity. They may precipitate glaucoma and cause xerostomia. Estrogens have occasionally been effective in women with uninhibited neurogenic bladders, particularly with an associated atrophic vaginitis (Brocklehurst 1973; Anderson 1976). Other medications are under investigation (Smith 1975; Anderson 1976).

The flaccid bladder is emptied if pressure is applied manually to the lower abdomen. The emptying is usually incomplete unless assisted by straining and bearing down as to void. When residual urine remains, it becomes a source of infection. Clients with flaccid bladder should be trained to void every 2 hours, and if a residual is present, they should be taught how to perform intermittent catheterization. A trial of medication may obviate the need for catheterization. Parasympatheticomimetics such as bethanecol chloride (Urecholine) 10 to 30 mg three to four times daily by mouth may initiate voiding and improve emptying of the bladder.

A number of external collection appliances are currently being introduced. One such incontinent brief is now being test-marketed by Proctor and Gamble and is suitable for both male and female clients. A similar pad is widely used in Great Britain. For some time external condom-type appliances, such as Paul's tubing, have been available for men. Nurses should familiarize themselves with these and attempt trial periods prior to resorting to an indwelling catheter.

The alternative to successful control of incontinence is the permanent placement of an indwelling catheter. This measure leads inevitably to urinary infection and eventual renal tissue destruction. The catheters must be changed periodically to prevent obstruction. The family must be taught how to avoid contamination and particularly to keep the collection bottle below the level of the bladder. Raising this container permits back flow of contaminated urine. The nurse must be alert to new techniques of catheter care.

Other techniques should be explored, including electrode implantation (Merrill et al. 1975) and prosthetic sphincter implantation (Scott et al. 1973). These techniques require evaluation by a urological surgeon.

URINARY TRACT INFECTIONS

Pathophysiology

In the presence of a bladder infection, urine may become alkaline; this condition in turn can cause the formation of inorganic salt precipitates, which can grow to the size of small stones. Calculi can form when use of a catheter is prolonged. The indwelling catheter also can predispose the client to bladder infection and result in precipitation of inorganic salts in urine. Stones known as secondary bladder calculi can also originate in the kidney and migrate to the bladder.

Frank and microscopic hematuria may be found in association with urinary tract infections. This disorder may originate in the kidneys and ureters but more commonly is associated with a breakdown of the mucosa and vessels of the bladder caused by stones, obstruction, ulcerating tumors, and infection.

417

Nonspecific infection of the urinary tract is a common problem in the elderly and may be found in as many as 20 percent of ambulatory clients over age 65 (Brocklehurst et al. 1968). Nonspecific infection is distinguished from the specific, often chronic, infections due to parasites, granuloma-forming organisms such as tuberculosis, and venereal diseases by the fact that a large number of gram-negative and gram-positive bacteria all present with the same nonspecific findings.

These bacteria enter the urinary tract from four sources: (1) they may be carried there by the blood stream; (2) they may be carried there by the lymphatics; (3) they may be directly implanted from another infected contiguous organ, as in acute diverticulitis; or, most commonly, (4) they may be introduced by the ascending route from the urethra (Hutch et al. 1963; Hinman 1966; Cox et al. 1968; Corriere et al. 1972; Stamey 1963). Thus one understands why women, with their shorter urethra and anatomical placement of the urethra close to the rectum, suffer urinary infection more frequently than men, particularly during childhood and the child-bearing years (Heldrick et al. 1967). The frequency of urinary tract infection rises in men after age 65, paralleling the development of urinary retention, which diminishes the effectiveness of their urethral protection (Brocklehurst et al. 1968; Hinman 1966).

Findings relate to the portions of the tract involved, the degree of systemic involvement, and the presence of obstructive disease or complications. Except in cases of urethritis, bladder symptoms of cystitis are usually present in acute urinary infections and in acute exacerbations of chronic urinary infections.

CYSTITIS

Nursing Assessment

The common subjective complaints of acute cystitis are burning on urination; frequency, often to the point of incontinence; nocturia or increased nocturia; and often terminal hematuria. Hematuria occurring at the end of voiding may cause staining of paper or underclothes with blood. Clients may complain of suprapubic pressure or mild low-back pain. Older clients may complain only of urinary incontinence without stress. Eneurisis (bed wetting) may occur. Tenderness over the bladder may be present. On rectal examination the prostate should be normal. If the rectal sphincter is relaxed, the nurse must consider the possibility of a neurogenic bladder with urinary retention. In chronic cases dysuria disappears and only urgency, incontinence, and nocturia may be present. Most cases, outside of acute exacerbation, are without findings. Fever is unusual, or is low grade at most, in the absence of renal or prostate infection.

Diagnostics

At the initial contact a midstream urine specimen is obtained for analysis, gram stain on the unspun specimen, culture, colony count, and sensitivity. While pure colony counts of 100,000 organisms or greater are diagnostic, colony counts between 50,000 and 100,000 pose a diagnostic dilemma. In such cases the colony count should be performed on a morning's first voided specimen. If the colony count is still below 100,000 organisms, the client should be referred to a physician. When cystitis occurs in a man, complete evaluation for obstructive uropathy should be performed. In women, treatment may be instituted without extensive evaluation.

Nursing Management

Unless the client's cardiac or renal status precludes large amounts of fluid intake, all clients with a urological disorder should be encouraged to drink fluids.

Acute Urinary Infections: Treatment. Appropriate treatment requires elimination of the infection and, if possible, elimination of the abnormality that initially precipitated the infection. In the older client with a neurogenic bladder and urinary stasis, such treatment may not be possible. The nurse may initiate appropriate antibiotic therapy, rendering the urine temporarily sterile, only to see a rapid recurrence with the same or another organism.

An appropriate antimicrobial agent is started at once. A short-acting sulfonamide, such as sulfisoxazole 4 g stat and 1 g four times daily for 10 days to 2 weeks, is often effective and is inexpensive. Also effective is nalidixic acid (Negram) 1 g four times daily for 7 to 10 days. If the urine bacterial stain reveals gram-positive cocci, penicillin "V" 250 mg four times daily for 2 weeks or Cloxacillin 500 mg four times daily for 2 weeks should be used. If gram-negative bacilli are seen, either tetracycline 250 mg four times daily or Ampicillin 500 mg four times daily, each for 10 to 14 days should be used. Nitrofurantoin tablets 100 mg four times daily for 2 weeks may also be tried. A urine culture and sensitivity will point to the appropriate drugs.

The *acute symptoms of cystitis* may be helped by hot sitz baths for 20 minutes three to four times daily and antispasmodics such as tincture of belladona 10 to 15 drops three or four times daily. The client is seen in 3 days and another urine obtained for gram stain. If bacteria are still seen, the urine is cultured and another colony count and sensitivity are obtained. The sensitivities of the first specimen are examined, and the appropriate alternative antibiotic is employed. However, if treatment does not eradicate the infection in 2 weeks or rapidly render the urine sterile, or if the client has a history of recurrent infection, complete evaluation for obstructive uropathy or other problems such as diabetes mellitus should be performed. These clients will probably require referral to a urologist.

Acute Urinary Infections: Evaluation of Care. Clients must be referred to a physician if treatment fails to eradicate infection within 2 weeks, if infection is frequently recurrent, if the colony counts are persistently less than 100,000 organisms in pure culture even when performed on the first voided specimen of the morning, and if the clients remain symptomatic and cultures are sterile. The further evaluation of a urinary infection includes a 2-hour postprandial blood sugar test, and intravenous pyelogram with postvoid films, and urine cultures for specific organisms. Other tests necessitate consultation with a urologist for special films taken during a voiding urethrocystogram as well as cystometric studies and even cystoscopy and retrograde pyelograms.

Chronic Urinary Infections: Treatment. *Chronic urinary infections* are often treated with long-term suppressive therapy. Appropriate antibiotics for 3 to 4 weeks, followed by a suppressive such as a sulfisoxazole 1 g four times daily or Methenamine mandelate 1 g four times daily with ascorbic acid, may be used for many years; consultation with a physician should be obtained prior to institution of chronic suppressive therapy.

Chronic Urinary Infections: Evaluation of Care. Urinary infections cannot be cured if an indwelling catheter, a stone, or a persistent bladder urine residual due to obstruction, reflux, diverticulum, or neurogenic bladder is present. An open colovesical fistula from ruptured colonic diverticulum will cause recurrent infection, which may be compounded by pneumaturia (gas in the urine) or occasionally fecaluria (stool mixed with urine). These cases are complex and require a complete evaluation by a urologist or nephrologist. Many older patients with cellular neurogenic bladders have urine that is chronically infected. Fortunately this condition is well tolerated by such clients (Brocklehurst 1974).

ACUTE PROSTATITIS

Nursing Assessment

Subjective Findings. Clients with bacterial prostatitis may have a history of alcohol abuse, heavy caffeine ingestion, abrupt change in sexual habits, or past gonorrhea or nonspecific stress prior to the onset of symptoms (Thompson and Edwards 1978).

Bacterial prostatitis may present with either systemic or nonsystemic findings. In the systemic form the disseminated infection produces chills, fever, and prostation.

The nonsystemic form involves the same symptom complex but without the fever or systemic symptoms.

In *acute prostatitis* clients complain of cystitis and low back pain. Perineal discomfort may be present. Hematuria is common; the hematuria and dysuria may be of the onset type or may be present during the entire episode of micturition. The urine is cloudy, and a urethral discharge may occur. Urinary obstruction with postvoiding dribbling, hesitancy, and incomplete voiding may be present. Urethral discharge may be manifested in the older client by anuria and a severe urge to void. Acute prostatitis infections frequently are associated with a history of increased sexual activity or after instrument examination or catheterization of the bladder.

Objective Findings. On rectal examination the prostate is usually exquisitely tender, enlarged, hot to touch, and sometimes firm. A soft, fluctuant gland indicates abscess. The examination must be gentle to avoid causing severe pain or seeding the infection.

Chronic prostatitis has few if any findings. This disorder is frequently due to an incompletely treated acute infection. Acute exacerbations are often associated with obstruction and bladder complaints. The prostate may be normal, boggy, or indurated to the examining finger. Massage reveals fluid with pus, but cultures are rarely useful (Mears and Stamey 1968).

Diagnostics

Laboratory studies again reveal an elevated white blood cell count. Prostatic secretion is purulent but cultures are usually

420

sterile. Bacteriuria may or may not be present. Diagnosis is confirmed with a positive culture of expressed prostatic secretions (EPS). Initially a microscopic examination of EPS should be performed because the presence of bacteria, red blood cells, or trichomonads is significant (Thompson and Edwards 1978).

Nursing Management

The most effective treatment for bacterial prostatitis is trimethoprin and sulfamethoxazole combination (Bactrim, Septra) 2 tablets twice a day for 6 to 12 weeks. Nonbacterial prostatitis may be treated with antimicrobials based on empirical trial for results. Acute prostatitis has a high frequency of chronicity if treatment is inappropriate or delayed and should also be evaluated by a urologist. Chronic prostatitis is difficult to eradicate and requires frequent prostatic massage and counseling regarding the salutary effects of intercourse in draining the prostate. This condition should be treated in collaboration with a urologist.

ACUTE URETHRITIS

Nursing Assessment

Subjective Findings. Acute nonspecific urethritis is predominately a disease of men. In women it is usually associated with gonorrhea (Cougar 1964). The single prevailing finding is a urethral discharge of variable consistency. It is present on arising and often causes staining of the pajamas or underwear. Clients may also complain of an itching or burning in the urethra. Onset dysuria may be present.

Objective Findings. The few objective findings vary with the site and nature of the infection. The external meatus is often red, swollen, and everted. The discharge may be thin or purulent.

Diagnostics

The laboratory findings are limited to the nature of the discharge. In the absence of secretion, the first few milliliters of a voided urine should be examined, as this portion contains the urethral contents. The next portion, or midstream specimen, should be devoid of pus and bacteria. Wet, unstained preparations should be examined for trichomonads or the lecithin bodies of prostatitis. The stained preparation may reveal *gonococcus*. Routine cultures and cultures for gonorrhea should be obtained.

Nursing Management

Acute urethritis does not respond well to treatment. Appropriate cultures for gonorrhea must always precede therapy. Intercourse aggravates the disorder, and clients should abstain from sexual intercourse and alcohol during treatment. Occasionally a combination of a sulfisoxazole 2 g at once and 1 g four times daily given along with tetracycline 250 mg or with erythromycin 250 mg four times daily for 10 days may be effective. Other combinations have been used with varying success.

PYELONEPHRITIS

Nursing Assessment

Clients with *acute pyelonephritis* have complaints of cystitis in addition to unilateral or bilateral midback and flank pain due to stretching of the capsule of the infected kidney. These clients are acutely ill, febrile, septic, and vomiting. The elderly client may be confused, agitated, and dehydrated. Tenderness is present over the involved kidney and its costovertebral angle (CVA). Abdominal distension, absent bowel sounds, and rebound abdominal tenderness may be present. Septicemia with shock may be present (Beeson 1971). Laboratory tests reveal an elevated white blood cell count with a left shift and an increased sedimentation rate. Urinalysis reveals a cloudy urine with protein, pus, and bacteria.

Chronic pyelonephritis is often quiescent. Findings, if present, are those of a bladder infection. Symptoms may include tiredness, backache, anemia, weight loss, renal failure, or hypertension. In the chronic infection, outside of the acute exacerbations, bacilluria and cylindruria may be the only findings. Anemia and uremia indicate that renal tissue has been damaged. In these cases the electrolyte pattern and arterial blood pH are often abnormal. Acute exacerbations of chronic disease are indistinguishable from primary acute episodes.

Nursing Management

The medical management of a client who has acute pyelonephritis with its high risk of septicemia should be conducted by a physician, usually in a hospital. In clients exhibiting the vague complaints of a chronic problem, obtaining a clean-catch urine for microscopic examination is always wise. Clients with chronic pyelonephritis require extensive evaluation and prolonged therapy and should be referred or managed in close collaboration with a physician.

UPPER AND LOWER TRACT OBSTRUCTION

Obstruction of urinary flow is divided between upper and lower tract obstruction. Findings vary according to the level of the obstruction and may also be complicated by findings due to uremia, which indicates advanced disease.

Pathophysiology

Bladder tumor is frequently found during the sixth decade and is found in males three to four times more often than in females (Robbins 1974). When the tumorous growth causes bleeding, the growth is usually a malignant, ulcerated, papillary carcinoma. Tumorous growths can also lead to urinary tract obstruction. However, the most common cause of obstruction is calculi, which, if large enough, can obstruct the kidney pelvis. Smaller stones formed in the kidney pelvis can pass on and obstruct any portion of the lower urinary tract. Tumors can also obstruct any part of the urinary tract, depending on their location. Strictures of ureter and urethra are other causes of obstruction. Pain, hematuria, and obstruction of urinary flow can result in all of these disorders. When clients develop urinary obstruction, initial hypertrophy of the detrusor muscle occurs, followed by decreased tone and cellularity, leading to stasis and bladder diverticuli with residual urine.

In the older male, obstruction of the neck of the bladder occurs when the prostate gland becomes enlarged, extends upward into the bladder, and compresses the vesical orifice. The enlargement can be up to ten times normal size. Initially the bladder wall hypertrophies and the trigone rises. The hypertrophied and trabeculated bladder then progressively decompensates and finally dilates passively. Most often prostatic enlargement is due to the presence of a benign tumor. In such cases one finds ". . . irregular, multifocal hyperplasia of the fibromuscular stroma, with a varying amount of secondary invasion by glandular elements" (Lytton and Epstein 1974, p. 1416).

The prostate gland is also subject to carcinomatous growth, usually adenocarcinoma. Most growths occur in the posterior lobe, and urinary symptoms appear only late in the course of the disease. Another, but not common, cause of prostatic hyperplasia is inflammation. Cocci such as *staphylococci, streptococci,* or *gonococci* are usually the offending organisms.

Carcinoma of the prostate is the fourth most common cause of cancer in men and has been estimated to be present in 30 percent of those over 70 and 80 percent of those in their eighties. However, it is rare in men under the age of 50. Benign prostatic hypertrophy usually occurs at an earlier age. Carcinoma of the prostate frequently presents with no symptoms (Anderson 1975, p. 315).

UPPER TRACT OBSTRUCTION

Nursing Assessment

Subjective Findings. Clients who have an upper tract obstruction complain of flank pain, which usually radiates along the course of the ureter and into the back. Hematuria, if present, is total and usually indicates a stone. Nausea and vomiting are often present. Passage of the stone to the lower ureter may cause urinary and rectal urgency. Chills, fever, cloudy urine, and dysuria indicate infection. Uremic symptoms indicate bilateral disease, even though uremia is present, the client may have no complaints.

The subjective uremia complaints consist of weakness and apathy. Clients often are confused at night and sleepy during the day. As the urea levels (BUN) rise, headache, loss of appetite, nausea, and vomiting appear along with pruritus, diarrhea, and involuntary skin twitching. Uremic gastritis may cause hematemesis. Findings of congestive failure are common in the older client. With further progression the client becomes comatose.

Objective Findings. The objective findings serve to determine the degree of illness, confirm the presence of obstruction, and identify the etiologic factors. Abdominal palpation may disclose an enlarged kidney. Renal tenderness or CVA tenderness usually indicates infection.

Pelvic examination helps reveal a cervical or uterine carcinoma, which may invade up along the ureters or directly to the bladder where it either may obstruct the ureterovesical orifices or interfere with micturition.

LOWER TRACT OBSTRUCTION

Nursing Assessment

Subjective Findings. The elderly male usually does not report symptoms spontaneously until the lower tract obstruction has reached a late stage. Therefore, the nurse must carefully elicit data concerning urinary functioning during the history. Initial symptoms include hesitancy, lowered

423

stream force, frequency, and nocturia. Later symptoms are related to obstruction: dribbling, poor control, overflow incontinence, an irritated outlet, and even sepsis may occur. Hematuria is more often found in the client with benign prostatic hypertrophy (BPH) than with a malignant prostate. The hyperplastic gland may be the instigator in a now chronically infected bladder (Jaffe 1978, p. 231).

Objective Findings. Urethral palpation may reveal a stricture. On rectal examination, prostatic hypertrophy can be palpated and the firm benign gland may be distinguished from a rock-hard carcinoma. Approximately 50 percent of all hard nodules felt on rectal examination of the prostate are malignant (Brocklehurst 1973). The size of the gland on rectal examination is frequently unrelated to the symptoms and only minimally related to residual volume and degree of obstruction.

Neurogenic bladder dysfunction, found in older clients of either sex, is another cause for the same problems of stasis and obstruction. Persistence of these problems for any length of time inevitably leads to hydronephrosis and loss of renal tissue. Also the stasis inevitably results in urinary infection, which causes more destruction. Prompt recognition of the problem will limit the damage and prevent renal insufficiency. Additionally fecal impaction may cause obstruction in older clients, particularly women.

Diagnostics

A midstream urine specimen should be examined microscopically. Complete examination requires cystoscopy and panendoscopy, which permit visualization of the bladder and urethra, respectively. Blood studies include blood counts, blood sugar, blood urea nitrogen, serum creatinine, acid and alkaline phosphatase, calcium, phosphorous, and uric acid. For several hours following rectal examination, acid phosphatase can be elevated. The incidence of elevated acid phosphatase is low in benign disease and only moderate when malignancy is present (Jaffe 1978). Metastasis may be detected by x-ray or radioisotope scans.

Stones must be analyzed to determine their crystalline substance base. Most stones (90%) are composed of calcium, uric acid and cystine stones comprising the rest. X-rays are usually diagnostic. The plain abdominal film may reveal renal enlargement. The IVP or drip infusion IVP reveals the level of obstruction and usually defines the cause.

Nursing Management

The nurse's primary concern lies in initial screening and tentative diagnosis in the case of early symptoms. Clients who have evidence of progressive bladder decompensation due to prostatic obstruction require referral to a urologist, as do those who have a suspected carcinoma of prostatic origin.

Management consists of relief of obstruction and stasis. Infection, if present, cannot be irradicated until normal, complete emptying occurs. Indeed, infection in the presence of obstruction or stasis is an absolute indication for referral to a urologist.

Clients with noncancerous, intermittent lower tract obstruction should be followed. They should be cautioned not to allow the bladder to overdistend and encouraged to void when they feel the urge. Health instructions specify the necessity of avoiding medications containing anticholinergics and antihistamines, including most commercial cold remedies and sleeping pills. Clients who tend to form calcium stones need dietary instructions. Many of these individuals are ingesting water that has high levels of calcium. Clients may be advised to purchase bottled water or install a water softener in areas where the mineral level of water is high.

GYNECOLOGICAL PROBLEMS

Pathophysiology

In the absence of surgical removal of the ovaries, menopause usually occurs in women between the ages of 45 and 55. Although all factors are not known, the progressive decline in ovarian follicles evidently accelerates suddenly around age 40. This change is associated initially with a progressive and eventual sharp decrease in measurable estrogen levels. It is presumably due to a decline in follicles, which are the primary source of the hormone (Paulsen et al. 1958). The associated secondary amenorrhea may begin abruptly or occur progressively.

Subjective and Objective Findings. Findings show a high degree of variation, and only a portion of all women are affected. Subjective vasomotor phenomena include "hot flashes," chills, sweating, and palpitations, which are usually accepted as symptoms of menopause. Other complaints may be related to hormonal menopausal changes or are of a psychosocial origin (Timiras 1972; Kase 1971). Such complaints include headaches, dizziness, irritability, emotional lability, memory

loss, feelings of ill health, and depression. Objective findings are directly related to the effect of hormone deprivation on the primary and secondary sex characteristics. These findings include breast thinning and sagging, changing hair pattern and hair thinning, irritation of the vagina and vulva, and involution and atrophy of the uterus and cervix.

In elderly females the vulva become pallid and the labia and vagina progressively atrophy. The thinning wall leads to vascular fragility and may be a common cause of postmenopausal staining or bleeding. The vaginal wall becomes flaccid, and subcutaneous atrophy may cause shortening and narrowing of the vaginal canal; the cervix also becomes narrowed and stenosed. Suspensory ligaments become increasingly weaker, with resulting cystocele, cystourethrocele, enterocele, and rectocele. Vaginal secretions are greatly diminished. Atrophic changes are also exhibited in the uterus and ovaries.

When atrophic changes occur in the vagina, the mucosa loses much of its resistance to infection. This lowered resistance is due to the loss of commensal organisms that protect the canal by creating an acid environment. With the loss of these organisms, pathogens such as *Pseudomonas aeruginosa* and *Staphylococcus aureus* can more easily invade the vagina and cause the production of an irritating vaginal discharge and pruritus.

ATROPHIC VAGINITIS

Vaginal atrophy may become so severe as to take on an inflammatory appearance. The thin, flat vaginal mucosa becomes less acidic and has a lowered resistance to bacterial invasion. Atrophic vaginitis is a com-

425

mon cause of postmenopausal bleeding. Bleeding may occur with or without recurrent infections and more commonly follows douching or coitus (Glowacki 1978). Uterine bleeding in any client who is known to have completed menopause is an indication for thorough examination.

Nursing Assessment

Trichomoniasis is usually associated with an abundant green discharge, but this sign may be lacking in the postmenopausal client. Subjective complaints include dyspareunia, perineal pruritus, and vaginal burning. The urethra may be involved, and urgency and onset dysuria often occur. The objective findings show a discharge that is foul or may be bloody. The vaginal mucosa is smooth, flat, and friable. The redness of the vaginal inflammation often extends onto the vulva. The discharge of monilia infection is usually white, with the appearance of curdled milk. Uterine, cervical, and vaginal carcinoma are excluded by careful physical examination and by cytologic examination of the cervical and vaginal material. Uterine cells may be obtained by sampling the endocervix with a cotton-tipped applicator dampened in saline and inserted through the external os. The cervix and vagina are scraped with the usual wooden spatula. Only 5 to 10 percent of cervical cancer cases are reported in women over the age of 70, whereas 60 percent of such cases are reported in women under 60. Carcinoma of the uterus, however, is more frequent in women over 60 (Soule 1976).

Diagnostics

A 10% solution of potassium hydroxide (KOH) smear will confirm the presence of candida. A gram stain and culture may disclose gonorrhea. The pap smear reveals a predominance of basal cells. These cells may be the only ones found and are caused by an absence of estrogen. Confirmation of the menopausal condition is obtained by an elevated serum follicular stimulating hormone (FSH), which indicates ovarian failure.

Nursing Management

The use of oral estrogen therapy as prophylaxis in postclimacteric women has come under controversy in recent years because of factors indicating a carcinogenic effect on the breasts and endometrium. However, the long-term benefits of oral estrogen therapy, such as maintenance of collagen integrity of the skin, decreased osteoporosis, and prevention of atrophic vaginitis, seem to warrant its use. The immediate benefit is the prevention of thermal reactions. Clients on long-term estrogen therapy should be informed of the potential risks and long-term benefits. The need for oral estrogens should be considered in terms of the need to relieve menopausal symptoms, the support of skin and mucosal metabolism, and the potential of endometrial and breast cancer (Glowacki 1978). Initiation of such therapy should be in collaboration with a physician. Oral estrogen may be given as conjugated equine estrogens (Premarin, Ogen) and should be given in small dosages (0.3 to 0.625 mg daily) for 3 weeks of each month (Glowacki 1978).

For the client who has atrophic vulvitis and vaginitis, an estrogen cream is applied in the morning and evening until symptoms subside. Then the applications may be decreased in frequency to maintain a healthy mucosa.

Nonspecific vaginitis usually responds to acidic douches. Lactic acid 30 ml in a liter of warm water (1 ounce in 1 quart) or clear, white distilled vinegar 15 ml in 1 liter of water provide effective douches. These douches are used nightly for 1 to 2 weeks. Topical sulfonamide cream or antibiotics give variable success.

Candidiasis is effectively treated by nystatin vaginal suppositories or cream, inserted twice a day for 14 days. A number of preparations are available, such as Mycostatin or Nilstat suppositories and Monostat, Vanobid, or Sporastacin creams. When vaginal intertrigo is a problem, the client should be instructed to use a mild medicated powder such as Caldescene or Diaperene as a prophylaxis.

Women who have recurrent monilial infections should be instructed to wear cotton underwear. Sexual partners may be harbingers of the infection and should also receive therapy.

Symptomatic trichomonas vaginalis responds to metronidazole (Flagyl) 250 mg three times daily for 7 days, provided the sexual partner is also treated and the couple refrains from intercourse for the treatment period. Women with trichomonas infection should have a repeat cervical smear 2 months after treatment, because the infection may give a falsely positive smear.

The client with gonorrhea is managed with full dosage of the appropriate antibiotic—usually 4.8 million U of procaine penicillin intramuscularly with 0.1 g Probenecid orally. Resistant strains are appearing and are being treated with tetracycline 1.5 g at once and .5 g four times daily for 4 days by mouth, or streptomycin 1 g daily intramuscularly for 3 days.

Clients with evidence of tumor or with a vaginitis not responding to treatment should be referred to a gynecologist.

MISCELLANEOUS CONDITIONS

A variety of conditions present with a common complaint of pruritus vulvae. Among these conditions are vaginitis, lichen sclerosis, leukoplakia, kraurosis vulvae, and vulvar carcinoma.

Nursing Assessment

Subjective complaints involve refractory itching. Examination usually reveals excoriation with one or another associated problem. Leukoplakia presents as a whitish gray, hyperkeratotic lesion, which in later stages becomes thin and forms the lesion of kraurosis. Lichen sclerosis is characterized by subepidermal edema without fibrosis, which gives a thin parchmentlike appearance to the vulvar area. Vulvar carcinoma generally is characterized as a flat infiltrative or ulcerated lesion. At times it may appear exophytic (Soule 1976).

Diagnostics

The diagnostic considerations include generalized dermatoses with vulval manifestations as well as vulvovaginal conditions. As with atrophic vaginitis, examination of the body and the genitalia along with appropriate fungal, bacteriological, and cytological samples must be performed. All clients with suspicious lesions are referred to a physician for biopsy since the peak incidence of vulvar carcinoma occurs in the elderly woman (Glowaki 1978).

Nursing Management

Pruritus vulvae may be exceedingly difficult to treat. Precipitating causes such as

427

atrophic vaginitis and specific or nonspecific infections should be treated appropriately (see the discussion above on the management of atrophic vaginitis). Resistant cases or cases in which the diagnosis is in doubt should be referred to a physician or managed in close collaboration with one.

SEXUAL PROBLEMS

Sexuality is a broad and complex dimension of human life from birth to death. Reared in an age when sexual topics were considered taboo, the elderly person is often reluctant to discuss readily such an intimate topic. Unfortunately nurses may have little knowledge concerning sexual functioning and even poorer attitudes concerning the need for sexual information (Lief and Payne 1975). Sexual impairment is not the result of aging in itself but is secondary to health disorders. Certain age-related physiological changes do occur, however, and affect male and female sexuality.

Male Physiological Changes

More direct stimulation is required as well as more time to achieve erection; the erection may be softer until right before ejaculation.

Preejaculatory lubrication is often absent.

Ejaculation is collapsed into one stage instead of two, and the amount of ejaculate is decreased.

Loss of erection is more rapid following ejaculation.

Focus on genital pleasures is diminished as sensuality becomes more diffused and generalized (Berman and Lief 1975, p. 127).

Female Physiological Changes

A thinning of the vaginal wall occurs.

Longer and more direct stimulation is necessary to produce vaginal lubrication.

The orgasmic phase is shorter and decreased in intensity.

Particularly when estrogen levels are lower, irritability of vaginal tissues and dyspareunia, or painful intercourse, may occur.

Nursing Assessment

Nurses must be aware of their feelings about their own sexuality, they must know how aging affects sexuality, and they must feel at ease in initiating an assessment of sexual problems with the older client. Often clients may only want to discuss or reminisce about past sexual activities and thus require an empathetic listener. On the other hand, the elderly may consider any discussion of sexuality to be unwanted and even sinful. In all instances the limitations that the client sets for discussion must be respected.

Sexual problems can be overt, such as coital pain in Peyronie's disease, retrograde ejaculation, and atrophic vaginitis; or they may present as subtle variations of lifelong habits or as unmet needs for intimacy. The most prevalent problem is the lack of sexual partners for aging females. In cohabiting older couples, one partner may use aging as an excuse to cease an activity that brings up negative memories and uncomfortable feelings, while the other partner may maintain an active interest in sex.

The need for intimacy and social support may outweigh familial and societal sanctions: some of the elderly choose to live

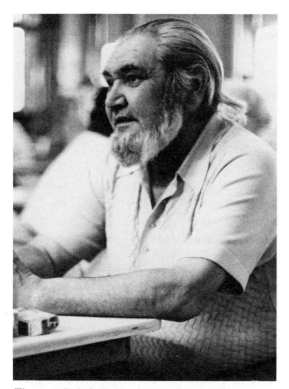

The gerontological nurse can help the elderly adapt to the aging process by encouraging open discussion of age-related changes that affect human sexuality; elderly clients not only need to understand their sexual capabilities and limitations but to maintain positive masculine or feminine self-images.

together without a legal matrimonial attachment. In the past this living arrangement was often caused by discriminating social security laws whereby the elderly stood to receive less income as a married couple. Such a relationship may bring concomitant feelings of guilt and inadequacy.

Masters and Johnson have written about the "widower's syndrome": typically the husband has nursed his wife of many years through a terminal illness; after a period of mourning and abstinence, the widower finds he has difficulty obtaining an erection, a problem that may be compounded by grief and guilt. This unfortunate occurrence may lead the male to question his virile ability and to avoid any further sexual contact (Masters and Johnson 1970).

Secondary sexual impairment results from a number of health problems that cause fatigue and lower the capacity to engage in sexual activities. These problems include cardiovascular, respiratory, endocrine, neurological, urological, and gynecological disorders as well as any type of debilitative surgery. Sedatives, hypotensives, and alcohol can cause secondary impotence. Tranquilizers tend to decrease sexual interest or desire. Some studies indicate that psychological influences have a gender-linked reaction. Depression may precede sexual withdrawal for women, whereas sexual dysfunction tends to precede depression for men (Boyarsky 1976). Boredom and routine often lead to cessation of sexual activity in the elderly.

Nursing Management

The nurse must never assume that interest is no longer present in any older person of either sex. The primary nursing role often revolves around the nurse's ability to be a counselor and educator. For the client who fears that sexual activity will affect some health problem, simply allaying the client's fear through sex education may be sufficient. Specific suggestions are often indicated, such as using a less tiring position, like side lying, or engaging in sexual activities after a nap or in the morning after the night's rest. For the arthritic client the nurse may suggest the use of pillows and the ingestion of aspirin 30 minutes before engaging in sexual activity.

429

The nurse should inform the client about the potential side effects of drugs on sexual functioning. Particularly information and clarification about normative changes in sexual functioning related to aging is necessary, as these may often be interpreted as impairment.

The nurse should not be reticent in bringing up the question of alternative forms of sexual functioning for the client who has no partner, providing both the nurse and client feel comfortable enough to participate in such a discussion. Included in sexual alternatives are masturbatory activity, fantasy, or even dreams. Masters and Johnson (1970), for example, report the cases of a number of elderly women who learned to masturbate for the first time in their later years and thus achieved sexual satisfaction and release. But for some, sexual outlet may be met simply through closer interpersonal relationships.

Adequate vaginal lubrication in elderly females can considerably assist intercourse. While vaginal creams or oral estrogen will help atrophic changes, the use of K-Y jelly can provide additional lubrication to prevent irritation and pain.

The elderly male's need for increased penal stimulation may be achieved by self-masturbation, partner masturbation, or oral stimulation, the mode being determined by whatever the client feels comfortable with. Again K-Y jelly application can be used to facilitate hand stimulation.

SUMMARY

Genitourinary and gynecological disorders of the older client are common and disabling problems. The gerontological nurse should not ignore these complaints, as proper management can alleviate many related psychosocial manifestations. Such management can restore dignity and often prevent institutionalization of the client.

REFERENCES

ANDERSON, W. F. 1975. "Diseases of the Genito-Urinary Tract." In H. P. von Hahn, ed., *Practical Geriatrics*. New York and Basel: Karger, A. G.

ANDERSON, F. 1976. *Practical Management of the Elderly*. Oxford: Blackwell Scientific Publications.

BEESON, P. B. 1971. "Pyelonephritis." In P. B. Beeson and W. McDermott, eds., *Cecil-Loeb Textbook of Medicine*. Philadelphia: W. B. Saunders.

BERMAN, E., and H. I. LIEF. 1976. "Sex and the Aging Process." In W. W. Oaks, ed., *Sex and the Life Cycle*. New York: Grune and Stratton.

BOYARSKY, R. E. 1976. "Sexuality." In F. U. Steinburg, ed., *Cowdry's The Care of the Geriatric Patient*. St. Louis: C. V. Mosby.

BROCKLEHURST, J. C. 1973. *Textbook of Geriatric Medicine and Gerontology*. Edinburgh: Churchill Livingstone.

_____, et al. 1968. "The Prevalence and Symptomatology of Urinary Infection in an Aged Population." *Gerontology Clinics* 10:242–56.

_____. 1971. "The Urinary Tract." In I. Rossman, ed., *Clinical Geriatrics*. Philadelphia: J. B. Lippincott.

_____, et al. 1971. "Dysuria in Old Age." *Journal of American Gerontological Society* 19:582–92.

BROWER, H. T., and L. TANNER. 1979. "A study of Older Adults Attending a Program in Human Sexuality." *Nursing Research* 28:36–39.

CAPEL, P., and D. CASE. 1976. *Ambulatory Care Manual for Nurse Practitioners*. New York: J. B. Lippincott.

COMARR, A. E. 1972. "Intermittent Catheterization for the Traumatic Cord Bladder Patient." *Journal of Urology* 108:79–91.

CORRIERE, J. N., J. M. MELLURE, and L. T. LIPSCHULTZ. 1972. "Contamination of Bladder Urine by Urethral Particles during Voiding: Urethrovesical Reflux." *Journal of Urology* 107:399–409.

COUGAR, K. B. 1964. "Gonorrhea and Nonspecific Urethritis." *Medical Clinics of North America* 48:767–89.

COX, C. E., S. S. MACY, and F. HINMAN, JR. 1968. "The Urethral Flora of the Female with Recurrent Urinary Infection." *Journal of Urology* 99:632–40.

GLOWACKI, G. 1978. "Geriatric Gynecology." In W. Reichel, ed., *Clinical Aspects of Aging.* Baltimore: Williams and Wilkins.

GREEN, T. 1977. *Gynecology: Essentials of Clinical Practice,* 3rd ed. Boston: Little, Brown.

HELDRICK, W. P., R. F. MATTINGLY, and J. R. AMBERG. 1967. "Vesico-Ureteral Reflux in Pregnancy." *Obstetrics and Gynecology* 29:371–79.

HINMAN, F., JR. 1966. "Mechanism for the Entry of Bacteria and the Establishment of Urinary Tract Infection in Female Children." *Journal of Urology* 96:546–54.

————. 1968. "Bacterial Elimination." *Journal of Urology* 99:811–17.

HUTCH, J. A., E. R. MILLER, and F. HINMAN, JR. 1963. "Perpetuation of Infection in Unobstructed Urinary Tracts." *Journal of Urology* 90:88–97.

JAFFE, J. W. 1978. "Common Lower Urinary Tract Problems in Older Persons." In W. Reichel, ed., *Clinical Aspects of Aging.* Baltimore: Williams and Wilkins.

KASE, N. 1971. "The Ovaries." In P. B. Beeson and W. McDermott, eds., *Cecil-Loeb Textbook of Medicine.* Philadelphia: W. B. Saunders.

LIEF, H., and T. PAYNE. 1975. "Sexuality, Knowledge, and Attitudes." *American Journal of Nursing* 75(11):2026–29.

LYTTON, B., and F. EPSTEIN. 1974. "Tumors of the Urinary Tract." In M. W. Wintrobe et al. *Harrison's Principles of Medicine.* New York: McGraw-Hill.

MASTERS, W. H., and V. W. JOHNSON. 1970. *Human Sexual Inadequacy.* Boston: Little, Brown.

MEARS, E. K., and T. A. STAMEY. 1968. "Bacteriologic Localization Patterns in Bacterial Prostatitis and Urethritis." *Investigational Urology* 5:492–508.

MERRILL, D. C., C. CONWAY, and W. DeWOLF. 1975. "Urinary Incontinence: Treatment with Electrical Stimulation of the Pelvic Floor." *Urology* 5:67–80.

NEWMAN, J. L. 1969. "The Prevention of Incontinence." *8th International Congress of Gerontology Proceedings.* Washington: Federation of American Societies for Experimental Biology. Vol. 2, pp. 75–100.

PAULSEN, C. A., et al. 1958. "Function of the Post-Menopausal Ovary, Comparison of Urinary Estrogen and Gonadotrophins Excretion and Response to Administration of FSH in Post-Menopausal and Ovariectomized Women." *Journal of American Geriatrics Society* 6:803–13.

PERKASH, I. 1974. "Intermittent Catheterization: The Urologist's Point of View." *Journal of Urology* 111:356–57.

ROBBINS, S. L. 1974. *Pathologic Basis of Disease.* Philadelphia: W. B. Saunders.

SCOTT, F. B., W. E. BRADLEY, and G. W. TIMM. 1973. "Treatment of Urinary Incontinence by Implantable Prosthetic Sphincters." *Urology* 1:252–68.

SMITH, D. R. 1975. *General Urology,* 8th ed. Los Altos: Lange Medical Publications.

SOULE, S. C. 1976. "Gynecological Disorders." In F. U. Steinberg, ed., *Cowdry's The Care of the Geriatric Patient.* St. Louis: C. V. Mosby.

STAMEY, T. A. 1963. "The Role of Introital Bacteria in Recurrent Urinary Infections." *Journal of Urology* 109:467–75.

THOMPSON, L. W., and L. M. EDWARDS. 1978. "Genitourinary Disorders." In C. J. Leitch and R. V. Tinker, eds., *Primary Care.* Philadelphia: F. A. Davis.

TIMIRAS, P. S. 1972. *Developmental Physiology and Aging.* New York: Macmillan.

431

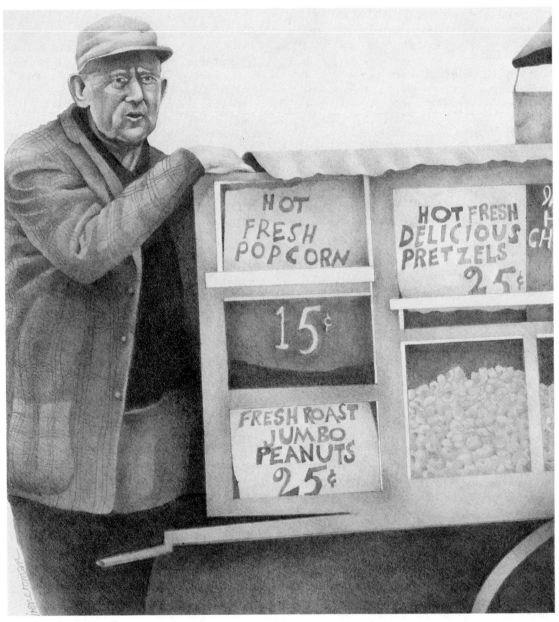

Chapter 18

GERONTOLOGICAL NURSING MANAGEMENT
THE ELDERLY CLIENT WITH A HEMATOLOGICAL PROBLEM

Clinical or experimental data do not support the assumption that anemia is common in the aged. However, its occurrence is frequent enough to warrant the gerontological nurse's attention. Pernicious anemia as well as iron and folic acid deficiency anemias are discussed here. Because of their increased incidence with age, several neoplastic disorders of the blood are also reviewed in this chapter.

THE ANEMIAS

Clients with sudden blood loss have dramatic findings related to the loss of circulating blood volume. In contrast, clients with slowly progressive anemias have findings that are unnoticed by them until the point where the hemoglobin content of each 100 ml of blood, or the oxygen-carrying capacity of the blood, has fallen below the ability of the homeostatic reserve to compensate. Thus findings in clients with anemia are related to the diminished tissue oxygen levels (anemic anoxia). Prior to this point anemias are often discovered from a complete blood count (CBC) performed during routine testing. The blood indices, derived from the blood hematocrit, hemoglobin, and red cell count, permit classification of the anemia by cell size, cell iron content, and cell iron concentration. This classification fortunately permits a certain etiologic division of the anemias.

Pathophysiology

Nutritional anemia can develop at any age when the diet is deficient in substances essential to the production and development of normal red blood cells. Among the food substances required are proteins, iron, folic acid, and vitamin B_{12}. Protein is an essential substance of all protoplasm, including that of erythrocytes and the hemoglo-

433

bin molecule. Iron, present in hemoglobin, binds oxygen (and carbon dioxide) to the molecule. Both folic acid and vitamin B_{12} are necessary for synthesis of chromosomal deoxyribonucleic acid (DNA) in red blood cells as well as in the other cells of the body.

Normal American diets contain approximately 15 mg of iron; of this quantity approximately 1.5 mg, or 10 percent, is absorbed. In the presence of iron-deficiency anemia, absorption is increased to about 20 percent of ingested iron. However, in an iron-poor diet—that is, one with insufficient meat, liver, fruit, and vegetables—individuals may not ingest even enough iron to meet the body's needs—that is, enough to replace the daily iron loss of 0.6 to 2 mg. The red blood cells will be hypochromic and microcytic.

Iron-deficiency anemia can develop secondarily to conditions in which chronic blood loss occurs. Again, circulating red blood cells will be hypochromic and microcytic. The conditions could include gastrointestinal bleeding in which chronic blood loss is inapparent. Chronic renal disease with uremia can also lead to iron-deficiency anemia.

In folic acid deficiency anemia, the abnormal blood cell is macrocytic but normochromic. The red blood cell (RBC) count, hemoglobin, and hematocrits are abnormally low. The clinical symptoms exhibited mimic those of pernicious anemia.

Pernicious anemia is more often found in the older than in the younger adult; the average time of onset is in the sixth decade, and both sexes may be equally affected. The condition is caused by a failure of the lower portion of the small intestine to absorb vitamin B_{12}. This failure is due to atrophy of gastric mucosa and subsequent fail-

ure of the mucosa to secrete an intrinsic factor that possesses strong vitamin B_{12}-binding capacity. Once bound to intrinsic factor, vitamin B_{12} is protected from gastric and intestinal enzymes and also cannot be utilized by bacteria in the small intestines. In the absence of the factor, the vitamin is utilized by the bacteria and thus is not available for assimilation (Sodeman and Sodeman 1970). Intrinsic factor also facilitates vitamin B_{12} absorption, which occurs in the distal ileum.

MICROCYTIC ANEMIA: IRON-DEFICIENCY ANEMIA

Authorities disagree about the incidence of iron-deficiency anemia in the elderly. Research studies give conflicting reports, some reporting a higher incidence and some a lower incidence in this age group (Hyams 1973). This anemia occurs when iron is lost from the body in greater amounts than it is absorbed. The imbalance may be due to increased loss or diminished replenishment. Iron-lack anemia is the most common anemia. It affects all ages and is more commonly found in women than in men (Brown 1971; Wintrobe 1974). In the initial stages iron-deficiency anemia may be normochromic and normocytic, but as body iron stores continue to fall, the true hypochromic and microcytic picture develops.

Nursing Assessment

In iron-deficiency anemia cases, the nurse must determine the etiology of the anemia. This disorder is due either to insufficient replenishment of iron stores or to an excessive iron loss, which surpasses the capacities of normal ingestion. Insufficient replenishment may be due to dietary deficiency. The older client with a limited income may be consuming a markedly deficient diet. The client's nutritional history should ascertain whether adequate amounts of leafy vegetables, legumes, fruit, and meats are being consumed.

Other conditions may interfere with iron absorption. The progressive achlorhydria of aging may interfere with the ability of gastric juice to liberate iron from ingested myoglobin in meat. The iron is thus unavailable for absorption. A subtotal gastrectomy with Billroth II anastomosis not only reduces gastric acid but also bypasses the duodenum and proximal jejunum, where iron is most readily absorbed (Jones et al. 1962; Hines et al. 1967).

Subjective Findings. The majority of clients have no complaints. When present, the most common complaints are easy fatigability, exertional dyspnea, palpitations, headache, and irritability. Anemia can easily be overlooked in the aged client by interpreting a complaint of exertional dyspnea as one caused by cardiopulmonary dysfunction. Also the typical signs of anemia, such as pale blepharal conjunctiva, may actually appear hyperemic in the anemic elderly person who has chronic conjunctivitis (Maekawa 1976). Less frequent are a variety of nonspecific complaints, such as indigestion, flatulence, heartburn, anorexia, and constipation. Dysphagia is also a rare subjective finding.

Objective Findings. The most striking objective finding is pallor. Clients who are edentulous and even those with teeth may have a stomatitis of the corners of the mouth. A peculiar glossitis associated with a smooth tongue may be noted. Clients who have dentures should be asked to remove them so that the oral cavity may be adequately viewed. Pharyngeal erythema and friability may be seen in clients with dysphagia. The nails may be brittle, ridged, and rough and may have a concave appearance, called spooning. The hair is often dry and lifeless, the skin dry and rough. Older clients often develop congestive heart failure with an enlarged heart, jugular distension, and peripheral edema.

The source of the increased iron loss is potentially a serious threat. All clients with a hypochromic anemia deserve evaluation for chronic blood loss. Gastrointestinal lesions are the most common source of difficulty. The nurse must always consider the possibility of a gastric or colonic carcinoma. Peptic ulceration may be asymptomatic in the elderly client (Vilardell 1974). Hiatal hernia with reflux esophagitis will usually cause heartburn, which typically occurs when the client lies down.

Diagnostics

Blood studies reveal the anemia; in typical cases the indices are microcytic and hypochromic. The mean corpuscular volume (MCV) is below 80 $c\mu$ and the mean corpuscular hemoglobin concentration (MCHC) below 30 percent. The peripheral smear reveals microcytosis. The serum iron is low, and the total iron-binding capacity is usually increased.

All clients with hypochromic anemia should have three stool examinations for occult blood while on a high-roughage, meat-free diet for 3 days. Rectal examination should always be performed and a

435

stool specimen obtained for examination for occult blood. If blood is found, appropriate barium and air-contrast x-rays of the entire gastrointestinal tract should be taken. If these x-rays are negative and blood has been found in at least one stool specimen, the client should be referred to a gastrointestinal endoscopist for examination. Achlorhydria is demonstrable by means of a gastric analysis. The history, physical examination, and x-rays of the stomach should reveal the presence of any prior gastric surgery.

Occasionally carcinoma of the uterus or cervix may cause the anemia. Women with such carcinoma are usually aware of the blood loss. Pelvic examination and appropriate cervical cytology specimens (Pap smears) should allow a diagnosis.

In very rare cases paroxysmal hemoglobinuria may be the source of blood loss. In such cases a urine test for *hemoglobin* will be positive in the morning specimen.

Nursing Management

Treatment requires restoration of iron stores and correction, if possible, of the primary disease. Most clients will tolerate ferrous sulfate tablets 300 mg three times daily. Best results are obtained if these are given 1 hour before meals. If clients complain of anorexia or nausea from the medication, tablets may be given after the meal if milk and calcium products are avoided at that time. These foods tend to bind to the iron and render it unabsorbable. Gastrointestinal side effects of ferrous sulfate ingestion include nausea, constipation, or diarrhea. Vomiting is rare. Clients should be instructed to increase dietary roughage and fluid intake to thwart constipatory effects.

Such clients should keep a daily meal plan for a week, writing down all they ingest. The nurse will use this dietary history to determine areas of nutritional deficiency and the need for nutritional counseling. Clients should be informed of the color change in their stools so that they do not become alarmed. Because ferrous sulfate can deposit on gums and teeth, clients should be instructed to perform frequent oral hygiene care. For clients using a liquid preparation, the use of a straw is indicated.

If oral ingestion is intolerable, an intramuscular iron-dextran preparation may be indicated. When oral iron is used, a total of 100 to 200 tablets usually are necessary to replete the iron stores of the body. Frequent rest periods are prescribed until blood levels return to normal. Hemoglobin and hematocrit levels should be monitored. The hematocrit and hemoglobin levels should be normal within 6 weeks. Hemoglobin levels increase at a rate of 1 g every 7 to 10 days.

Correction of the primary disease usually requires prolonged treatment and collaboration with a physician. Clients with severe anemias or evidence of congestive failure usually need to be hospitalized. The client should be told that fatigue is due to the anemic condition and will be alleviated when the anemia is corrected.

MACROCYTIC ANEMIA:
PERNICIOUS ANEMIA

The fundamental cause of pernicious anemia is vitamin B$_{12}$ deficiency. The true disease is rare before age 35 and its incidence progressively rises with increasing age (Jandl 1971; Cantor 1963). The blood indices characterize this disorder as a macrocytic, normochromic anemia. It is complicated by the neurological complications of *combined-system* disease induced by the vitamin deficiency's effect on the central nervous system.

The most common cause is an atrophy of the acid-producing cells of the gastric fundus, which also produce the intrinsic factor essential for B_{12} absorption in the distal ileum. This disorder appears to be linked to genetic factors: a family history of pernicious anemia is common. Total gastrectomy or a large subtotal gastric resection also reduces the number of intrinsic factor secreting cells (Cox et al. 1964; Johnson et al. 1969). Other disorders prevent B_{12}–intrinsic-factor complex absorption at the ileal-binding site. These disorders include a variety of malabsorptive ones, such as nontropical sprue, chronic pancreatitis, multiple jejunal diverticulosis, and the blind loop syndrome. Regional enteritis or resections of the distal ileum also remove the absorptive sites and interfere with B_{12} absorption.

Nursing Assessment

Subjective Findings. Pernicious anemia is slowly progressive in nature. When subjective findings appear, the disease is well advanced and clients have difficulty pinpointing the time of onset. Early complaints are similar to those found in the client with an iron-deficiency anemia. Complaints relating to the anemia are nonspecific and include easy fatigability, weakness, faintness, palpitations, irritability, and effort-related dyspnea. Neurological complaints are bilateral and include symmetric paresthesias in the fingers and toes, which progress to frank numbness; diffi-

culty in walking; and difficulty in the coordinated use of the fingers, with stiffness and spasticity. Older clients lose their ability to concentrate and, if the disorder is severe enough, may become psychotic.

Objective Findings. The objective findings include pallor and an odd waxy or jaundiced appearance. The client often appears somewhat obese. Fever may be present. A glossitis causing a smooth, red tongue, particularly along the sides and at the tip, is often found. Older clients may

The gerontological nurse can help the elderly adapt to the aging process by encouraging interest in the world around them; elderly clients need to keep mentally active despite their increased need for physical rest.

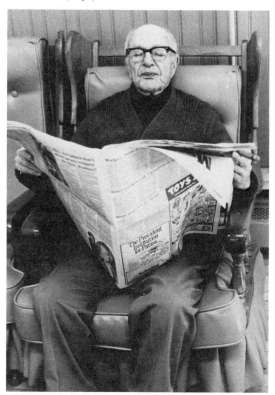

show evidence of congestive heart failure with jugular distension, an enlarged heart and liver, and peripheral edema. The spleen may be slightly enlarged. The neurological findings involve the lateral and posterior columns of the spinal cord. Loss of vibration and position sense occurs. The Romberg sign is positive, deep tendon reflexes are hyperactive with spasticity, and the Babinski sign is present.

Diagnostics

Blood studies reveal a macrocytic anemia, which may be quite severe. The peripheral smear of the blood demonstrates the macrocytes and large multilobed polymorphonuclear leukocytes. Serum lactic dehydrogenase (LDH) is usually elevated, and serum B_{12} levels are low. In true pernicious anemia, gastric analysis reveals no free hydrochloric acid even after stimulation with histamine (0.01 mg per kg), betazole (50 mg to 100 mg per kg), or pentagastrin (6 mg per kg). Gastrointestinal barium x-rays of the stomach and small bowel should demonstrate evidence of G.I. tract surgery, regional enteritis, or malabsorption. In malabsorption syndromes, stool fat content is increased and clients usually complain of diarrhea. A two-part Schilling test can distinguish between gastric and intestinal causes. In part 1 of the test, the client ingests 2 mcg of radioactive vitamin B_{12} and then is given a large "flushing dose" of the vitamin (1,000 mcg). The urine is collected for 24 hours and the level of excreted radioactivity is measured. In part 2, the test is repeated, using radioactive B_{12}–intrinsic-factor complex by the oral route. If urine radioactivity is low in part 1 and normal in part 2, the problem is a lack of intrinsic factor secretion by the stomach. If this radioactivity remains low in part 2, the problem is in the intestine.

Nursing Management

The correction of pernicious anemia with parenteral vitamin B_{12} is both diagnostic of the condition and an effective form of treatment. Crystalline, pure vitamin B_{12} is the only form that should be used. It is inexpensive and has few, if any, side effects. The basic daily need is 1 mcg. Initially, to replenish hepatic stores, one administers daily injections of 100 mcg over a 1-week period. Lifelong therapy is then instituted with a dosage of 100 mcg per month. Clients must be impressed with the fact that this is a lifelong illness requiring health care attention for continuing observation and medication treatment. The client can be assured that prognosis is excellent when therapy is maintained. Treatment is rewarded by an almost immediate improvement in the client's sense of well-being. The anemia responds rapidly and is corrected over the next several weeks. Mental changes and psychosis respond more slowly. Peripheral nerve changes improve, but spinal cord lesions may only partially regress. Cardiovascular improvement also occurs as the anemia is corrected. Clients with very severe anemias or with evidence of congestive heart failure should be hospitalized. Regional enteritis and malabsorption syndromes require specific treatment.

In addition to checking the blood count and neurological findings every 6 months, clients with treated, controlled pernicious anemia should have complete reevaluation annually. The incidence of gastric carcinoma in persons with pernicious anemia is twenty-two times greater than in the normal population (Hitchcock et al. 1957). The nurse must inquire not only about general complaints and diet but also about the presence of any gastric problems. Annual stool examinations for occult blood are mandatory.

FOLIC ACID DEFICIENCY ANEMIA

Nursing Assessment

The subjective complaints of folic acid deficiency anemia are those of any anemia. No neurological findings appear. The objective findings are similar to those of pernicious anemia, but without any evidence of combined-system disease. Clients are pale and in severe cases may show evidence of congestive heart failure with peripheral edema and dilated jugular veins. The peripheral blood smear is identical to that of B_{12} deficiency.

Nursing Management

The proper treatment of folic acid deficiency anemia is folic acid 5 mg three times daily by mouth. This treatment is rewarded by a prompt normalization of the hemogram within a few weeks. As this vitamin is abundantly present in the normal diet, clients usually suffer from malnutrition with multiple deficiencies that must also be corrected. The association of this illness with chronic alcoholism is acknowledged, and a history of alcoholism must be sought by the nurse.

The danger of folic acid is that it will correct the anemia of B_{12} deficiency but has no effect on the progressive neurological aspect of this disorder. Thus all clients with macrocytic anemia must be evaluated for a B_{12} deficiency before treatment is initiated.

NEOPLASTIC DISORDERS OF THE BLOOD

Neoplastic diseases appear with increasing frequency with advancing years. An altered immunologic state and a long period of contact with causative agents are likely contributing factors. Chronic leukemias, lymphoma, and myeloma have a special predilection for the aged: these disorders are rarely found before age 40.

Pathophysiology

White blood cell disorders include leukemia, lymphoma, and myeloma. Myeloma involves the plasma cell. Fortunately these blood disorders are not common in the aged, although they do affect some of the elderly. A common feature of all these blood diseases is unregulated, excessive development and accumulation of the white cell in bone marrow and in the spleen, liver, and lymph nodes (Rappaport 1971).

Leukemia, when it occurs in the adult, is usually seen after age 50. The cause is unknown, but viruses, environment, and genetic factors are all suspect. In leukemia bone marrow and organs of the reticuloendothelial system become overcrowded due to the wildly growing leukocyte. This state of affairs results in diminished red blood cell, platelet, and granulocyte production; anemia, thrombocytopenia, and granulocytopenia develop (the last disorder does not occur if the leukemia is chronic granulocytic leukemia).

439

Lymphoma is a neoplasm of lymphoid tissue cells that can appear at any age, but a peak incidence occurs in the sixth decade (Robbins 1974). Both viruses and immunological defense deficiencies have been proposed as the cause of lymphoma. In lymphoma proliferation of the stem cell of the lymphoreticular system, the lymphocytes, or the histiocytes, is uncontrolled.

Myeloma is a neoplasm of the lymphoreticular system in which the plasma cell is the neoplastic cell. Although the evidence is not conclusive, the cause of myeloma is thought to be immunologic. In this situation the plasma cell proliferates uncontrollably, and antibody synthesis, a normal function of plasma cells, becomes excessive. However, the immunoglobins produced do not function as antibodies in myeloma. In clients thus affected, susceptibility to bacterial infections increases and anemia, bleeding tendencies, and renal disorders, which are symptomatic, occur (Robbins 1974).

CHRONIC LYMPHOCYTIC LEUKEMIA

Chronic lymphocytic leukemia is the most common leukemia of the elderly. It represents 28 percent of all leukemic diseases (Clifford 1971). Chronic lymphocytic leukemia is characterized by a marked increase in the numbers of lymphocytes in the peripheral smear as well as in the bone marrow.

Nursing Assessment

Subjective Findings. The onset of the disease is insidious. The presenting complaint is usually an enlarged lymph node. Occasionally the client has the findings of an anemia, with easy tiring, paleness, and effort-induced dyspnea. The client may be febrile and may present with bleeding from mucous membranes. Other possible complaints include easy bruising or bleeding; itching skin and rash; herpes zoster; or pressure symptoms due to lymph node enlargement in the mediastinum, which causes pain in the ribs or muscles. Gastrointestinal complaints are anorexia, flatulence, and diarrhea. Occasionally gastrointestinal bleeding and abdominal pain may occur.

Objective Findings. Physical assessment reveals painful symmetric adenopathy of the neck, axillae, and groin. The nodes vary from pea size to 3 to 4 cm in diameter. Occasionally, large masses of nodes may occur. The tonsils may be involved and enlarged. The spleen is often enlarged, and if infarction of the spleen occurs, the client will complain of left upper quadrant pain and a friction rub may be heard. Hepatomegaly is frequent, and the liver is smooth and firm. Cardiac enlargement is usually associated with congestive heart failure; however, a pericardial leukemic infiltrate can cause pericarditis and a pericardial effusion. Hemorrhage and lymph node enlargement can cause cranial nerve palsies or appear as strokes or meningitis. Retinal hemorrhages may be seen. Recurrent infections such as pneumonia or herpes zoster are related to altered resistance and to the infections that occur in the advanced stages of the illness. Skin lesions are variable and pruritic. Exfoliative dermatitis and a diffuse, itching, fiery erythema are particularly troublesome complications.

Diagnostics

The diagnosis is often suggested by a peripheral blood smear where large numbers of circulating lymphocytes are found. Counts of 50,000 to 5,000,000 with 90 percent lymphocytes are not unusual (Wintrobe 1974). Anemia and decreased platelets are often described. A bone marrow aspiration or biopsy by a physician is necessary for diagnosis. Occasionally a lymph node biopsy must be performed.

Nursing Management

The average client will live over 5 years. Occasional cases have a fulminant course. Some clients, however, have lived for 20 years with little treatment. Differences in survival rate may relate only to the time of discovery in the natural course of the illness (Wintrobe 1962; Clifford 1971). Treatment is symptomatic and should be in collaboration with a hematologist or oncologist. The client should be instructed to avoid stress, eat well, take frequent rests, and avoid situations that are potentially infection-producing, such as large crowds. Any infection requires prompt attention and appropriate treatment by the nurse. Chemotherapy with chlorambucil, an aromatic mustard, and corticosteroids can induce remissions for variable periods. These medications can improve the quality of life but do not change the survival rate. Such therapy should therefore await the appearance of the following conditions: (1) painful enlargement of lymph nodes or spleen, (2) significant anemia of less than 10 g per 100 ml, (3) progressively increasing white blood cell counts, (4) the occurrence of hemorrhages, and (5) marked skin infiltration (Anderson 1976). Any of the above conditions is reason to refer the client to a physician for consultation for treatment. Localized, painful adenopathy may be treated by radiation. If infections are recurrent and serum gamma globulin levels are low, the client may benefit from gamma globulin injections.

Eventually the disease process becomes resistant to all treatment. In this final stage one must be wise enough to avoid the now useless chemotherapeutic agents that will only serve to sicken clients in their last days. Supportive, symptomatic, caring therapy is the best regimen to follow.

LYMPHOMA AND MYELOMA

Lymphoma and myeloma are often seen in older clients, in whom Hodgkin's lymphoma may be particularly aggressive (Clifford 1971).

Nursing Assessment

Subjective Findings. Lymphomas may present as a localized, painless lymph node involvement, usually unilateral and progressive. Other findings are related to the organ infiltrated by the disease. Intestinal lymphoma will cause obstructive phenomena; mediastinal lymph nodes may cause complaints due to painful pressure on nerves or vertebrae or due to obstruction of blood vessels and air passages. At times fever may be the only finding. Myeloma is usually a painful disease, and the complaints usually relate to vertebral compression and long-bone fractures.

Objective Findings. The physical findings in lymphoma relate to the presence or absence of a discoverable adenopathy. Prolonged fever with periods of remission followed by recurrence is typical of the Pel-Epstein fever and is found in Hodgkin's disease. In myeloma evidence of fracture or vertebral collapse may be noted. Occasionally clients with myeloma have an enlarged tongue.

Diagnostics

X-rays may show typical myeloma lesions or may only reveal diffuse osteoporosis. Anemia may be present in lymphoma and is usually present in myeloma. Indeed, osteoporosis in association with an anemia points to myeloma. The diagnostic laboratory studies in myeloma involve immunoelectrophoretic studies of serum and urine. These studies show the production of abnormal forms of gamma globulin, which may pass into the urine where they form the Bence-Jones protein. Lymphoma diagnosis requires biopsy of lymph nodes or bone marrow. Early diagnosis is important, so any suspicious swelling of the lymph gland must be biopsied.

Nursing Management

Lymphoma, particularly Hodgkin's lymphoma, requires staging to determine the progress of the disease and the possibility of cure. Staging often requires abdominal laparotomy and splenectomy. X-ray and a variety of combination antimitotic agents are used with certain degrees of success in attaining some cures and many prolonged remissions. Malignant lymphoma can be cured if treatment is begun when

the disease is in the localized stage (Maekawa 1976).

These diseases are best managed in close collaboration with a hematologist or oncologist; however, the nurse must continue to provide moral support and empathetic care to clients throughout their illness.

SUMMARY

In this chapter we have discussed the anemias and blood-related tumors of the older client. Assessment of these conditions often requires some type of medical measure procedure, and management frequently requires medical attention. The nurse working with clients who have hematological disorders should establish a close, collaborative relationship with the medical specialists providing the various aspects of care. The gerontological nurse can contribute information about the client's response to treatment and also help the client through the many phases of what is often an uncomfortable and frightening experience.

REFERENCES

ANDERSON, F. 1976. *Practical Management of the Elderly.* Oxford: Blackwell Scientific Publications.

BROWN, E. B. 1971. "Hematologic and Hematopoietic Disease." In P. B. Beeson and W. McDermott, eds., *Cecil-Loeb Textbook of Medicine.* Philadelphia: W. B. Saunders.

CANTOR, A. M. 1963. "A Study of Pernicious Anemia in Elderly Patients." *Gerontological Clinic* 5:23–30.

CLIFFORD, G. 1971. "Hematologic Problems in the Elderly." In I. Rossman, ed., *Clinical Geriatrics.* Philadelphia: J. B. Lippincott.

COX, A. G., et al. 1964. "Aspects of Nutrition after Vagotomy and Gastrojejunostomy." *British Medical Journal* 1:465–72.

HINES, J. D., A. V. HOFFBRAND, and D. L. MOLLIN. 1967. "The Hematologic Complications Following Partial Gastrectomy: A Study of 292 Patients." *American Journal of Medicine* 43:555–62.

HITCHCOCK, C. R., L. D. MacLEAN, and W. A. SULLIVAN. 1957. "Secretory and Clinical Aspects of Achlorhydria and Gastric Atrophy as Precursors of Gastric Cancer." *Journal of National Cancer Institute* 18:795–801.

HYAMS, D. E. 1973. "The Blood." In J. C. Brocklehurst, ed., *Textbook of Geriatric Medicine and Gerontology.* London: Churchill Livingston.

JANDL, J. H. 1971. "Megablastic Anemia." In P. B. Beeson and W. McDermott, eds., *Cecil-Loeb Textbook of Medicine.* Philadelphia: W. B. Saunders.

JOHNSON, H. D., T. A. KHAN, and R. SRIVATSA. 1969. "The Late Nutritional Effects of Vagal Section." *British Journal of Surgery* 56:4–15.

JONES, C. T., J. A. WILLIAMS, and E. V. COX. 1962. "Peptic Ulceration: Some Hematologic and Metabolic Consequences of Gastric Surgery." *Lancet* 2:423–32.

MAEKAWA, T. 1976. "Hematological Diseases." In F. U. Steinberg, ed., *Cowdry's The Care of the Geriatric Patient,* 5th ed. St. Louis: C. V. Mosby.

RAPPAPORT, S. 1971. *Introduction to Hematology.* New York: Harper and Row.

ROBBINS, S. L. 1974. *Pathologic Basis of Disease.* Philadelphia: W. B. Saunders.

SHAFER, K., et al. 1975. *Medical Surgical Nursing,* 6th ed. St. Louis: C. V. Mosby.

SODEMAN, W. A., and W. A. SODEMAN, JR. 1970. *Pathologic Physiology.* Philadelphia: W. B. Saunders.

VILARDELL, F. 1974. "Chronic Gastritis." In H. L. Bockus, ed., *Gastroenterology,* 3rd ed. Philadelphia: W. B. Saunders.

WINTROBE, M. M. 1974. "Disorders of the Hematopoietic System." In T. R. Harrison et al., eds., *Principles of Internal Medicine,* 4th ed. New York: McGraw-Hill.

IV

RESOURCES

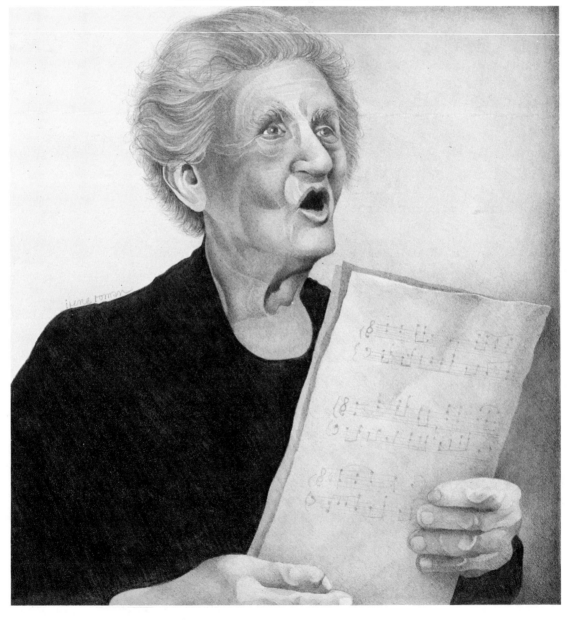

Chapter 19

COMMUNITY RESOURCES FOR THE OLDER ADULT

Atchley (1977, p. 261) defines a community as " . . . a group of people who interact with one another frequently, who share their location in space, who depend on one another—even if indirectly—to fill their needs, and who share an identity with the place where they live." Most communities differ from each other according to the needs of the individuals who inhabit the specific areas. Many of the elderly do not want to move to a new community because of their familiarity with ways of doing things in their present community, their low-income status, and their lack of mobility. Others may remain because they have no choice rather than because they consciously desire to stay. Thus elderly individuals are usually long-term residents and have a commitment to the community. The community in turn should have a commitment to its elderly inhabitants.

Depending on the size of the community, this commitment may be expressed by the types and numbers of facilities and services offered to the elderly. Larger and more complex urban communities with greater resources can offer a greater variety of facilities and services. However, Taietz (1975) found that the larger the rural area, the less the older person knows about available facilities because transportation is often lacking and communication in many rural areas tends to be by word of mouth. (Refer to chapter 2 for demographic information regarding geographic distribution of the elderly.)

In order to more effectively serve older people in both urban and rural communities, nurses need to update their knowledge of available resources. Information and referral services are available from the Social Security office, the Department of Public Health, and the local Area Agency on Aging (AAA) in each state. In addition many communities have published booklets and directories describing programs, services, and facilities available to the elderly. Making the proper referral from the outset is important because it will minimize frustration and costs for both the consumer and the provider. This chapter discusses some of the major programs, health services, and facilities available to the elderly.

PROGRAMS FOR THE ELDERLY

The four major programs affecting the elderly are: (1) Social Security Income, (2) Medicare and Medicaid, (3) Supplemental Security Income (SSI), and (4) programs under the Older Americans Act.

SOCIAL SECURITY INCOME

The Social Security Administration administers the monthly Social Security checks that go to workers and their dependents when the workers retire, become severely disabled, or die. This is the United States' method of providing a continuing supplement to income when family earnings are reduced or stopped because of retirement, disability, or death. Unfortunately it may often be the *only* income. Although the usual age of retirement is 65, the elderly can retire as early as 62; however, in these instances the retirement check is less than what would be available at age 65. This differential is permanent.

Social Security is the largest and fastest growing component of the cash transfer expenditures of the federal budget (Gold, Kutza, and Marmor 1976, p. 12). The growth of Social Security is causing policy makers concern about future financing of the program. The viability of the Social Security system is now a public issue and is the center of political debate. For more information regarding Social Security eligibility and benefits, obtain booklets at the nearest Social Security office.

MEDICARE

Medicare is a health insurance program for people 65 or older and some people under 65 who are disabled. It is a federal program run by the Health Care Financing Administration under Social Security. Medicare has two parts: one is called hospital insurance and the other, medical insurance.

The *hospital insurance* (part A) can help pay for inpatient hospital care and, after a hospital stay, for inpatient care in a skilled nursing facility and for limited care in the home by a home health agency. However, it is important to know that Medicare does not provide for services furnished primarily to assist people in meeting personal, family, and domestic needs, such as household services, meal preparation, shopping, assistance in bathing and dressing, and the like. (These services may be covered by other sources—see section on home health services.)

The *medical insurance* (part B) can help pay for doctors' services, nurse practitioners' services in rural health clinics, outpatient hospital services, outpatient physical therapy and speech pathology services, and a number of other medical services and supplies not covered by the hospital insurance described above.

Hospital and medical insurance coverage is limited in that Medicare does not pay the full cost of some services. In addition, Medicare sets time limits for hospital and skilled nursing facility stays and for the visits of professionals who treat the elderly person. Medicare does not cover custodial care (personal needs), psychiatric care, or emotional/psychosocial care of the elderly. If government reimbursing agents decide the service is not needed or not covered, the client must pay the entire cost. For information regarding the specifics of Medicare and its coverage, ask at the nearest Social Security office or refer to *Your Medicare Handbook,* available at Social Security offices.

MEDICAID

The Medical Assistance Program (Medicaid), authorized under title XIX of the

Social Security Act, is a federal-state program that finances medical services for public assistance recipients and for those deemed medically indigent. To be eligible for Medicaid, an older person must meet the eligibility criteria for SSI or reside in a state that exercises the option of including persons with incomes higher than the SSI limit whose medical expenses threaten them with indigency.

The Medicaid program pays about 60 percent of the nation's $7.5 billion nursing home bill, with Medicare paying 7 percent (Gold, Kutza, and Marmor 1976, p. 16). Because Medicaid can finance certain services when they are provided within the in-

TABLE 19.1
Eligibility Criteria for Supplemental Security Income

Basic Eligibility Conditions

Aged	65 or over
Blind	Vision no better than 20/200 even with glasses, or tunnel vision (limited visual field of 20 degrees or less)
Disabled	A physical or mental impairment that prevents a person from doing any substantial work and that is expected to last at least 12 months or result in death
Income	Below $189.40 a month for an individual, $284.10 for a couple*
Resources	$1,500 for an individual, $2,250 for a couple**

Additional Eligibility Factors

Citizen or lawfully admitted immigrant

U.S. residence

Disabled must accept vocational rehabilitation if offered

Disabled addicts and alcoholics must accept treatment if offered

* *Not counting $20 a month of unearned income and $65 plus half of remainder of earned income. (A person may have income above these levels and possibly be eligible for a state supplement only, but the income levels vary with each state.)*

** *Not counting a home regardless of its value; not counting a car, personal effects, household goods of reasonable value.*

Source: A Guide to Supplemental Security Income, *DHEW Publication No. (SSA) 78–11015, Washington, D.C., July 1978, p. 5.*

stitution but not when rendered outside it, Gold, Kutza, and Marmor feel the program is a decided incentive to institutionalization of the elderly.

SUPPLEMENTAL SECURITY INCOME

Supplemental Security Income is available for people in financial need who are 65 or older or who are blind or disabled (see table 19.1). Individuals are eligible if they have little or no regular income and few assets. Money for SSI comes from the general funds of the U.S. Treasury and *not* from Social Security funds. Individuals may be eligible for both Social Security payments and SSI if they are classified below the poverty level.

Under SSI the federal, state, and local governments work together. On the national level the federal government administers the program through the Social Security Administration. It makes the basic payments to recipients, determines eligibility of claimants, and maintains a master record of beneficiaries. On the local level the states, in addition to supplementing the federal payments, provide Medicaid, food stamps, and/or various social and rehabilitation services. Also some states and local subdivisions make interim assistance payments to SSI claimants who are waiting for a decision on their eligibility for federal payments. The state or local government can be reimbursed out of the beneficiary's first SSI check.

PROGRAMS UNDER THE OLDER AMERICANS ACT

The Older Americans Act of 1965 and its recent amendments provide additional benefits for the elderly.

The Older Americans Act
To provide assistance in the development of new or improved programs to help older persons through grants to the states for community planning and services and for training, through research, development, or training project grants, and to establish within the Department of Health, Education, and Welfare an operating agency to be designated as the "Administration on Aging." [Older Americans Act of 1965, as amended, March 1978, p. 1]

This act also established a fifteen-member Federal Council on the Aging. The members are appointed by the president, and their functions are listed in the law.

In 1971 a White House Conference on Aging was held. Recommendations from this conference pointed to the lack of coordination among organizations that provide services for the elderly. The 1973 amendments to the Older Americans Act created new community organizations in each state, called Area Agencies on Aging (AAA), designed to improve the original act and to help plan and coordinate services for the elderly. The effectiveness of these agencies cannot be determined at this time since most of the agencies were not created in 1974. Because they are new, they do not yet have the status, influence, or resources necessary to effectively represent the elderly in planning, coordination, and delivery of services, but they do have access to the resources that are available and can be used as a resource by practicing nurses to enter the client into the Social Service system. Some states have avoided problems associated with new agencies by designating existing agencies as their local AAA.

Nurses and other health care workers can call the AAA for information and referral services. Furthermore, gerontological nurses should know where the AAAs are in their states and who is in charge of administering each organization. The needs and priorities of older people are usually met at the local level. Local AAAs have advisory councils that are made up of older people and professionals in gerontology. They serve the AAA in identifying needs and planning services.

As noted above, the Older Americans Act authorized funds (1) for the establishment of state and substate agencies that are to plan and coordinate services for the elderly within a given geographic area (title III), (2) for the training of professionals and support of research in the field of aging (title IV), (3) for the construction of multipurpose centers (title V), (4) for the development of congregate meal programs (title VII), and (5) for employment opportunities for the elderly (title IX).

Senior Centers

Senior centers established through the Older Americans Act allow the elderly to remain in contact with the community. For some of the elderly, however, transportation to these centers may present a problem. In such cases, elderly persons can get to these centers by utilizing any one of the many transportation services that may be available to them. The local Regional Transportation Authority by law must provide transportation for the elderly and handicapped. Dial-a-Bus Service and Dial-a-Ride-Taxi Service are two examples of new, innovative ideas for improvement of transportation for the elderly. Reduced fares, public subsidy, use of volunteers in private automobiles, and nonprofit trans-

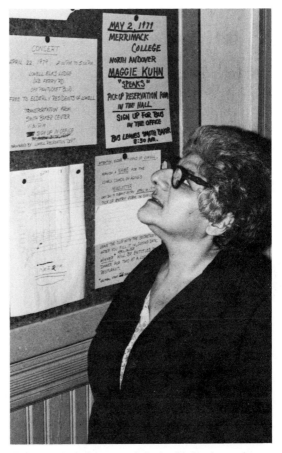

The gerontological nurse can help the elderly adapt to the aging process by promoting awareness of local programs and services; elderly clients need to utilize the full range of community resources in order to maintain their maximum level of wellness.

portation services operated by senior centers are other solutions that have been tried with some success. Transportation is a very important service, as it brings older people to senior centers, congregate meals, and Social Security offices. Nurses and other health care workers should check with the Regional Transportation Authority, Council on Aging, or AAA for specific information.

451

Volunteers or paid staff at senior centers supervise activities and teach painting, ceramics, sewing, knitting, and other handicrafts. They also accompany members of the center to various activities, exhibits, and museums. Many senior members themselves become volunteers and visit the sick elderly in hospitals, write their letters, and do their errands. Counseling services, "hot-lines," and outreach programs have been very successful at some senior centers.

Meal Programs

Title VII provides for congregate meal programs and operates the Meals-on-Wheels program. Elderly individuals who are housebound can have hot meals delivered to their homes (if they qualify and if no waiting list exists) through Meals on Wheels, which is part of the nutrition program for the elderly. Many of these community programs have long waiting lists. A national Meals on Wheels Act is at present being considered by Congress. Some states allow meals to be served to the elderly in high school cafeterias; senior centers also may provide meals at a much reduced rate.

Employment Opportunities

Efforts also have been made both to involve the elderly in providing community services and to employ the talents of the elderly. Foster Grandparents is a program designed to use the elderly to provide care for institutionalized children. The elderly are paid a small fee and paid for transportation costs. Senior Companions is a program that uses older people to help adults with special needs, such as the handicapped or disabled. RSVP (Retired Senior Volunteer Program) is another example of

a program involving the elderly in community services. Elderly volunteers in this program serve in mental hospitals, elementary schools, day care centers for children and the aged, museums, and libraries. They tutor children in areas where they need help and also teach English to minorities. Lunch and transportation are provided for the volunteers. Senior Aides employs older people to work with other older people in a variety of settings. In addition, many senior centers have elderly volunteer programs.

OTHER PROGRAMS THAT AFFECT THE ELDERLY

Other programs also affect the elderly, although their impact is not as great as that of the ones described above. Several of these programs will be discussed in this section.

Housing Subsidies

The government has at least two approaches to housing: one is to subsidize demand, the other is to subsidize suppliers of housing. In 1974 a new housing bill was passed that authorized 45,000 units of public housing, with at least 20 percent set aside for the elderly (Gold et al. 1976, p. 17). Tax relief also has been suggested as an aid to housing problems.

Generally each community has a public corporation or housing authority that maintains, owns, and operates public housing for the elderly. Funds for housing may be federal or state. Many public housing "projects" also offer other social, health, and support services to residents. In addition, funds provided by section 8 of the 1974 housing bill may subsidize private apartments. Generally the elderly pay 25 percent of their income for housing. Many communities unfortunately have long waiting lists. Eligibility for public housing is based on income and assets. Nurses should check with the local housing authority or AAA for information.

Food Stamps

Eligibility for participation in the food stamp program is similar to eligibility requirements for SSI. Little information is available regarding participation of the elderly in the program. The program in general has grown more rapidly than expected and major reform and evaluation of this program are needed.

Legal Aid

Many communities have regional legal programs called Legal Service Corporations. These programs are established to assist low-income people obtain needed legal aid. Although not geared directly toward the elderly, they can assist with wills, tax abatements, divorces, and the like. In addition, many have expanded services to include programs just for the elderly (noncriminal). Many local bar associations offer legal assistance and referral programs. Nurses and other health care workers should check local resources and AAAs.

Community Action Programs (CAP)

Community Action Programs are designed to serve low-income people in areas such as housing, advocacy, and welfare rights. Many agencies operate programs that affect the elderly either directly or indirectly. Health care workers need to be aware of these local agencies and should use them as a resource for the elderly.

Emergency Financial Aid

Many local communities provide emergency funds for rent or food. Contact for assistance from the Salvation Army, Red Cross, churches, and community fund organizations is usually a simple matter. Property tax abatements may be available through local tax offices and represent effective emergency financial aid.

Home Health Services

Home health services can provide care at home to the elderly. Services such as skilled nursing provided by the Visiting Nurses Association (VNA), personal care assistance (home health aide), occupational therapy, and physical therapy can be provided seven days a week and reimbursed to some extent by Medicare and Medicaid.

Many of these home health services are arranged by the discharge planner or home care unit personnel of the hospitals. Requests for care may also go directly to the Visiting Nurses Association. In addition, many VNAs offer clinics and health screening programs for the elderly. These services may be offered in conjunction with public health nurses or hospitals and are generally held at locations accessible to the elderly (e.g., senior centers, nutrition sites, hospitals). These programs may be supported through funds from the AAA (title III) or local funds.

Proprietary Home Health Corporations are appearing in greater numbers in most states. Nurses should evaluate the quality of care as well as the availability or lack of third-party payments to these corporations before making referrals.

Homemaker services are also available. Although these services are social rather than health related, they are often used in conjunction with home health aides. Services include meal preparation and housekeeping, although the socialization aspect of the service may have a major impact on recovery. Homemaker services may be available separately and are usually funded with local or title XX funds (Social Security).

Health Systems Agency

The Health Systems Agency (HSA) is a regional system for coordinating health care resources. The National Health Planning and Resources Development Act of 1974 (P.L. 93–641) made provisions for an agency to plan and to review and comment on hospital changes, nursing home construction, and the overall delivery of health care in the community. These agencies are relatively new and offer little direct service other than planning, coordination, and approving certificates of need to agencies seeking to expand their services. All federal funding for health services must first be approved by the HSA.

Councils on Aging and State Level Offices

Councils on Aging or Offices on Aging are located in many towns, cities, and counties. These local councils offer programs that meet many needs of the elderly that cannot be met with federal or state funds, such as recreational activities and trips. Generally the services are locally supported and operated out of a senior center or drop-in center. Many centers also offer health, nutrition, and counseling services and serve as a focal point for the elderly in each community.

Most states now have a Division or Department of Elder Affairs. These departments function as planners and as information and referral sources, they disperse both federal and state funds to local agencies for services to the elderly, and they also act as advocates for the elderly.

AMBULATORY HEALTH SERVICES

Many ambulatory health care services are now available to the elderly in the community, but few communities provide specific services geared to comprehensive health care for elderly people.

DAY CARE SERVICES

The development of day care centers for the elderly is recent. These facilities provide a wide range of services available to older people who have some mental and/or physical impairments but who can remain in the community with supportive services. Care usually is offered on an eight-hour-a-day, five-day-a-week basis, with transportation and meals sometimes provided.

Day care centers differ in the emphasis they place on health versus social functioning. At least four types of day care facilities exist, according to Rathbone-McCuan and Elliott (1976–1977): (1) medical day care centers, (2) health-related day care centers,

(3) psychosocial day care centers, and (4) social day care centers.

Medical day care centers provide health care and supervision for individuals recovering from acute illnesses who do not need hospitalization. Health-related centers provide health services for chronically ill persons who require nursing and other kinds of support. Psychosocial day care centers offer a protective environment for individuals with mental health and psychiatric problems. Social day care centers provide social experiences for those not capable of independent social functioning.

All of the above centers provide services to elderly individuals who are at risk. Nurses can serve in these centers in several capacities: they can provide management of health problems (physical and mental) and offer health teaching and counseling. Costs for the services vary, and reimbursement funding is needed to use some of the centers more fully.

PHYSICIAN/NURSE PRACTITIONER OFFICES

Physicians and nurses can have independent offices or they can practice as a team (Zahourek et al. 1976; Roueche 1977) when providing primary care for the elderly. Either the client goes to the practitioner or the practitioner goes to the client's home or nursing home. Both kinds of professionals provide preventive, maintenance, and restorative aspects of physical and emotional health care.

HOSPITALS—OUTPATIENT DEPARTMENT

Most hospitals in larger cities have clinics that offer services to the total public. Some hospitals provide a clinic specifically for the elderly. In either case, medical residents, nurse practitioners, and outpatient physicians provide the care on a walk-in or appointment basis.

SCREENING CLINICS

More and more communities periodically offer screening clinics for preventive care. These clinics may not be established specifically for the elderly, but the elderly are welcomed, as are all age groups.

This method of disease detection is sponsored by the Visiting Nurses Association and/or public health department, fraternal organizations like the Lions Club, or voluntary groups like the Cancer Society. Blood pressure clinics, breast cancer clinics, vaginal examinations, and glaucoma/cataract screening clinics are examples of clinics whose services the elderly should be encouraged to use.

HEALTH MAINTENANCE ORGANIZATIONS

Health maintenance organizations (HMOs) constitute a form of health care delivery that is essentially a prepaid group practice. These organizations employ nurse practitioners, physicians, surgeons, and other personnel and offer services twenty-four hours a day, seven days a week. Many HMOs do not own their own hospitals but use the services of hospitals through contractual agreements. Large industrial health programs, such as the Kaiser-Permanente Plan, are more successful than smaller HMOs. However, the elderly have been excluded from participation in many HMOs because of the high cost of services and lack of access.

455

MENTAL HEALTH CENTERS

The Community Mental Health Act of 1963 made provision for services for the elderly in community mental health centers. The elderly have tended not to go to mental health centers for reasons of cost, stigma, and lack of transportation. Some mental health centers are now providing outreach workers who go to the client's home or senior centers. Nurses with expertise in geropsychiatry can play an important role in the provision of services at these ambulatory sites or in the client's home.

NURSING HOMES

When elderly individuals can no longer care for themselves and/or their families cannot provide the assistance required to keep them at home, or when community services are inadequate or unavailable, consideration must be given to placing such individuals in an institution. This decision is an emotional and very difficult one to make, and careful analysis of the needs of the individual and the type of institution required is mandatory. The nurse can do a great deal in counseling the family to ease the transition and lower the guilt feelings.

Medicare and Medicaid legislation define three types of nursing home facilities that qualify for reimbursement provided that they meet certain standards of safety, staffing, and services. The different staffing and service requirements for various types of facilities have suggested the concept of "levels of care." Accordingly, the facilities eligible for federal reimbursement include extended-care, skilled-nursing, and intermediate-care facilities.

EXTENDED-CARE FACILITIES

Free-standing facilities and special units within hospitals can be certified as extended-care facilities (ECFs). Standards for this level of care require extensive professional nursing and supportive staffs. Changes made in 1969 by Congress imposed very strict controls on the type of claim that could be reimbursed by Medicare. Consequently many facilities have withdrawn from the program.

SKILLED-NURSING FACILITIES

Requirements for participation in either Medicare or Medicaid skilled-care reimbursement programs are now identical. Skilled-nursing facilities provide twenty-four-hour care, largely by registered nurses and practical nurses, as well as medical and dietary supervision. Designed to provide a lower level of care at lower costs than ECFs, they were to provide care for long-term convalescent and terminal clients rather than acute care clients. Much controversy centers around the care and the type of personnel needed for such facilities.

INTERMEDIATE-CARE FACILITIES

Federal standards for intermediate-care facilities (ICFs) were not issued until 1974; therefore, each state has different requirements for certification. The ICF is what most of us call a nursing home. It is for those who need help with problems of daily life and with administration of daily medications. These facilities require twenty-four-hour supervision by a registered nurse.

Many long-term facilities provide both skilled and intermediate levels of care.

Some facilities, however, offer no medical or nursing care and are largely unsupervised by government agencies. Such facilities, called *residential facilities,* include rest homes, church-related homes, old-age homes, boarding homes, adult congregate living facilities, and retirement homes.

Long-term care of the elderly at any level poses many problems. A major problem has been the difficulty of defining the need for nursing services. Another problem is the reimbursement factor for professionals who visit the client in the nursing home. Nurses must take an active role in improving the quality of long-term care through advocacy and management of care.

SELECTION OF A NURSING HOME

Nursing care is expensive, and a prolonged period in a nursing home can wipe out the savings of a lifetime. Consequently one of the immediate concerns of most families is the cost of nursing homes. Faced with the necessity of finding a nursing home for a parent or relative, a family should first find out what help is available from health insurance plans, fraternal orders, community-based home health services, family service agencies, unions, and private insurance plans. Eligibility for Medicare and Medicaid must be determined. Doctors' fees and prescribed medicines are not included in the cost of the nursing home. After gathering this information, the family must then select a nursing home.

Guidelines for Selecting a Nursing Home

1. Get a list of nursing homes in the area from the local health department, medical society, Social Security office, Area Agency on Aging, or clergy. Determine the rates per month and find out if the nursing home participates in Medicare/Medicaid.
2. Contact people with friends or relatives in a home or ask clergymen and volunteer agencies for recommendations.
3. Visit the homes under consideration. Go at noon to see how a meal is served, taste the food, and observe the environment in which the elderly are eating. How are residents treated? Do they have privacy and is the home cheerful? Talk to the residents and their families. Ask if the home provides a "Patient Bill of Rights." Check for unpleasant odors and determine whether the residents use the recreational and physical therapy facilities. Also note whether residents are active or are staring vacuously. Note whether the home is clean and tidy and the beds offer privacy. Also see if the toilet and wash facilities are convenient to the living area.

A quality nursing home has (1) registered nurses on duty twenty-four hours and responsible for all nursing services, (2) a ratio of one nurse to six patients, and (3) daily access to a licensed nutritionist and physical therapist as well as to equipment such as lamps, whirlpools, and walkers. In such a home residents are encouraged to walk and read newspapers, magazines, and books, and social and recreational programs are supervised.

Some obstacles to quality health care in long-term care facilities are a lack of physician services and a poorly trained staff.

457

Most homes lack staff prepared to take complete health histories and perform thorough physical examinations on admission. Not only do many homes lack the skilled staff needed to continually assess the residents' health status, but physician visits are also often inadequate.

The home itself, as well as the administrator, must have a license from the state. The family should determine whether the home is certified to participate in Medicare, Medicaid, and other publicly financed programs. Each home ought to provide special services such as preparing special diets and offering physical therapy programs. Assurance regarding the safety of the facility can be gathered by examining the recent report on fire safety inspection of the home. The nurse should advise the family of such documents. Families need assurance that they are making the right decision.

Institutions care for 5 percent of the older population (NCOA 1978), and the median age of the resident is 82. Women comprise 73 percent of all of the elderly; most of them (68 percent) have less than $3,000 annual income from all sources (Office of Nursing Home Affairs 1977). Because, in the future, a much larger percentage of persons at one time or another will enter such a facility and because an immense amount of money will be required for nursing home care, these institutions have received an ever increasing amount of attention from the public. However, the attention thus far has been insufficient to bring about enough positive change. Institutions are clearly needed. It is the *quality* of care rendered and the *utilization* of the institutions that are under question.

SUMMARY

Many resources are available to the elderly but go unused because many consumers and providers are unaware of their existence. The gerontological nurse's responsibility is to educate clients and the public about federal, state, municipal, and private health services. The nurse and other health care workers can be an invaluable link in providing the needed bridge between social services and health services.

REFERENCES

Administration on Aging. 1978. *Older Americans Act of 1965, As Amended.* Washington, D.C., Office of Human Development Services, U.S. Department of Health, Education, and Welfare, March.

ATCHLEY, R. 1977. *The Social Forces in Later Life,* 2d ed. Belmont, Calif.: Wadsworth.

BUCKLEY, M. 1972. *The Aged Are People Too.* New York: Kennikat Press.

BUTLER, R. 1975. *Why Survive? Being Ald in America.* New York: Harper and Row.

Citizens for Better Care and the Institute of Gerontology (University of Michigan/Wayne State University). *How to Choose a Nursing Home.* 960 E. Jefferson Avenue, Detroit, Michigan 48207.

Comptroller General of the United States. 1977. *Home Health—The Need for a National Policy to Better Provide for the Elderly.* Report to Congress. Washington, D.C.: General Accounting Office, December 30.

GOLD, B., E. KUTZA, and T. MARMOR. 1976. "United States Social Policy on Old Age: Present Patterns and Predictions." In B. Neugarten and R. Havighurst, eds., *Social Policy, Social Ethics, and the Aging Society.* Washington, D.C.: National Science Foundation.

GUSTAFSON, E. 1974. "Day Care for the Elderly." *The Gerontologist* 14:46–49.

KART, C., E. METRESS, and J. METRESS. 1978. *Aging and Health: Biologic and Social Perspectives.* Menlo Park, Calif.: Addison-Wesley.

KNOPF, O. 1975. *Successful Aging—The Facts and Fallacies of Growing Old.* New York: Viking Press.

LOPATA, H. 1975. "Support Systems of Elderly Urbanites: Chicago of the 1970's." *The Gerontologist* 15:35–41.

MATALACK, D. 1975. "The Case for Geriatric Day Hospitals." *The Gerontologist* 15:109–11.

McCOY, J., and D. BROWN. 1978. "Health Status among Low-Income Elderly Persons: Rural-Urban Differences." *Social Security Bulletin* 41(6):14–26.

McCUAN, E. 1975. "Impact of Socialization Therapy in a Geriatric Day-Care Setting." *The Gerontologist* 15:340–42.

National Council on the Aging. 1978. *Fact Book on Aging: A Profile of America's Older Population.* Washington, D.C.: NCOA.

Office of Nursing Home Affairs. 1977. *Long-Term Care Facility Improvement Study: Introductory Report.* 5600 Fishers Lane, Rockville, Md.

PERCY, C. H. 1974. *Growing Old in the Country of the Young.* New York: McGraw-Hill.

RATHBONE-McCUAN, E., and M. ELLIOTT. 1976–77. "Geriatric Day Care in Theory and Practice." *Social Work Health Care* 2(2):153–70.

ROUECHE, B., ed. 1977. *Together—A Casebook of Joint Practices in Primary Care.* Chicago: The National Joint Practice Commission.

Select Committee on Aging, U.S. House of Representatives. 1978. *Area Agencies on Aging and the Older Americans Act.* Washington, D.C.: U.S. Government Printing Office, Comm. Pub. No. 95–131, March 17.

Special Committee on Aging, United States Senate, 95th Congress. 1977. *Health Care for Older Americans: The "Alternative" Issue,* parts 1, 2, 3, 4. Washington, D.C.: U.S. Government Printing Office, May 16, 17; June 15; July 6.

TAIETZ, P. 1975. "Community Facilities and Social Services." In R. Atchley, ed., *Environments and the Rural Aged.* Washington, D.C.: Gerontological Society.

TERRIS, B. 1972. *Legal Services for the Elderly.* Washington, D.C.: National Council on the Aging.

TOWNSEND, C. 1971. *Old Age: The Last Segregation.* New York: Grossman Publishers.

TURBOW, S. 1975. "Geriatric Group Day Care and Its Effect on Independent Living." *The Gerontologist* 15:509–10.

ZAHOUREK, R., D. LEONE, and F. LANG. 1976. *Creative Health Services—A Model for Group Nursing Practice.* St. Louis: C. V. Mosby.

INDEX

469

INDEX OF AUTHORS

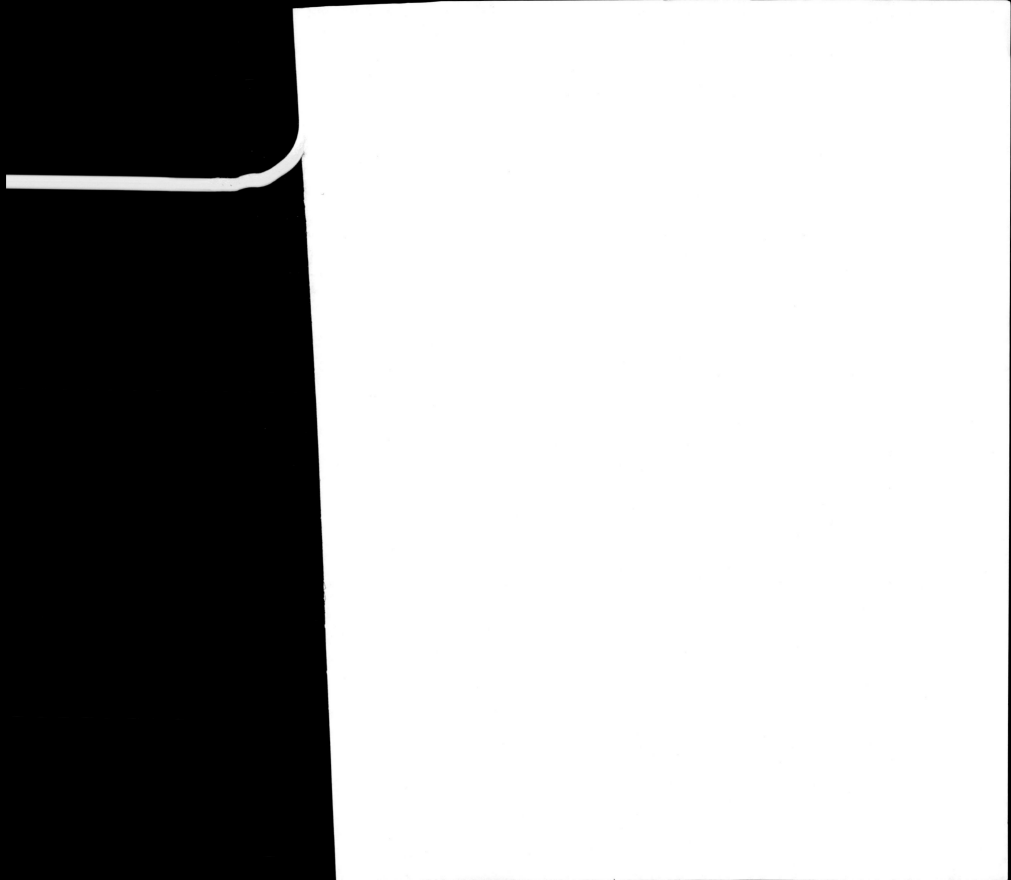

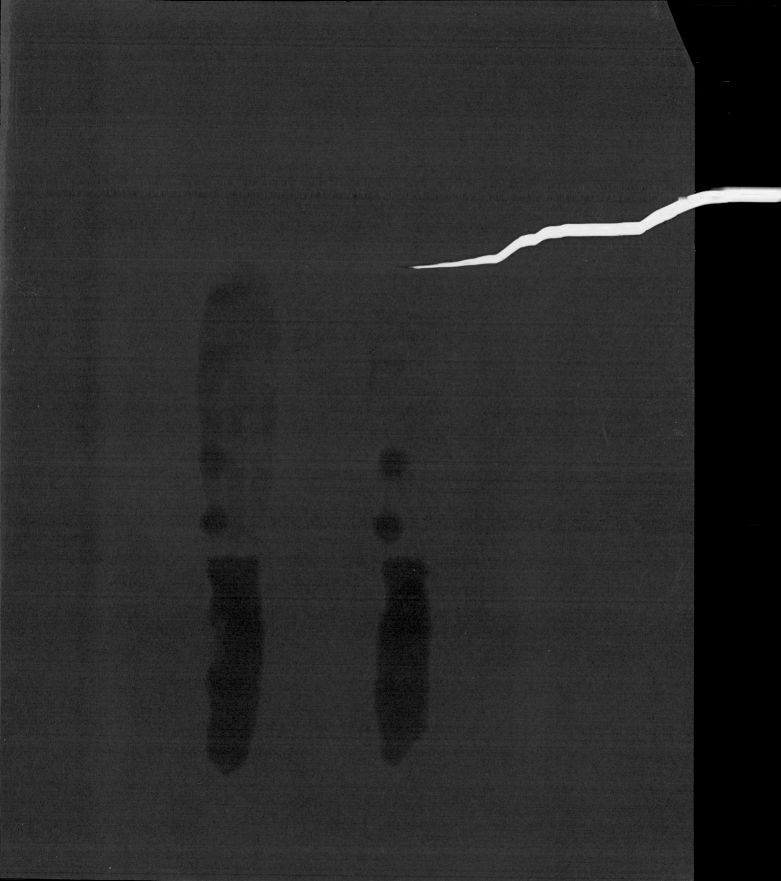

DATE DUE

GAYLORD   PRINTED IN U.S.A.